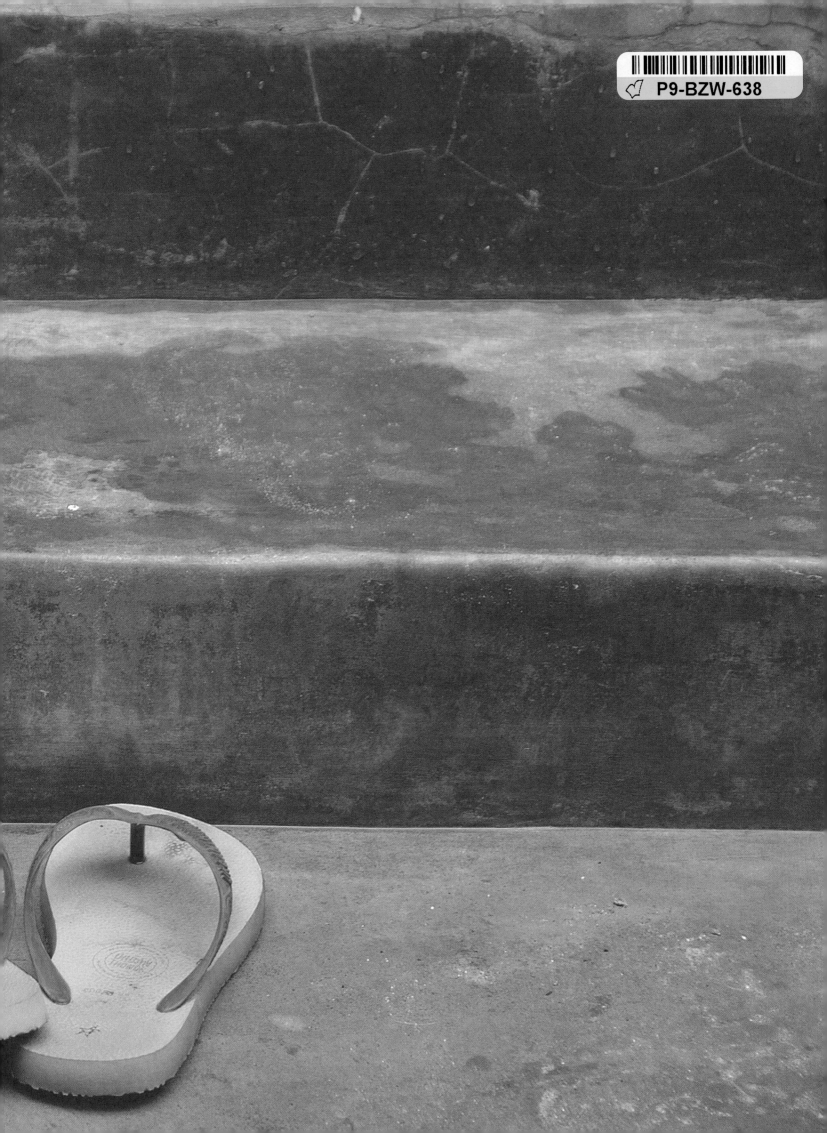

Great Yoga
Retreats

Edited & compiled by Angelika Taschen   *Texts by* Kristin Rübesamen

Great Yoga
Retreats

TASCHEN

HONG KONG KÖLN LONDON LOS ANGELES MADRID PARIS TOKYO

Contents Inhalt Sommaire

Contents Inhalt Sommaire

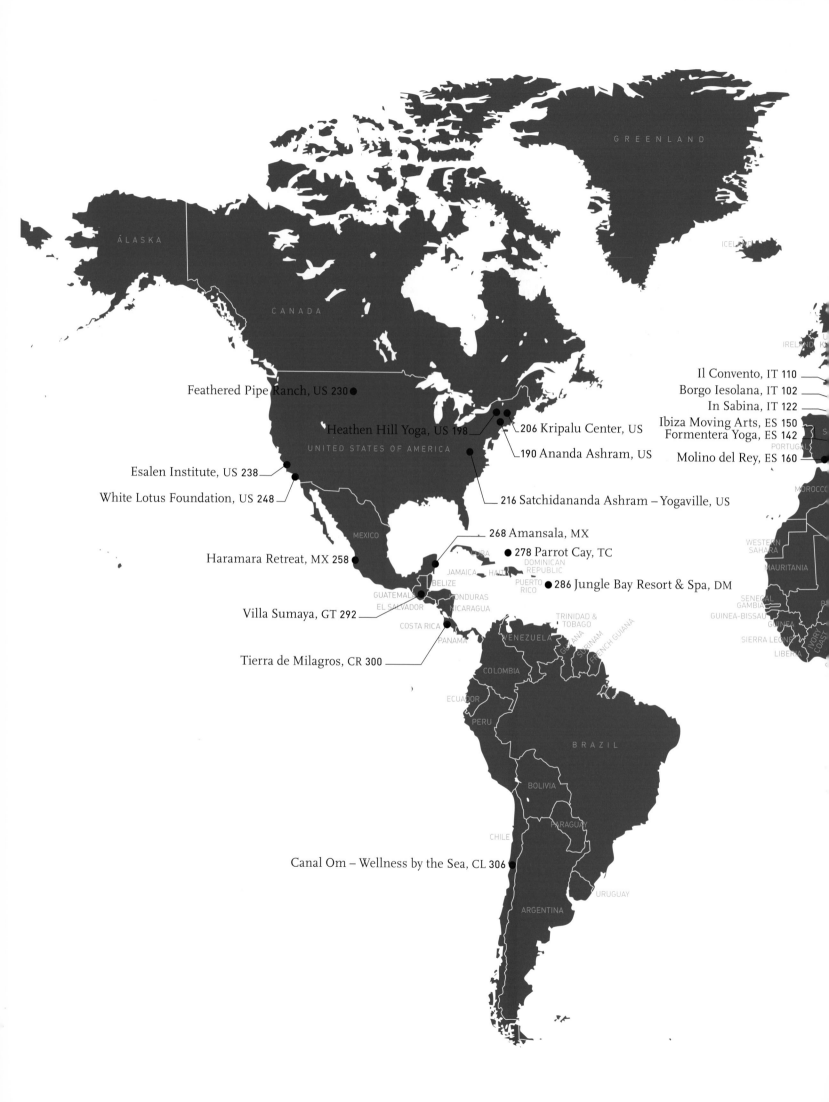

Il Convento, IT **110**
Borgo Iesolana, IT **102**
In Sabina, IT **122**
Ibiza Moving Arts, ES **150**
Formentera Yoga, ES **142**
Molino del Rey, ES **160**

Feathered Pipe Ranch, US **230**

Heathen Hill Yoga, US **198**

206 Kripalu Center, US

190 Ananda Ashram, US

Esalen Institute, US **238**

White Lotus Foundation, US **248**

216 Satchidananda Ashram – Yogaville, US

268 Amansala, MX

278 Parrot Cay, TC

Haramara Retreat, MX **258**

286 Jungle Bay Resort & Spa, DM

Villa Sumaya, GT **292**

Tierra de Milagros, CR **300**

Canal Om – Wellness by the Sea, CL **306**

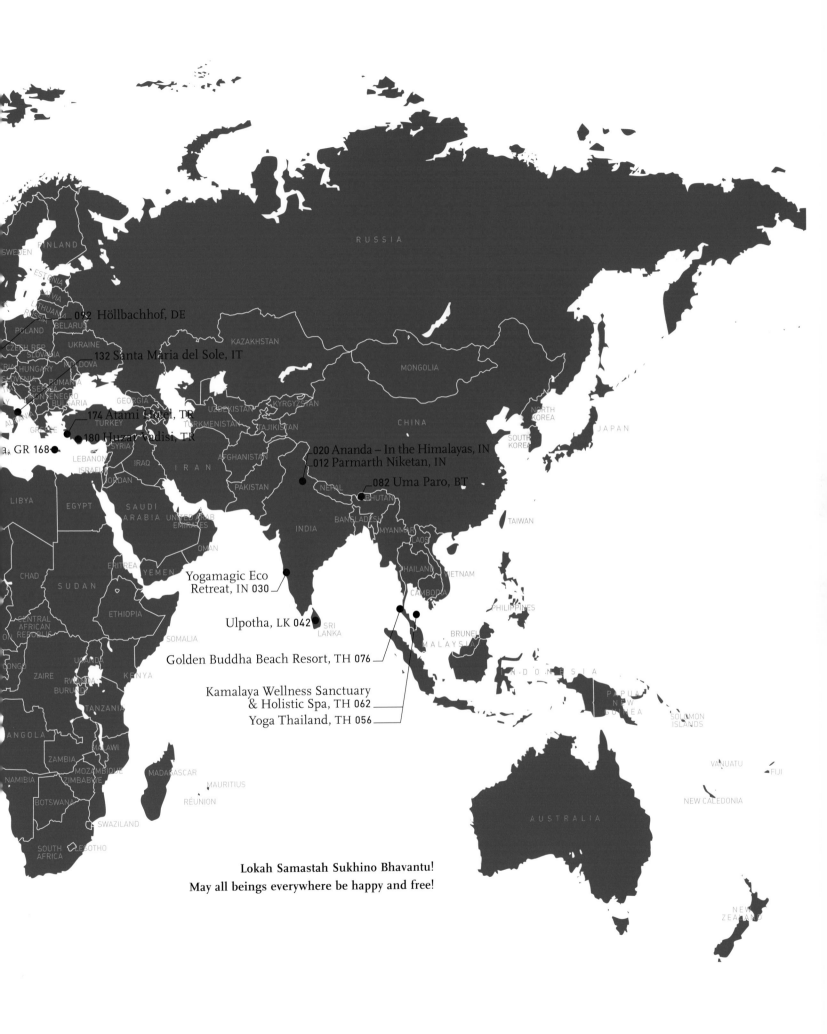

092 Höllbachhof, DE

132 Santa Maria del Sole, IT

174 Atami Hotel, TR

180 Huzur Vadisi, TR

a, GR 168

020 Ananda – In the Himalayas, IN
012 Parmarth Niketan, IN

082 Uma Paro, BT

Yogamagic Eco
Retreat, IN 030

Ulpotha, LK 042

Golden Buddha Beach Resort, TH 076

Kamalaya Wellness Sanctuary
& Holistic Spa, TH 062

Yoga Thailand, TH 056

Lokah Samastah Sukhino Bhavantu!
May all beings everywhere be happy and free!

Preface   Vorwort   Préface

Holistic Yoga Holidays

After more than 10 years of intensive Yoga practice, I plan not only my day around the daily Yoga session but also my holidays, and I visit a Yoga retreat once or twice a year. I can but warn you: Yoga is addictive and will make you high. As such, this book could be your introduction to the Yoga drug, so please proceed with caution.

This is because Yoga is not just a kind of gymnastics that strengthens the back and maintains general flexibility, but far more a comprehensive way of living that embraces the body, spirit and soul in equal measure.

Modern life is often very stressful: constant overstimulation, unhealthy food, little exercise, insufficient sleep. Often a couple of Yoga sessions a week are not enough to provide a real balance to this. Thus a Yoga retreat offers a chance to relax completely and to recharge your batteries, because above and beyond the daily Yoga sessions there is also healthy, mostly vegetarian food and beautiful, inspiring surroundings and nature -- the Yogis know a thing or two about real beauty. All this helps you find new energy in next to no time. It is also nice that you can go alone, with a partner or together with friends, and you are sure to meet like-minded people.

For this book I have selected the world's most beautiful places where instruction is provided by the best Yoga teachers internationally. According to need and experience, you can choose either a spiritually oriented ashram or a luxury resort where you can book daily Yoga sessions. Among the retreats you will find an ashram in Rishikesh, the birthplace of Yoga, an exotic luxury hotel in Bhutan, a farmstead in Tuscany and

Holistic Yoga Holidays

Seit mehr als zehn Jahren mache ich Yoga. Ich plane nicht nur meinen Alltag um die täglichen Yogastunden herum, sondern auch meinen Urlaub. Ein- bis zweimal im Jahr besuche ich ein Yoga Retreat, und ich kann nur warnen: Es macht high und süchtig. Deshalb kann die Lektüre dieses Buches der Einstieg in die Droge Yoga sein. Also bitte Vorsicht!

Yoga ist nicht nur eine Gymnastik, die den Rücken stärkt und beweglich hält, sondern ein umfassender Lebensstil, der Körper, Geist und Seele umfasst. Das moderne Leben stresst uns durch ständige Reizüberflutung, ungesundes Essen, fehlende Bewegung und zu wenig Schlaf. Deshalb genügen ein paar Stunden Yoga in der Woche oft nicht mehr, um diese negativen Einflüsse auszugleichen. Ein Yoga Retreat bietet die Möglichkeit, vollständig zu entspannen und die Batterien wieder aufzuladen. Neben täglichen Yogastunden gibt es gesundes, meist vegetarisches Essen, und die umgebende Natur ist inspirierend, da Yogis Spezialisten für wahre Schönheit sind. Das alles verhilft in kurzer Zeit zu neuer Energie. Ein weiterer Pluspunkt ist, dass man wahlweise allein, mit Partner oder Freunden reisen kann und stets auf Gleichgesinnte trifft. Für dieses Buch habe ich die schönsten Orte in aller Welt gesucht, wo die international besten Yogalehrer unterrichten. Je nach Bedürfnis und Erfahrung kann man wählen zwischen rein spirituell ausgerichteten Ashrams und luxuriösen Resorts, die täglich Yoga anbieten. In meiner Auswahl finden Sie einen Ashram im indischen Rishikesh, dem Geburtsort des Yoga, ein exotisches Luxushotel in Bhutan, ein Bauerngut in der Toskana

Holistic Yoga Holidays

Aujourd'hui, après plus de dix années de pratique intensive du yoga, je n'organise pas seulement mon programme quotidien tout autour des séances de yoga, mais également mes vacances, et je me rends une à deux fois par an dans un lieu de séjour pour yoga. Mais attention : risque d'accoutumance et d'euphorie. Cet ouvrage peut donc être l'initiation à la drogue yoga, à consommer avec précaution.

Car le yoga n'est pas seulement un type de gymnastique destinée à fortifier le dos et assouplir le corps en général, il est surtout un mode de vie complet, impliquant à la fois le corps, l'esprit et l'âme. La vie moderne est souvent épuisante : trop-plein de sollicitations permanentes, alimentation malsaine, manque d'exercice physique, manque de sommeil. Souvent, quelques heures de yoga par semaine ne suffisent pas à compenser le stress. Un séjour yoga est alors une possibilité réelle de se relaxer entièrement et de recharger les batteries, puisque non seulement des séances quotidiennes de yoga sont proposées, mais aussi une alimentation saine, le plus souvent végétarienne, dans un environnement et une nature magnifiques et stimulants, car les yogis savent ce qu'est la vraie beauté. Tout ceci contribue en peu de temps à un regain d'énergie. L'avantage est aussi que l'on peut y aller seul et indépendant, avec son partenaire ou avec des amis et que l'on rencontre toujours des personnes ayant les mêmes goûts. Pour ce livre j'ai sélectionné les plus beaux endroits au monde où enseignent les meilleurs professeurs de yoga de la planète. Toutefois, l'on peut, selon les besoins et l'expérience acquise, choisir entre un âshram orienté vers le spirituel

a beach resort in Mexico. Highlights include Yogamagic, an eco retreat in Goa on the Indian Ocean. Il Convento in Tuscany and Santa Maria del Sole in Apulia unite the sometimes ascetic world of Yoga with the sensuous Italian way of life. In California's Big Sur the legendary Esalen Institute offers, in over 500 workshops, Yoga and much more for body and spirit. At the Amansala Bikini Boot Camp in Tulum, Mexico, meanwhile, you can combine beach life and Yoga lessons marvellously. Last but not least, at the Jungle Bay Resort & Spa on the Caribbean island of Dominica you will find Yoga teachers from all over the world who give their courses in the midst of the tropical rainforest.

Alas, I could not accommodate in this book all the wonderful retreats, ashrams, resorts and hotels, and I hope to be able to create a second volume soon. But I am confident that, worldwide, Yoga has a big future, because it seems there is a need for spiritual meaning and for counteracting day-to-day stress. The range of Yoga retreats on offer is set to grow and grow.

Namasté!

und ein Strandresort in Mexiko. Zu meinen Favoriten zählt das Yogamagic, ein ökologischer Retreat in Goa am Indischen Ozean. Il Convento in der Toskana und Santa Maria del Sole in Apulien vereinen die manchmal asketische Yogawelt mit der sinnesfreudigen Lebensweise Italiens. In Big Sur in Kalifornien bietet das legendäre Esalen Institute mehr als 500 Yoga-Workshops an und etliches mehr für Körper und Geist. Im Amansala Bikini Boot Camp im mexikanischen Tulum kann man Strandleben und Yogaunterricht auf herrlichste Weise kombinieren, und im Jungle Bay Resort & Spa auf der Karibikinsel Dominica finden Sie Yogalehrer aus aller Welt, die ihre Kurse mitten im tropischen Regenwald abhalten.

Leider konnte ich in dieses Buch nicht alle empfehlenswerten Retreats, Ashrams, Resorts und Hotels aufnehmen. Deshalb hoffe ich, bald einen zweiten Band zusammenstellen zu können. Ich bin überzeugt, dass Yoga weltweit eine große Zukunft hat, denn das Bedürfnis nach spiritueller Sinngebung und nach Ausgleich zum Alltagsstress wird immer größer – und diese steigende Nachfrage wird auch die Zahl der Yoga Retreats in die Höhe schnellen lassen.

Namasté!

ou un site de luxe, où l'on peut suivre chaque jour des séances de yoga. Vous trouverez, entre autres, un âshram à Rishikesh, le berceau du yoga, un hôtel de luxe exotique à Bhutan, une ferme en Toscane et une station balnéaire au Mexique.

Parmi les stars citons : le Yogamagic, un site écologique à Goa au bord de l'océan Indien. Le Il Convento en Toscane et le Santa Maria del Sole dans les Pouilles associent le monde parfois ascétique du yoga à l'art de vivre sensuel des Italiens. A Big Sur, en Californie, le légendaire Esalen Institute offre plus de 500 stages de yoga, et bien plus encore pour le corps et l'esprit. En revanche, dans le Bikini Boot Camp d'Amansala à Tulum, au Mexique, la vie de plage et les cours de yoga se complètent le mieux du monde et, last not least, vous trouverez dans le Jungle Bay Resort & Spa sur l'île des Caraïbes Dominique des professeurs de yoga du monde entier qui donnent leurs cours au cœur même des forêts tropicales.

Je n'ai malheureusement pas pu inclure dans cet ouvrage tous les merveilleux sites, âshrams, lieux de séjour et hôtels, et j'espère bientôt pouvoir écrire un second volume. Mais je suis certaine que le yoga a un grand avenir devant lui dans le monde, car il semble y avoir un besoin de spiritualisme et d'équilibre réel du stress quotidien, et ainsi l'éventail de lieux de séjour pour yoga est appelé à s'élargir de plus en plus.

Namasté!

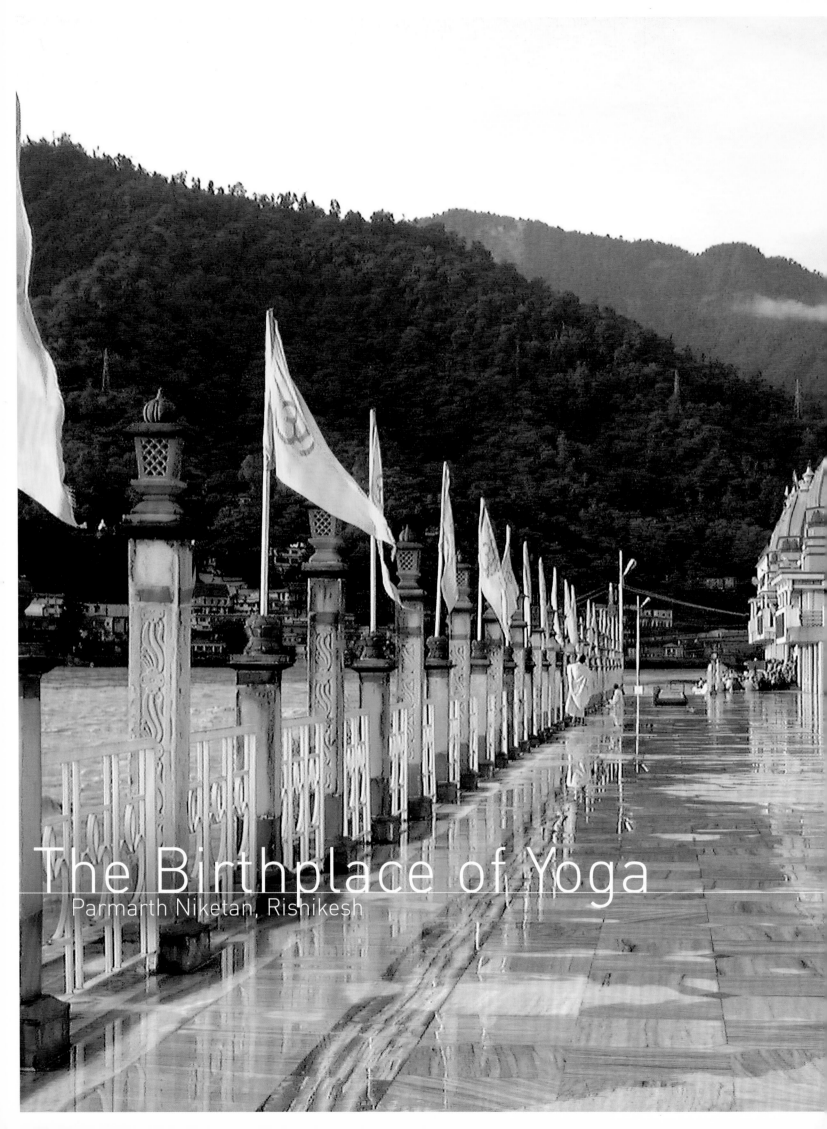

The Birthplace of Yoga
Parmarth Niketan, Rishikesh

Parmarth Niketan, Rishikesh

The Birthplace of Yoga

The cell-like rooms in the ashram are clean and well swept, the day's agenda clearly organised; in fact the whole concern is surprisingly disciplined in view of the fact that this, the birthplace of Yoga, is in India, in Rishikesh. Of the countless Yoga schools in Rishikesh the instruction given in the Parmarth Niketan is among the best, which is why many students register for the twice-yearly teacher-training course. As soon as the sun rises, the first of them begin to do their sun salutations and to meditate. Asana classes and readings on philosophy follow, and the day continues with Asanas until the evening. Then, with great spectacle, the chief guru of the ashram, Swami Chidanand Saraswatiji, conducts Ganga Aarti, the fire ceremony. Swamiji doesn't just have strikingly beautiful eyes and a hotline to God; he is also a man of the world. Every year at the beginning of March he organises an impressive international Yoga festival in the ashram, at which the best-known Indian stars as well as those from the West assemble. He is invited by the United Nations to speak on the subject of religion, and in the ashram itself he has founded an orphanage in which Indian orphans, in addition to receiving a school education, learn Yoga and Sanskrit and study the Vedas. When, in the evening, happy and close to a state of bliss, they start to sing while huddled up on cushions on the floor of the stone altar at the river, you understand why rich Indian families from London return every year to support the ashram. Even Ringo Starr would have liked it here – and he once had to leave Rishikesh, as his supply of baked beans had run out.

Books to pack: "The Bhagavad Gita" (2 volumes) by Paramahansa Yogananda and "Siddhartha" by Hermann Hesse.

Parmarth Niketan Ashram

P.O. Swargashram
Rishikesh (Himalayas)
Uttaranchal 249304
India
Tel. +91 35 244 0088
Fax +91 35 244 0066
parmarth@parmarth.com
www.parmarth.com

DIRECTIONS	Located on the bank of the Ganges, south of the Ram Jhula Bridge. 30 min from Jolly Grant Airport in Rishikesh/Dehradun. By train from Delhi to Haridwar, continuing by taxi or bus to Rishikesh.
YOGA	Traditional Hatha, advanced Vinyasa Yoga, Yoga Nidra.
TEACHERS	Swami Ramdevji, Swami Veda Bharati, Swami Yoganandaji, Bhava Ram, Gurmukh Kaur Khalsa and Gabriela Bozic come to the International Yoga Festival.
ROOMS	Over 1000 places to sleep in 2–4-bed rooms.
FOOD	Indian vegetarian, without onions or garlic.
TREATMENTS	Ayurveda.
RECREATION	Trekking, whitewater rafting.

Geburtsort des Yoga

Sauber und gefegt sind die zellenartigen Zimmer im Ashram, klar organisiert die Tagesordnung, überraschend diszipliniert der ganze Betrieb angesichts der Tatsache, dass man sich in Indien und in Rishikesh an der Geburtsstätte des Yoga befindet. Von den unzähligen Yogaschulen in Rishikesh zählt der Unterricht im Parmarth Niketan zu den besten, weshalb sich viele Schüler zur zweimal jährlich stattfindenden Lehrerausbildung anmelden. Sobald die Sonne aufgeht, beginnen die Ersten, ihre Sonnengrüße zu machen und zu meditieren. Asana-Klassen und Vorlesungen über Philosophie folgen, und weiter geht es mit Asanas bis zum Abend. Dann führt in großer Inszenierung der Chefguru des Ashrams, Swami Chidanand Saraswatiji, die Feuerzeremonie Ganga Aarti am Ganges durch. Swamiji hat nicht nur auffallend schöne Augen und einen heißen Draht zu Gott, er ist auch ein Mann von Welt. Er organisiert im Ashram jährlich Anfang März ein beeindruckendes internationales Yoga-Festival, an dem außer den bekanntesten indischen auch westliche Stars teilnehmen. Er wird von den United Nations als Redner zum Thema Religion eingeladen, im Ashram selbst hat er ein Waisenhaus gegründet, in dem indische Waisenjungen zusätzlich zu einer Schulbildung Yoga und Sanskrit lernen und die Veden studieren. Wenn sie abends vergnügt und geradezu selig, auf den Boden des steinernen Altars am Fluss auf Kissen gekauert, anfangen zu singen, versteht man, warum reiche Inderfamilien aus London jedes Jahr wiederkommen, um den Ashram zu unterstützen. Hier hätte es sogar Ringo Starr gefallen, der damals aus Rishikesh abreisen musste – ihm waren die mitgebrachten Dosen mit Baked Beans ausgegangen.

Buchtipps: »Die Bhagavad Gita« (2 Bände) von Paramahansa Yogananda und »Siddhartha« von Hermann Hesse.

Le berceau du yoga

Dans l'âshram, les chambres, ressemblant à des cellules, sont propres et nettes, l'emploi du temps clairement organisé, la maison tout entière étonnamment disciplinée vu que nous nous trouvons en Inde et à Rishikesh, berceau du yoga. Parmi les innombrables écoles de yoga de Rishikesh, l'enseignement donné au Parmarth Niketan compte parmi les meilleurs, raison pour laquelle nombre d'élèves s'inscrivent à la formation de professeurs qui se tient deux fois par an. A peine le soleil levé, les premiers commencent leurs saluts du matin et leurs méditations. Ensuite ont lieu les classes d'Âsanas et les cours magistraux, suivis d'exercices d'Âsanas jusqu'au soir. Puis, dans une mise en scène grandiose, Swami Chidanand Saraswatiji, Ganga Aarti, le gourou en chef, procède à la cérémonie du feu. En excellents termes avec Dieu, Swamiji n'a pas seulement des yeux magnifiques, c'est aussi un homme du monde. Chaque année, il organise début mars un brillant festival de yoga international auquel, outre les plus grandes célébrités indiennes, participent aussi des stars occidentales. Il est invité par les Nations Unies pour parler de la religion, dans l'âshram même il a fondé un orphelinat où les garçons, en plus de leur formation scolaire, apprennent le yoga, le sanskrit et étudient les Védas. Lorsque, le soir venu, sur le sol de l'autel de pierre au bord du fleuve, ils se mettent à chanter dans une joyeuse béatitude, accroupis sur des coussins, on comprend pourquoi de riches familles indiennes de Londres reviennent chaque année apporter leur soutien à l'âshram. Même Ringo Starr s'est senti à l'aise ici; à l'époque il avait dû quitter Rishikesh – sa réserve de boîtes de baked beans était épuisée.

Livres à emporter : « La Bhagavad Gîtâ » de Swami Chinmayananda et « Siddhartha » de Hermann Hesse.

ANREISE	Am Ganges, südlich der Brücke Ram Jhula gelegen, 30 min vom Jolly Grant Airport in Rishikesh/Dehradun entfernt. Mit dem Zug von Delhi nach Haridwar, weiter per Taxi oder Bus.
YOGA	Traditional Hatha, Advanced Vinyasa Yoga, Yoga Nidra.
GASTLEHRER	Zum International Yoga Festival kommen Swami Ramdevji, Swami Veda Bharati, Swami Yoganandaji, Bhava Ram, Gurmukh Kaur Khalsa, Gabriela Bozic.
ZIMMER	Über 1000 Schlafplätze in 2–4-Bettzimmern.
KÜCHE	Indisch-vegetarisch, ohne Zwiebeln oder Knoblauch.
ANWENDUNGEN	Ayurveda.
FREIZEIT	Trekking, Wildwasser-Rafting.

ACCÈS	Situé au bord du Gange, au sud du pont Ram Jhula. A 30 min de l'aéroport Jolly Grant de Rishikesh/Dehradun. Trajet en train de Dehli à Haridwar, puis en taxi ou bus à Rishikesh.
YOGA	Traditional Hatha, Advanced Vinyasa Yoga, Yoga nidra.
PROFESSEURS	Participent au Festival international de yoga Swami Ramdevji, Swami Veda Bharati, Swami Yoganandaji, Bhava Ram, Gurmukh Kaur Khalsa, Gabriela Bozic.
CHAMBRES	Plus de 1000 places dans des chambres de 2 à 4 lits.
RESTAURATION	Cuisine indienne et végétarienne, sans oignon ni ail.
TRAITEMENTS	Ayurveda.
ACTIVITÉS	Trekking, rafting en eau vive.

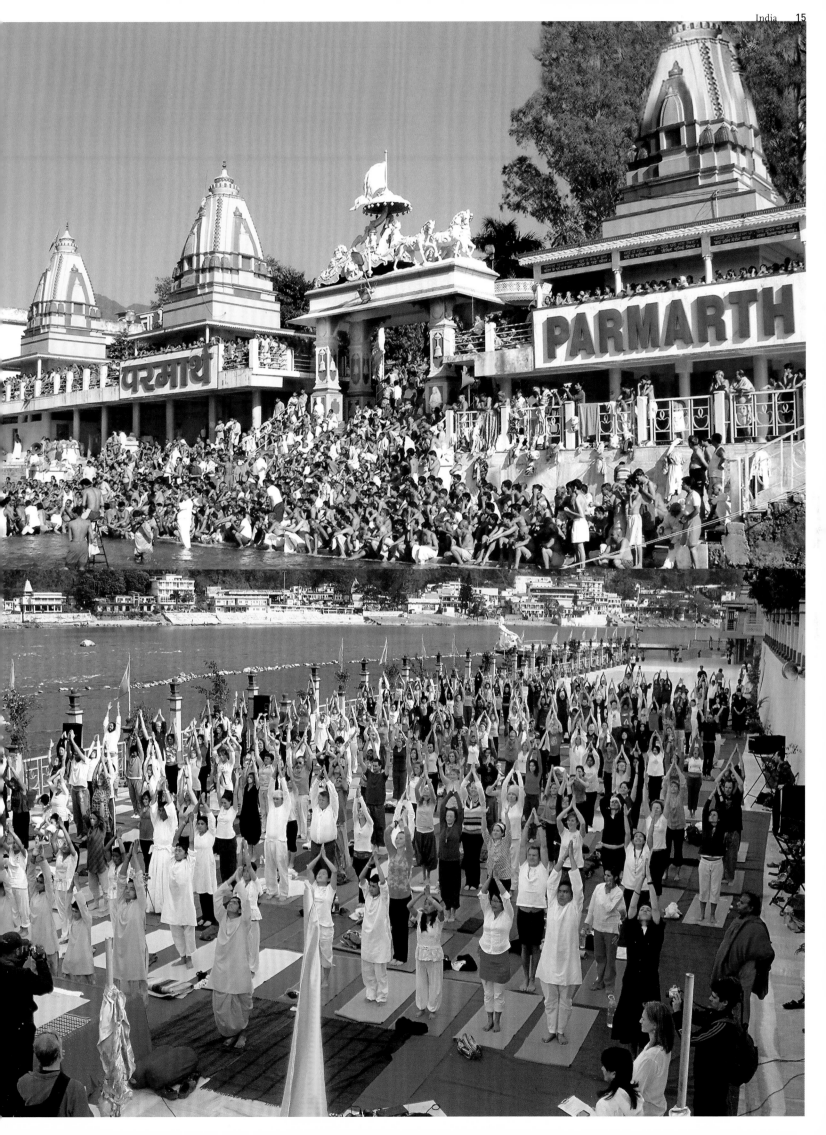

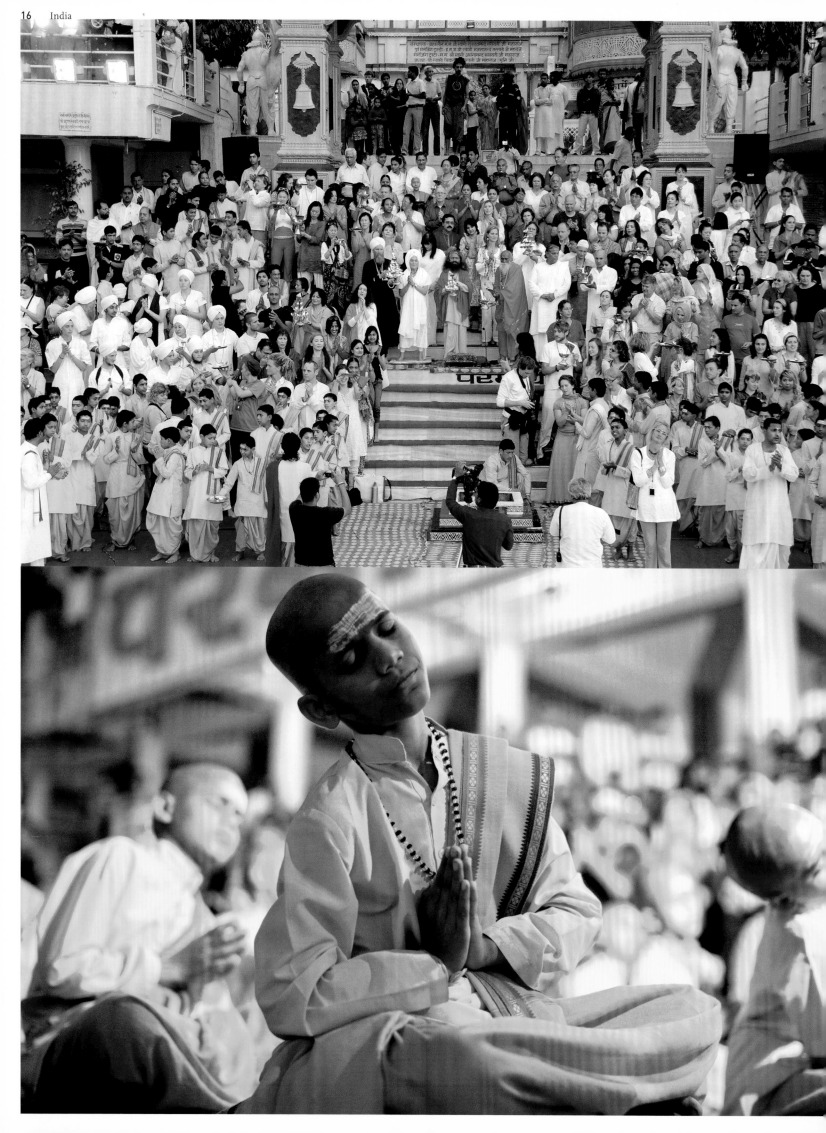

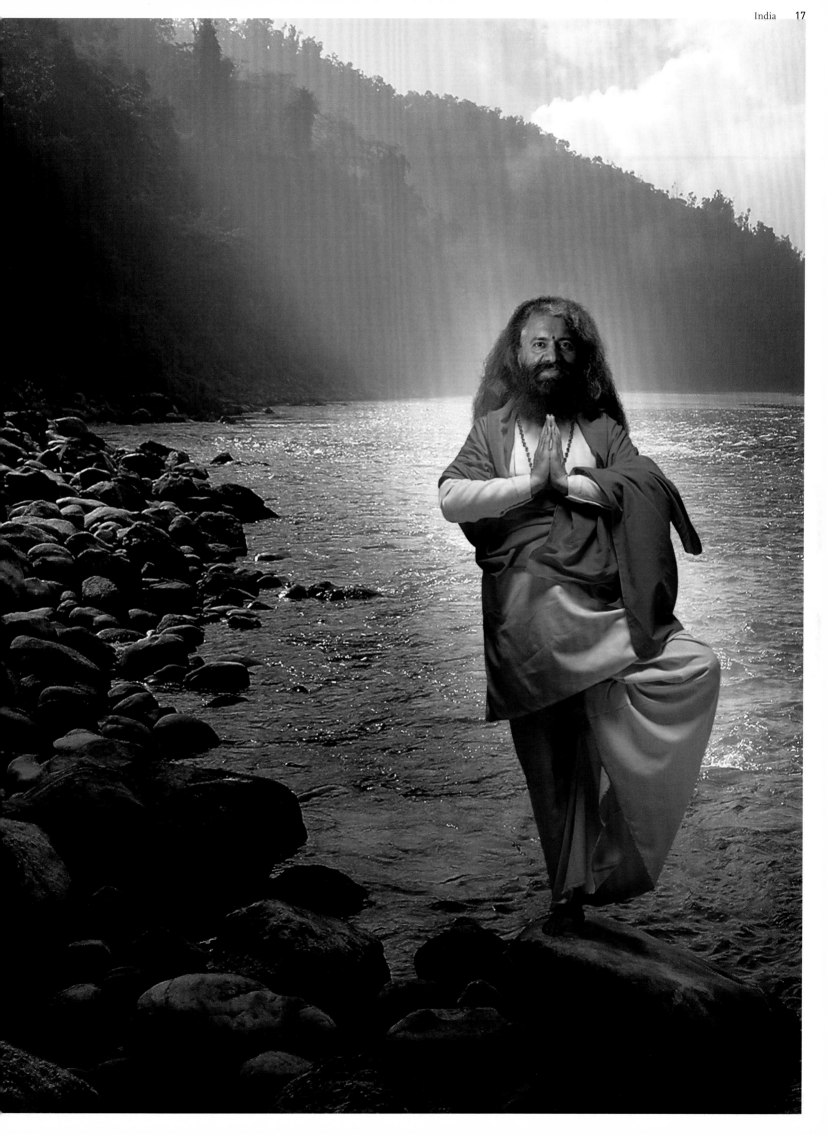

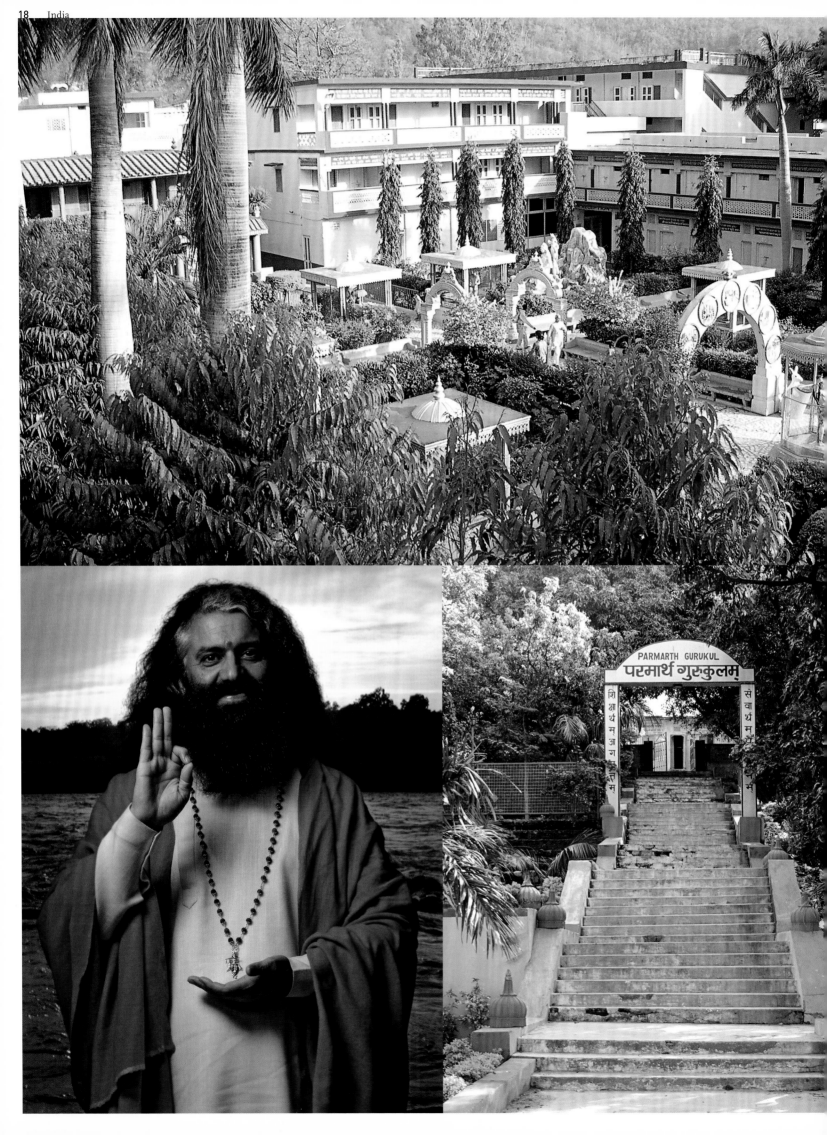

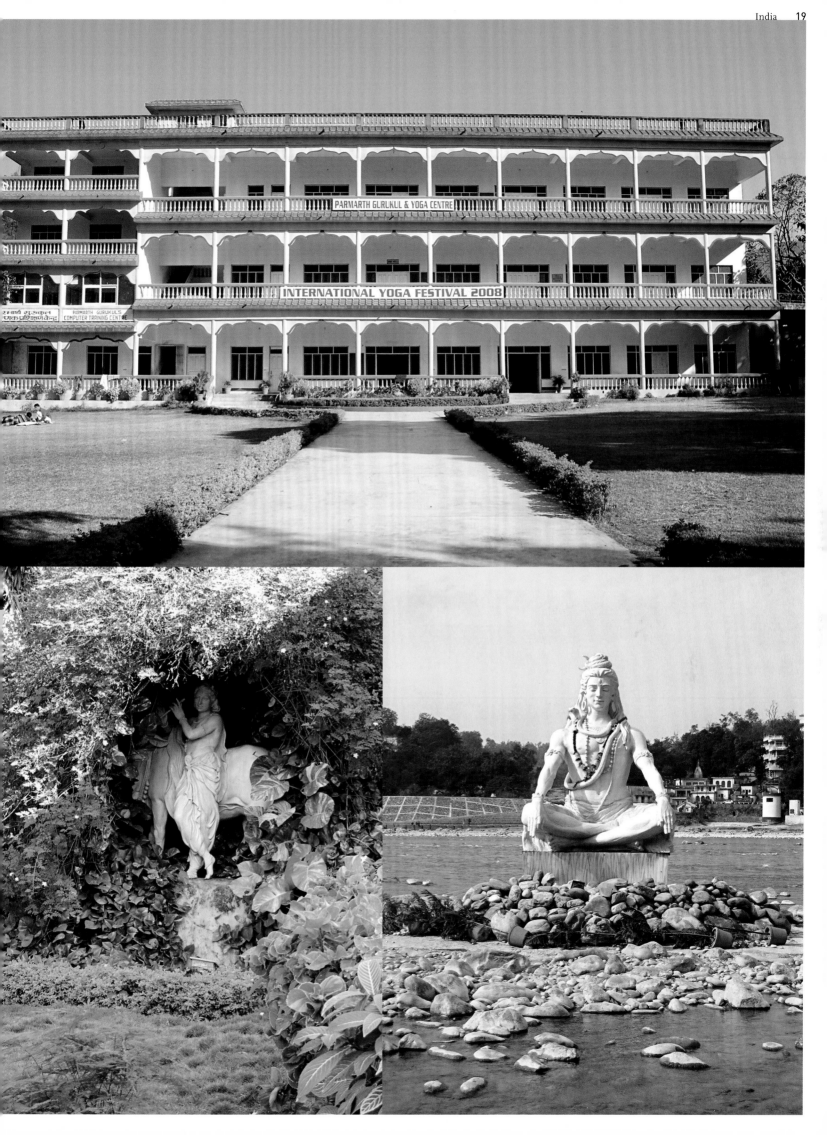

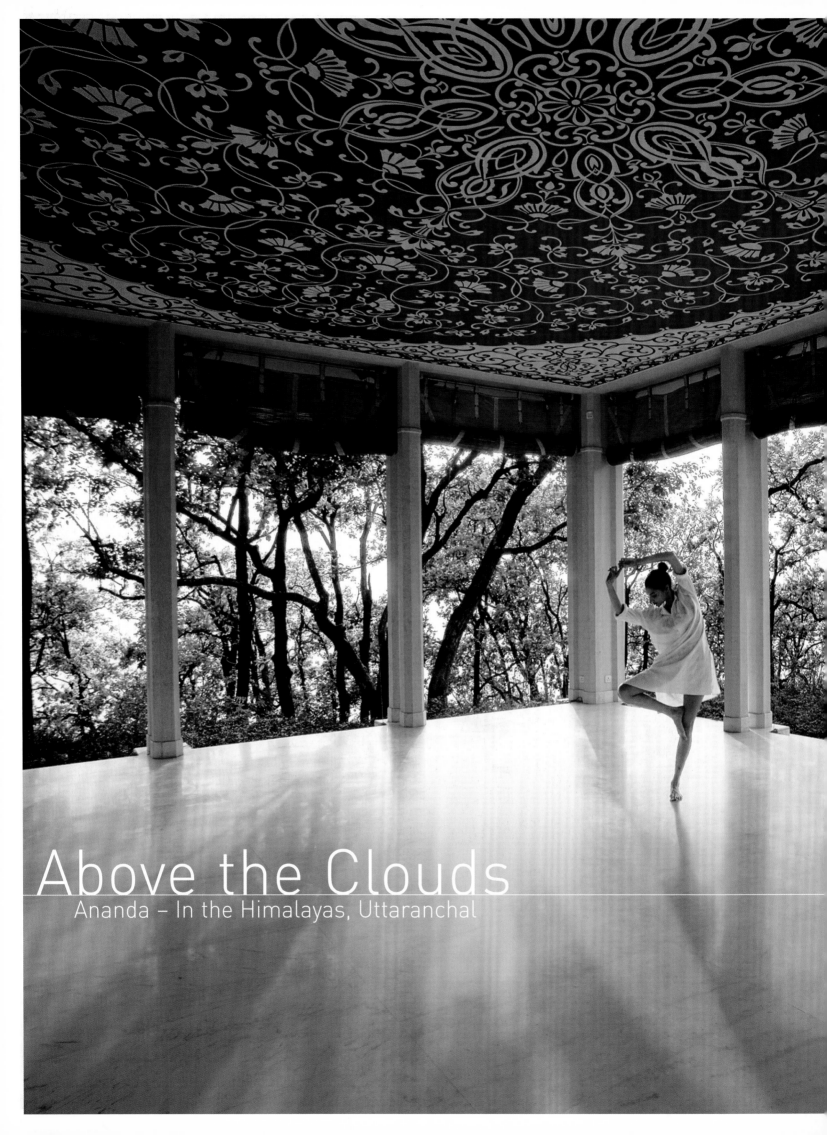

Above the Clouds

Ananda – In the Himalayas, Uttaranchal

Ananda – In the Himalayas, Uttaranchal

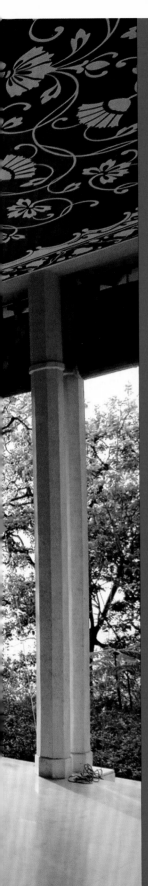

Above the Clouds

The palace lies high up in the mist. From the whitish veil of light, green hills emerge, more and more of them – the foothills of the Himalayas. Down in the valley the broad, turquoise Ganges winds southwards through the countryside. Up here you live like they did in the time of the maharajas, or would do if the stress that brings the guests to Ananda weren't so modern. Sirodhara treatments (hot oil poured onto the forehead) lasting for hours, sesame oil massages, a soothingly babbling waterfall, the scent of sandalwood and ginger tea await the guest after the Yoga sessions, which take place at least twice daily – in the palace, in the pavilion or in the amphitheatre in the marvellous park. The teachers who offer instruction here did not qualify with a mere weekend seminar. As a rule, they hail from nearby Rishikesh, the birthplace of Yoga, and teach a gentle Hatha Yoga in as natural a way as it has been passed down through the generations. Private tuition is available. Ananda is the Sanskrit word for "bliss". And it sets in easily after the morning's meditation and Yoga, even before you have been served your sweet toast, made of chickpea flour, with roasted melon seeds and fresh mango compote on the terrace built like a tree house into the ancient Sal trees.

Books to pack: "Life in Freedom" by Jiddu Krishnamurti and "Into Thin Air" by Jon Krakauer.

Ananda – In the Himalayas
The Palace Estate
Narendra Nagar, Tehri-Garhwai
Uttaranchal 249175
India
Tel. +91 1378 227 500
Fax +91 1378 227 550
sales@anandaspa.com
www.anandaspa.com

DIRECTIONS	162 miles north of New Delhi, 45-min flight to Jolly Grant Airport in Rishikesh/Dehradun, 5-hr train journey from Delhi to Haridwar, transfer by arrangement.
YOGA	Hatha, Kunjal Yoga.
TEACHER	Bhavini Kalan.
ROOMS	70 deluxe rooms, 5 deluxe suites, 3 separate luxury villas.
FOOD	Indian, Asian and Western organic food. Vata, Pitta and Kapha meals.
TREATMENTS	Over 79 different traditional Ayurveda treatments, detox, anti-aging, weight & inch loss, aromatherapy.
RECREATION	Teaching in Vedanta, swimming, temple trekking, white water rafting, safaris, billiards, golf, cooking courses.

Über den Wolken

Hoch oben im Nebel liegt der Palast. Aus dem weißlichen Schleier aus Licht tauchen grüne Hügel auf, immer mehr, die Ausläufer des Himalajas. Unten im Tal windet sich der Ganges breit und türkis durchs Land nach Süden. Hier oben lebt man wie zu Zeiten der Maharadschas, wäre der Stress, der die Gäste herbringt, nicht so modern. Stundenlange Stirngüsse, Sesamölmassagen, ein beruhigend plätschernder Wasserfall, der Geruch nach Sandelholz und Ingwertee erwarten den Gast nach den Yogastunden, die mindestens zweimal täglich stattfinden, im Palast, im Pavillon oder im Amphitheater im herrlichen Park. Die Lehrer, die hier unterrichten, haben sich nicht nur mit einem Wochenendseminar qualifiziert. Sie kommen in der Regel aus dem nahe gelegenen Rishikesh, dem Geburtsort von Yoga, und unterrichten ein sanftes Hatha Yoga so selbstverständlich, wie es von Generation zu Generation weitergegeben wurde, auf Wunsch auch im Einzelunterricht. Ananda heißt in Sanskrit Seligkeit. Die stellt sich leicht ein nach Morgenmeditation und Yoga, noch bevor einem auf der Terrasse, die wie ein Baumhaus in die uralten Sal-Bäume gebaut ist, süßer Toast aus Kichererbsenmehl mit gerösteten Melonensamen und frischem Mangokompott serviert wird.

Buchtipps: »Vollkommene Freiheit« von Jiddu Krishnamurti und »In eisige Höhen« von Jon Krakauer.

Au-dessus des nuages

Bien au-dessus des brumes resplendit le palais. Emergeant du voile blanchâtre de lumière, apparaissent de plus en plus nombreuses les collines vertes, contreforts de l'Himalaya. En bas, dans la vallée, le Gange traverse le pays en larges méandres turquoise en direction du sud. Dans les hauteurs on vit comme au temps des maharadjas, si ce n'était le stress moderne qui fait affluer les visiteurs. De longues affusions du front, des massages à l'huile de sésame, une cascade qui clapote doucement, l'odeur du bois de santal et une tisane au gingembre attendent le visiteur après les séances de yoga, qui se tiennent au moins deux fois par jour dans le palais, le pavillon ou l'amphithéâtre du magnifique parc. Les professeurs enseignant ici n'ont pas acquis leur qualification dans un séminaire de week-end. Le plus souvent, ils viennent de Rishikesh, berceau du yoga situé à proximité, et enseignent le Hatha-yoga doux avec le même naturel qu'on le leur a appris de génération en génération, en cours particulier sur demande. En sanskrit, ananda signifie béatitude. Celle-ci vous envahit agréablement après la méditation du matin et le yoga, avant même que l'on vous serve, sur la terrasse construite comme une maison-arbre dans les sals ancestraux, un toast sucré de farine de pois chiches aux graines de melon grillées, accompagné de compote de mangue fraîche.

Livres à emporter : « De la liberté » de Jiddu Krishnamurti et « Tragédie à l'Everest » de Jon Krakauer.

ANREISE	260 km nördlich von Delhi, 45 min Flug zum Jolly Grant Airport in Rishikesh/Dehradun, 5 Std. Zug von Delhi nach Haridwar. Transfer nach Absprache.
YOGA	Hatha, Kunjal Yoga.
GASTLEHRER	Bhavini Kalan.
ZIMMER	70 Deluxe-Zimmer, 5 Suiten, 3 separate Villen.
KÜCHE	Indisch-, asiatisch-, westlich-organisch. Vata-, Pitta-, Kapha-Mahlzeiten.
ANWENDUNGEN	Über 79 verschiedene Ayurveda-Anwendungen, Detox, Anti-Aging, Weight & Inch Loss, Aromatherapie.
FREIZEIT	Unterricht in Vedanta, Schwimmen, Tempel-Trekking, White Water Rafting, Safari, Billard, Golf, Kochkurse.

ACCÈS	Situé à 260 km au nord de Delhi, à 45 min de vol du Jolly Grant Airport à Rishikesh/Dehradun, à 5 h de train de Delhi à Haridwar, transfert peut être organisé.
YOGA	Hatha, Kunjal Yoga.
PROFESSEUR	Bhavini Kalan.
CHAMBRES	70 chambres de luxe, 5 suites, 3 villas de luxe.
RESTAURATION	Cuisine organique indienne, asiatique, occidentale. Repas de types Vata, Pitta et Kapha.
TRAITEMENTS	Plus de 79 traitements de l'Ayurveda, désintoxication, anti-aging, weight & inch loss, aromathérapie.
ACTIVITÉS	Cours en védânta, natation, tempel trekking, rafting en eau vive, safari, billard, golf, cours de cuisine.

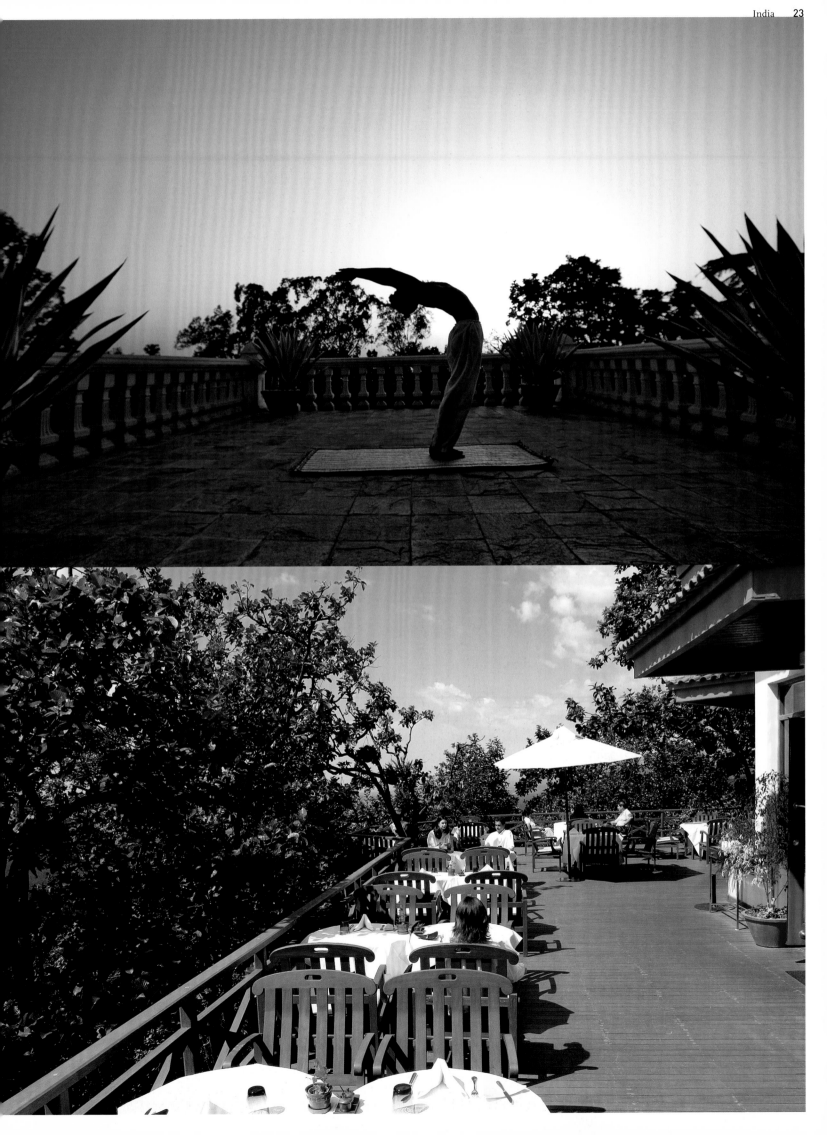

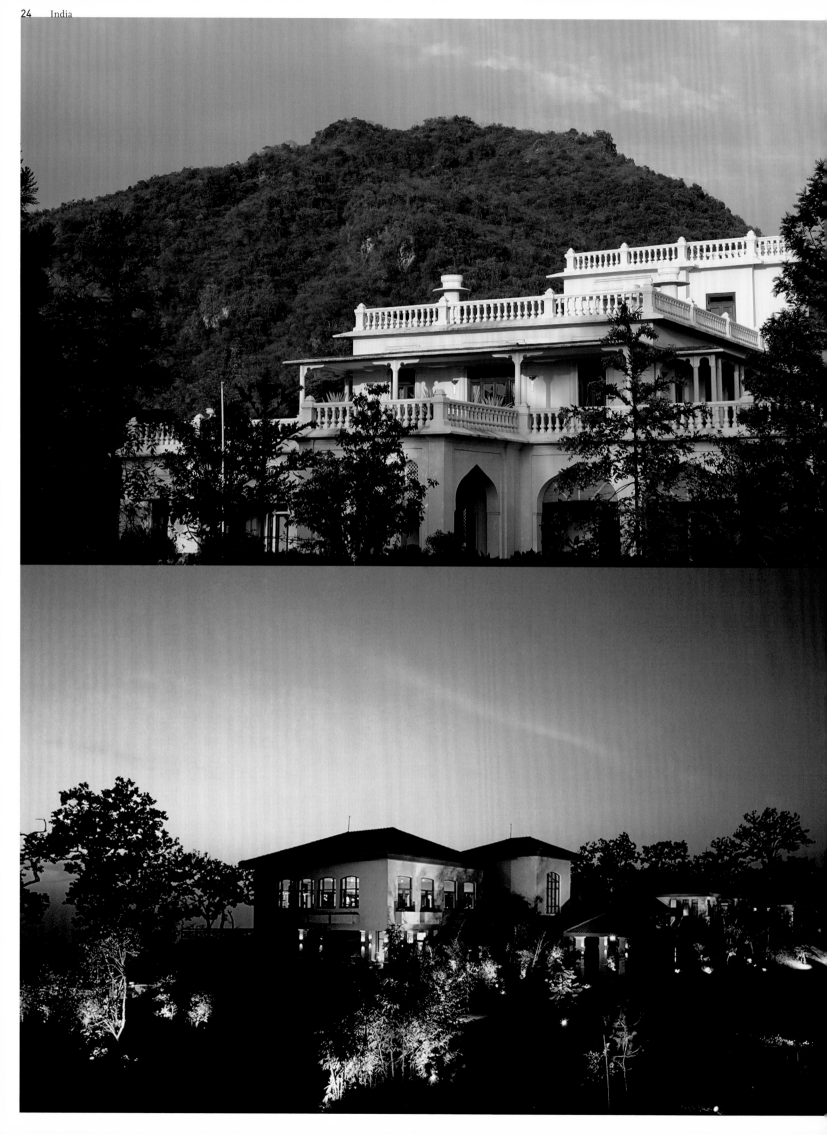

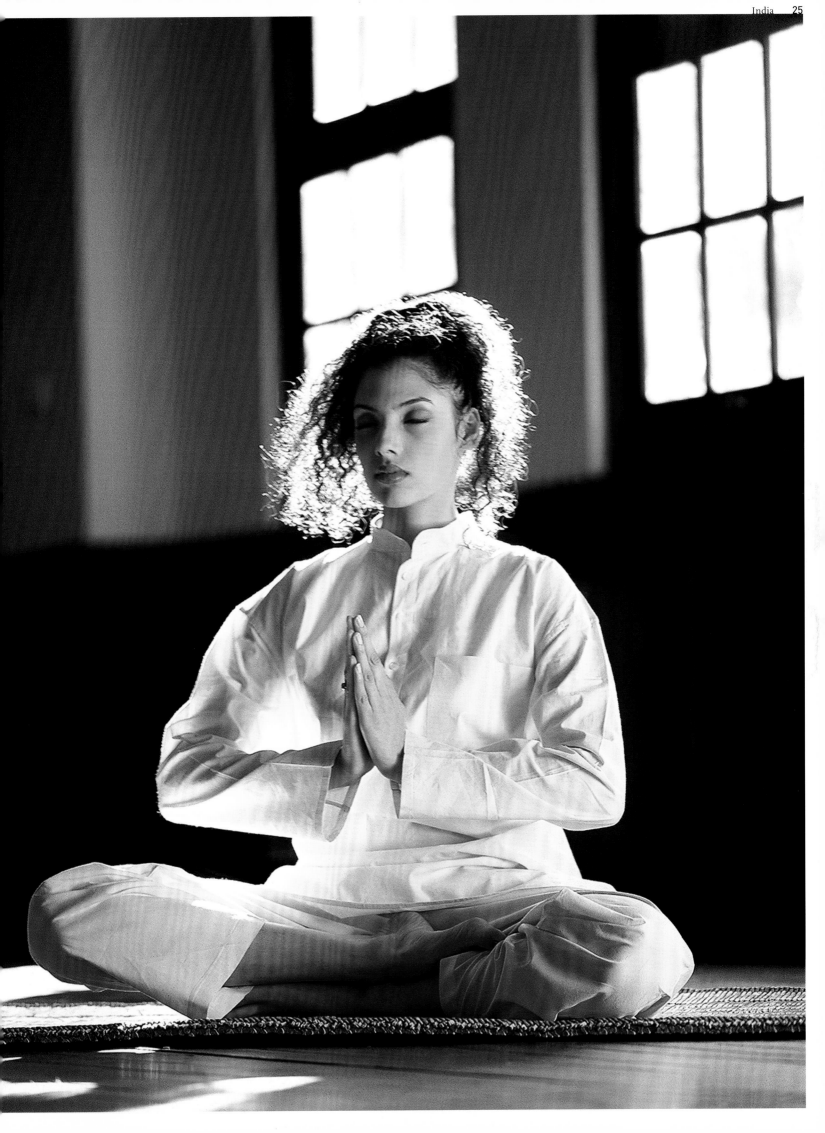

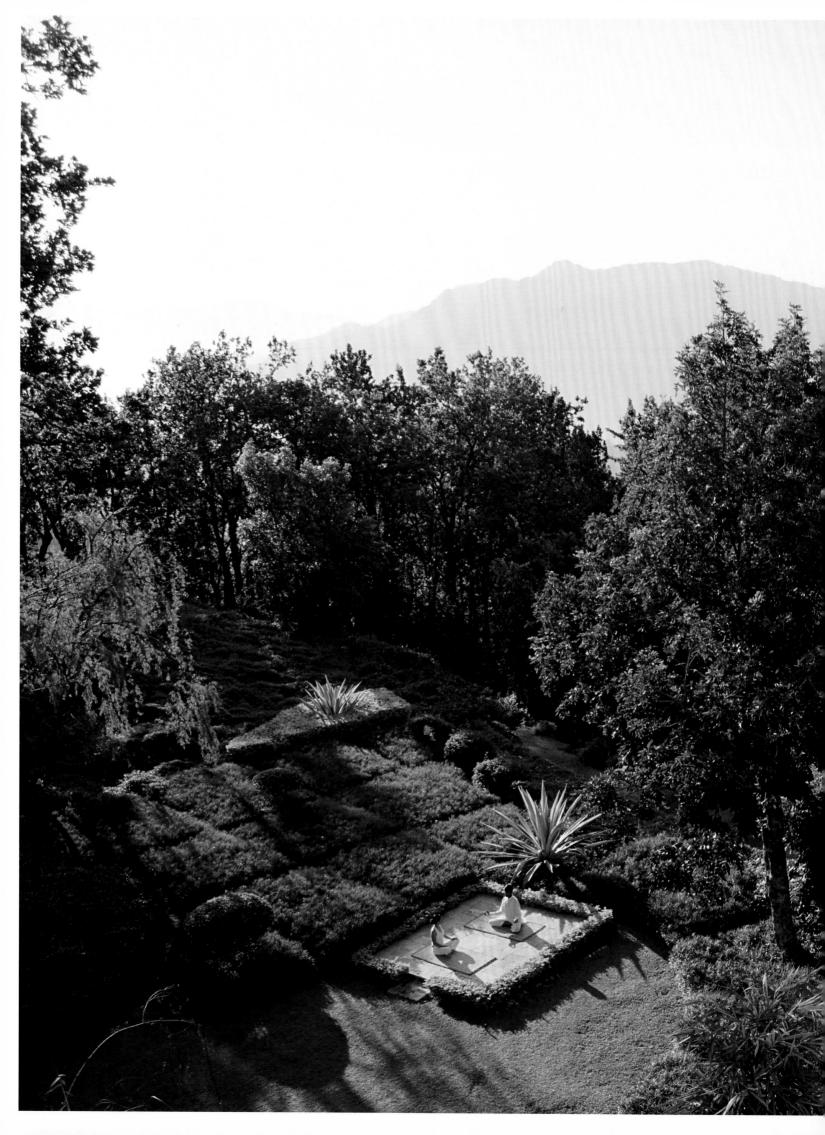

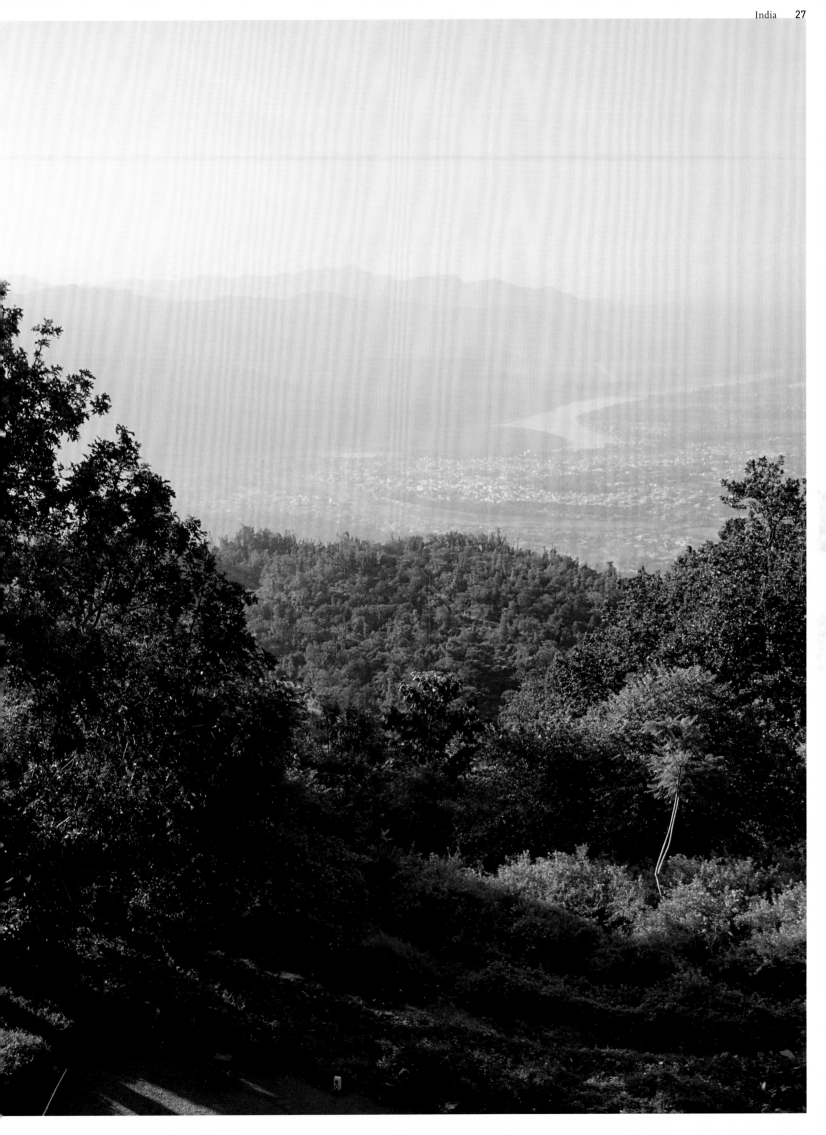

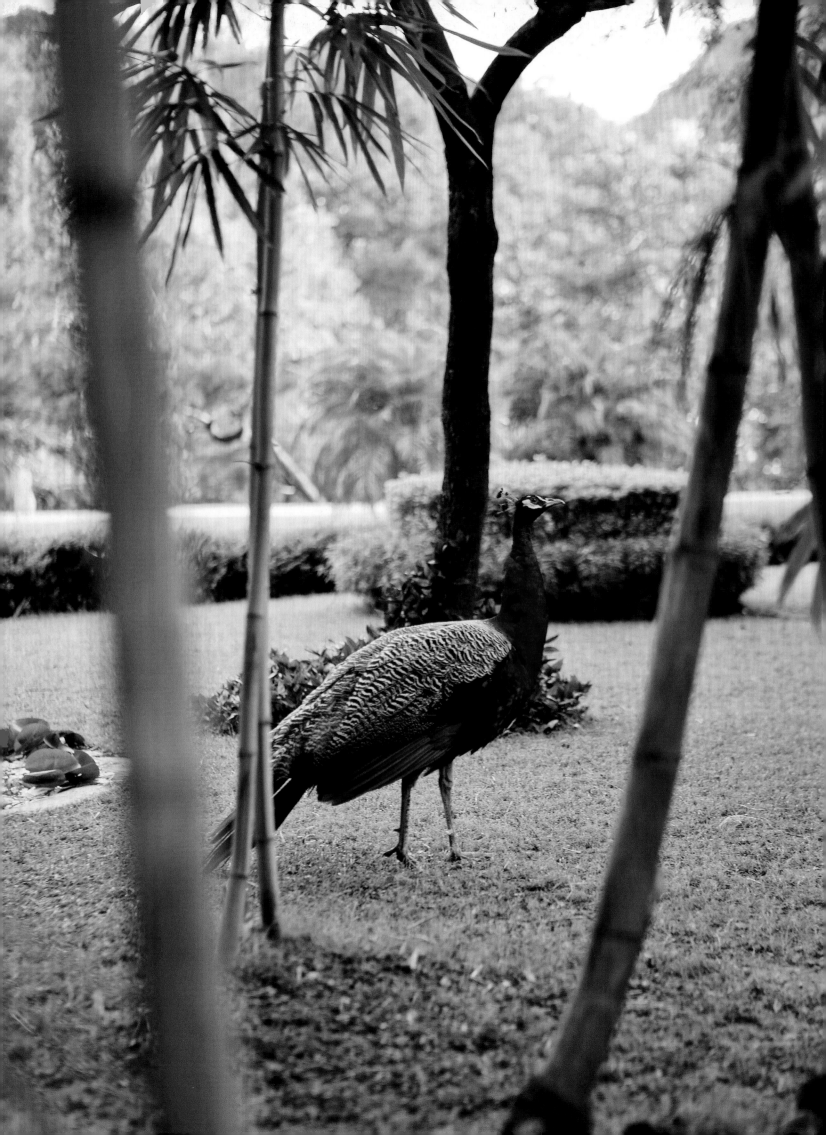

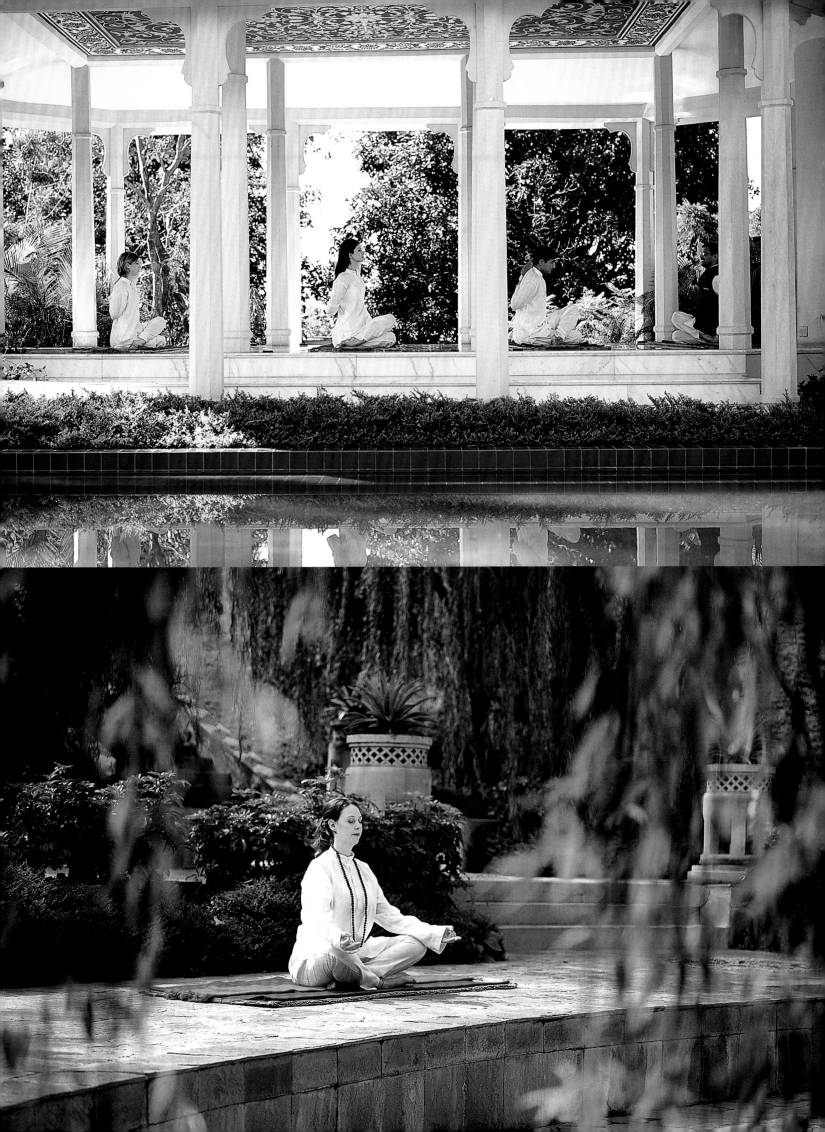

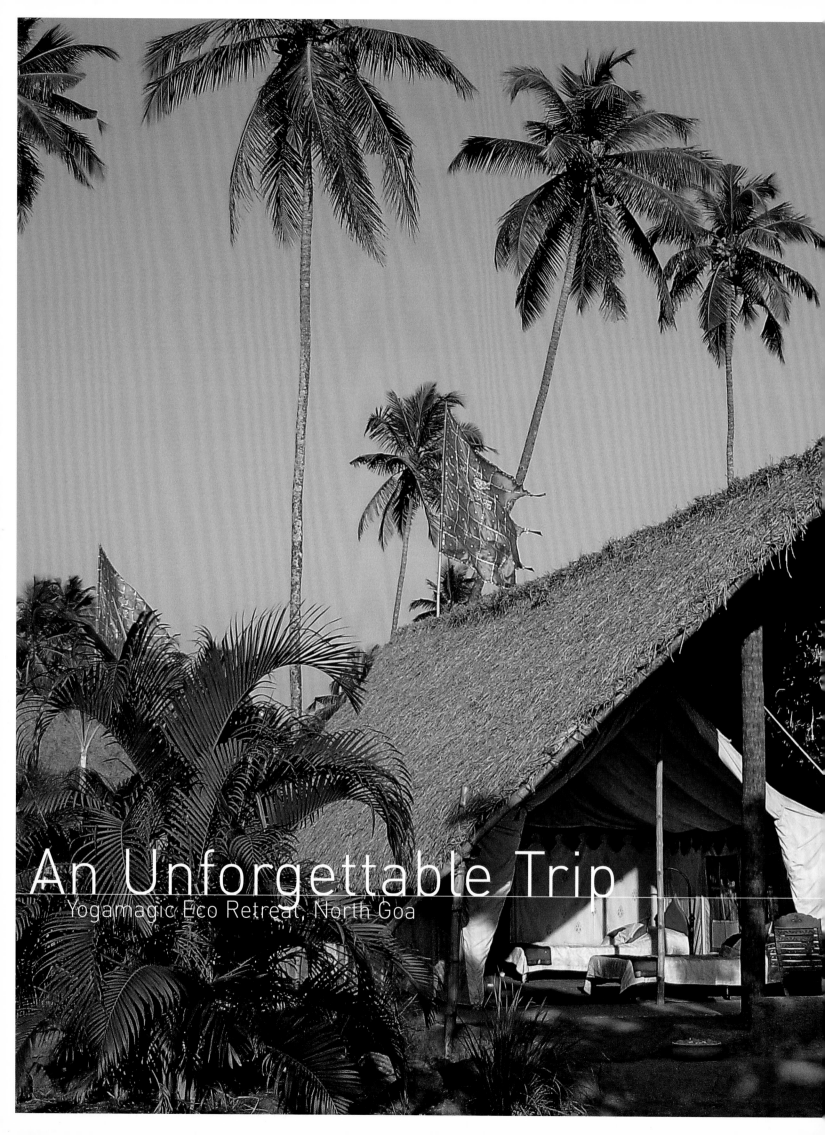

An Unforgettable Trip
Yogamagic Eco Retreat, North Goa

Yogamagic Eco Retreat, North Goa

An Unforgettable Trip

Rice fields and rainforest in the hinterland, whitewashed Catholic churches in the villages, enchanted 17th-century manor houses, endless white beaches on the Arabian Sea: no wonder that Goa was declared a paradise of free love by the hippies in the 1960s. The former Portuguese colony only survived the onslaught of stoned dropouts in a rather tarnished state. But beyond the party beaches, insiders' tips such as Yogamagic serve as reminders of the unmistakable appeal India's smallest state has always had for its visitors. Half an hour from the sea and built in a coconut grove, the magic of this eco resort comes purely from its natural resources. Those who, at the end of the morning Yoga session, lie on the floor of the Yoga temple, which has been conjured up using dried mud, cow dung and clay, and look above them to the high light roof made of bamboo and palm leaves will experience a fully legal trip. And if that's not enough, try Vishnu, the legendary masseur from Pune, to help you relax, or the delicious chai, served at sunrise on the veranda of the solar-powered luxury tents.

Books to pack: "Be Here Now" by Ram Dass, "A Son of the Circus" by John Irving and "The God of Small Things" by Arundhati Roy.

Yogamagic Eco Retreat	
1586/1 Grand Chinvar	
Anjuna, Bardez	
403509 North Goa	
India	
Tel. +91 832 652 3796	
info@yogamagic.net	
www.yogamagic.net	

DIRECTIONS	25 miles north of Dabolim Airport; just over a mile away from Anjuna Beach.
YOGA	Ashtanga, Vinyasa Flow, Scaravelli, Sivananda, Kundalini, Iyengar.
ROOMS	7 tents for 2–3 people, 2 suites for 2–3 people.
FOOD	Organic tropical vegetarian cuisine. Caramelised pumpkin couscous.
TREATMENTS	Ayurvedic massage, Reiki, Indian head massage, foot massage, nutritional advice.
RECREATION	Ayurvedic massage courses, swimming, art and music sessions.

Ein unvergesslicher Trip

Reisfelder und Regenwald im Hinterland, weiß getünchte
katholische Kirchen in den Dörfern, verwunschene Herren-
sitze aus dem 17. Jahrhundert, endlose weiße Strände an
der Arabischen See – kein Wunder, dass die ehemalige por-
tugiesische Kolonie von den Hippies in den 1960ern zum
Paradies der freien Liebe erklärt wurde und den jahrelangen
Ansturm bekiffter Aussteiger nur ziemlich angeschlagen
überlebte. Doch jenseits der Partystrände erinnern Geheim-
tipps wie Yogamagic daran, welchen unverwechselbaren
Reiz der kleinste Bundesstaat Indiens seit jeher auf seine
Besucher hat. Eine halbe Stunde vom Meer, in einen Kokos-
nusshain gebaut, gewinnt dieses Öko-Resort seinen Zauber
ganz aus natürlichen Ressourcen. Wer am Schluss der
morgendlichen Yogastunde auf dem Boden des Yoga-
Tempels liegt, der mit getrocknetem Schlamm, Kuhdung
und Lehm aus der Erde gestampft wurde, und den Blick
zum hohen lichten Dach aus Bambus und Palmblättern
hebt, erlebt einen völlig legalen Trip. Wem das nicht genügt,
dem hilft Vishnu, der legendäre Masseur aus Pune, bei der
Entspannung oder der köstliche Chai, der bei Sonnenaufgang auf der Veranda der mit Solarenergie versorgten Luxus-
zelte serviert wird.
Buchtipps: »Sei jetzt hier« von Ram Dass, »Zirkuskind«
von John Irving und »Der Gott der kleinen Dinge« von
Arundhati Roy.

Un trip inoubliable

Rizières et forêts vierges dans l'arrière-pays, églises catho-
liques aux murs blanchis dans les villages, manoirs féeriques
datant du 17e siècle, plages blanches longeant à l'infini la mer
d'Arabie : quoi d'étonnant si l'ancienne colonie portugaise
fut instituée paradis de l'amour libre par les hippies dans les
années 1960 et sortit bien éprouvée de la longue invasion de
ces fumeurs de hasch en quête d'aventure. Pourtant, au-delà
des plages festives, des endroits cachés, comme le Yogamagic,
rappellent le charme incomparable que le plus petit Etat
indien exerce depuis toujours sur ses visiteurs. Situé à une
demi-heure de la mer au cœur d'un petit bois de cocotiers,
ce site écologique tire toute sa magie de ressources natu-
relles. Celui qui, après une séance matinale, est étendu sur
le sol du temple de yoga, mélange de terre battue, de boue
séchée, de bouse de vache et d'argile, et qui lève très haut
les yeux vers le toit aéré fait de bambous et de feuilles de
palmiers, vit un trip entièrement légal. Celui qui recherche
davantage s'adresse pour sa relaxation à Vishnu, le masseur
légendaire de Pune ou déguste le succulent Chai, servi au
lever du soleil sur la véranda d'une des luxueuses tentes
chauffées à l'énergie solaire.
Livres à emporter : « Vieillir en pleine conscience » de Ram
Dass, « Un enfant de la balle » de John Irving et « Le Dieu des
petits riens » d'Arundhati Roy.

ANREISE	40 km nördlich vom Flughafen Dabolim, etwa 2 km von Anjuna Beach entfernt.
YOGA	Astanga, Vinyasa Flow, Scaravelli, Sivananda, Kundalini, Iyengar.
ZIMMER	7 Zelte für 2–3 Personen, 2 Suiten für 2–3 Personen.
KÜCHE	Organisch-vegetarisch-tropisch. Karamellisierter Kürbis-Couscous.
ANWENDUNGEN	Ayurvedische Massage, Reiki, indische Kopfmassage, Fußmassage, Ernährungsberatung.
FREIZEIT	Ayurvedische Massagekurse, Schwimmen, Kunst- und Musiksessions.

ACCÈS	Situé à 40 km au nord de l'aéroport de Dabolim, à environ 2 km d'Anjuna Beach.
YOGA	Ashtânga, Vinyasa Flow, Scaravelli, Shivananda, Kundalinî, Iyengar.
CHAMBRES	7 tentes pour 2–3 personnes, 2 suites pour 2–3 personnes.
RESTAURATION	Cuisine tropicale organique et végétarienne. Couscous caramélisé au potiron.
TRAITEMENTS	Massage ayurvédique, reiki, massage crânien de tradition indienne, massage des pieds, conseils de diététique.
ACTIVITÉS	Cours de massage ayurvédique, natation, sessions artistiques et musicales.

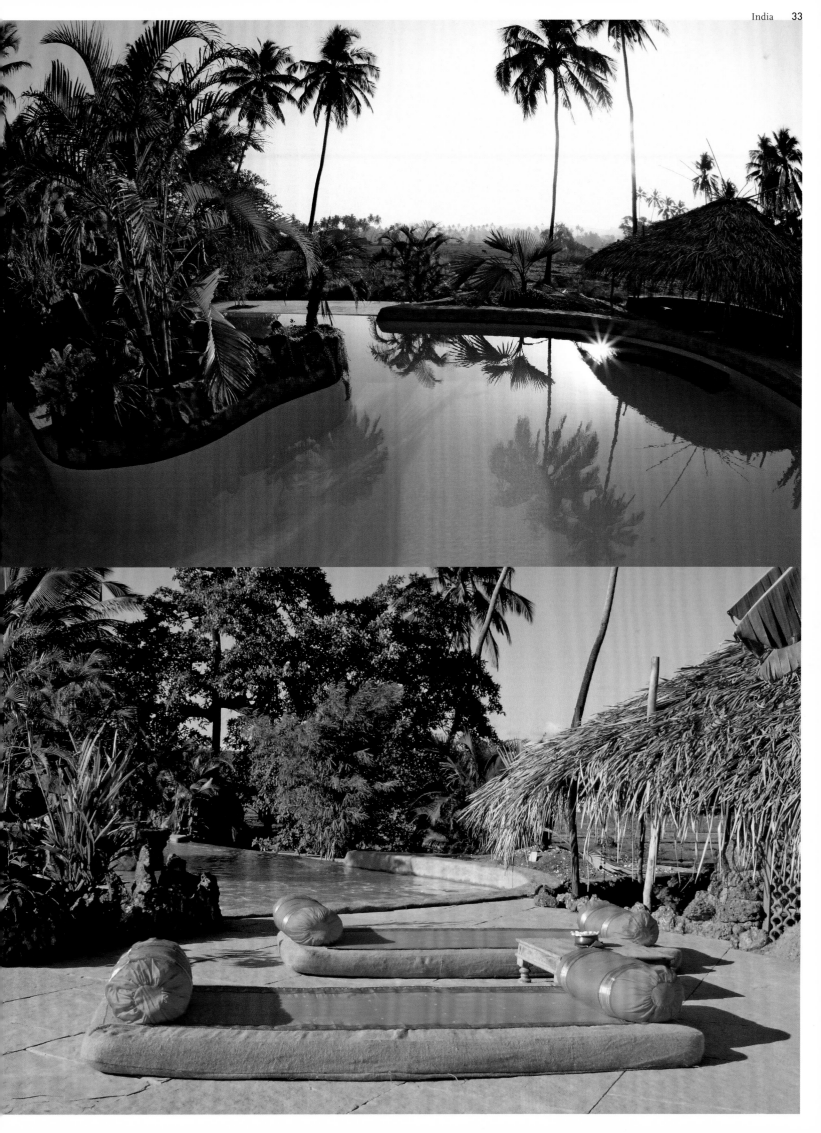

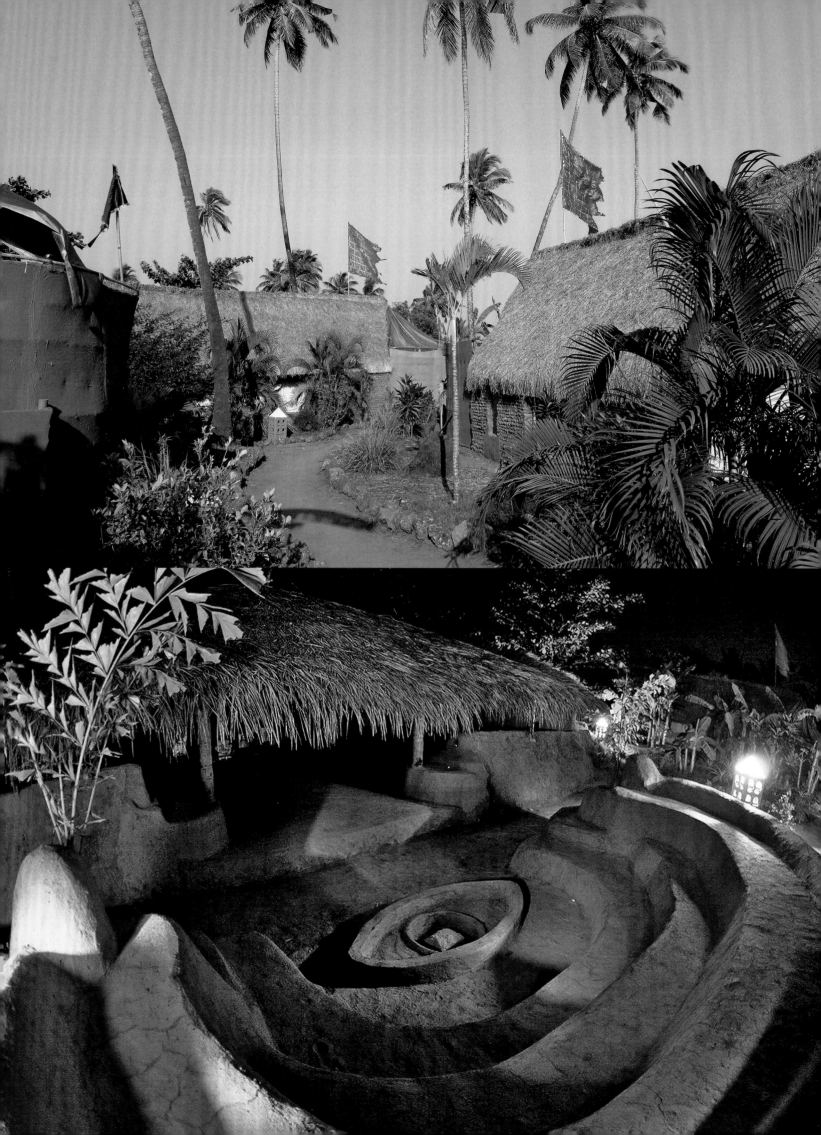

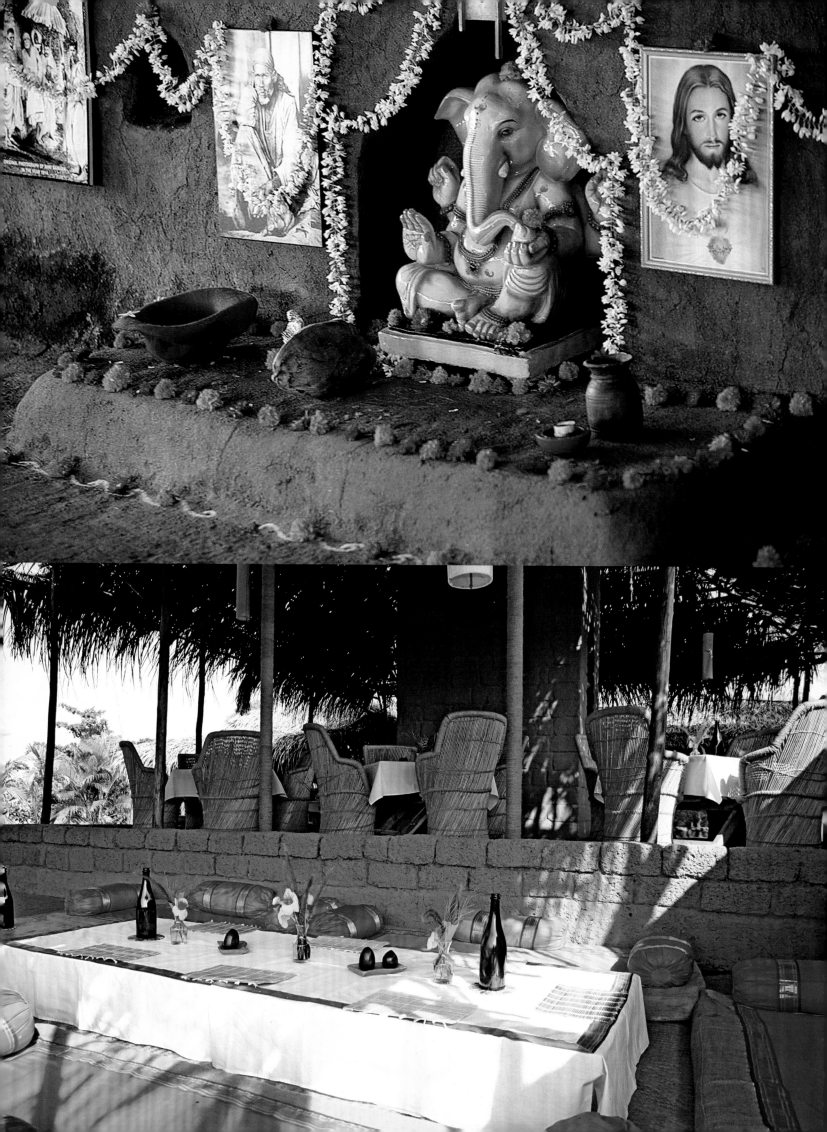

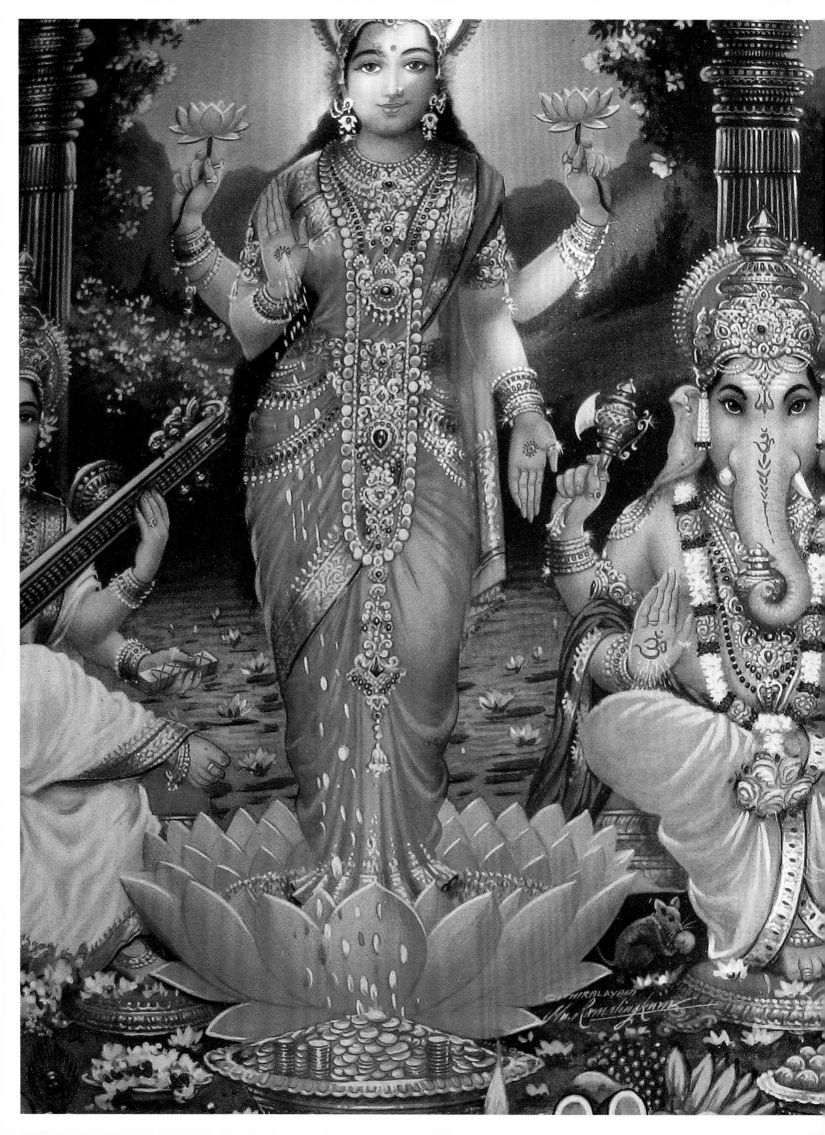

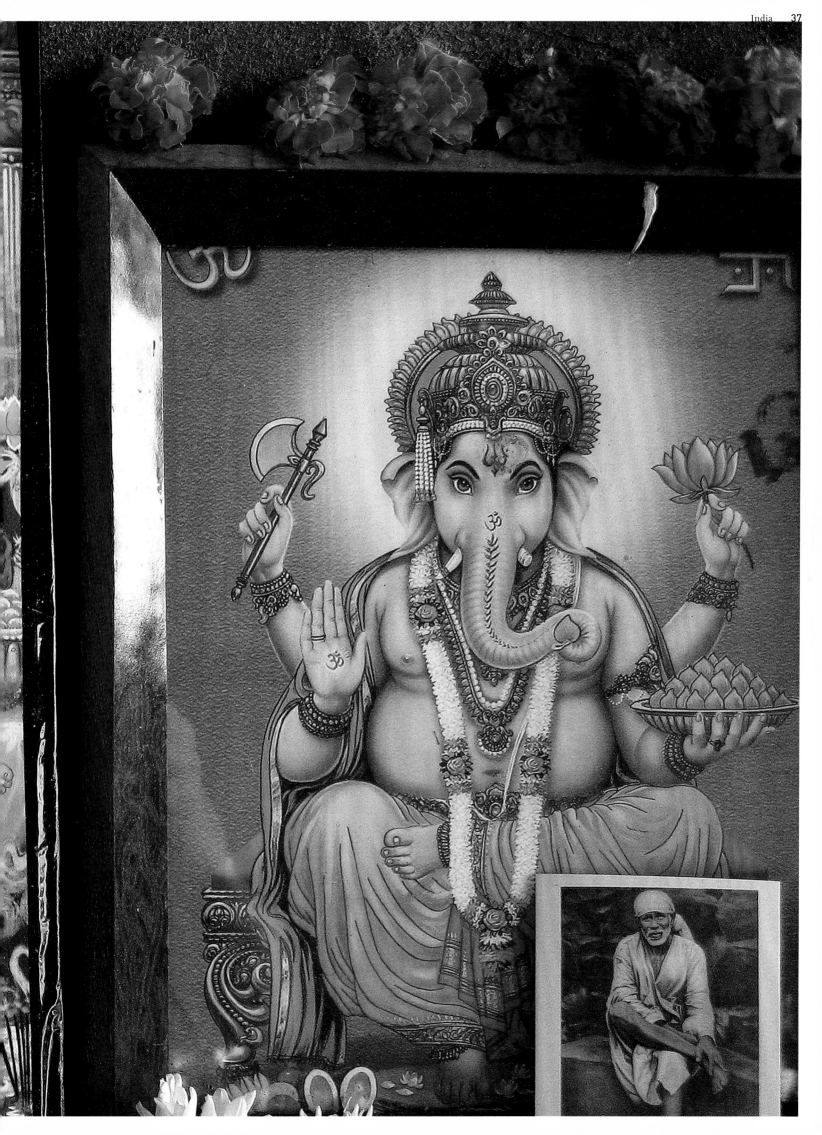

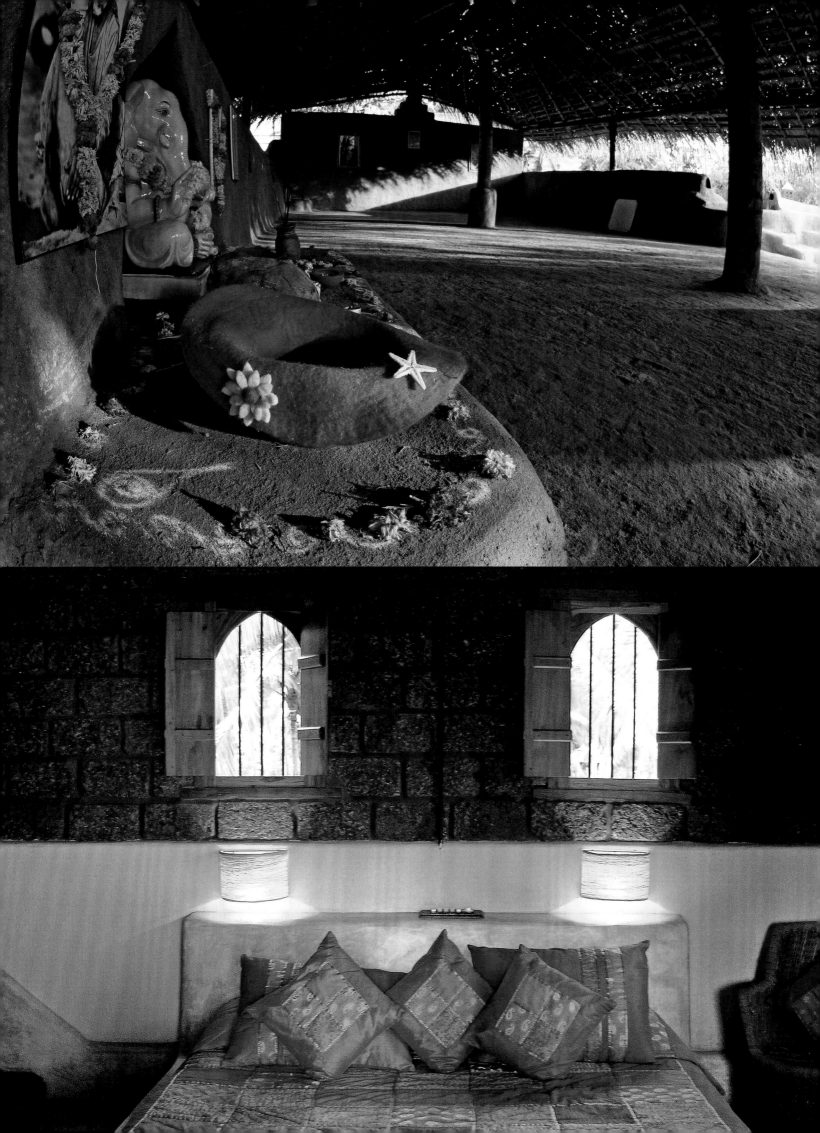

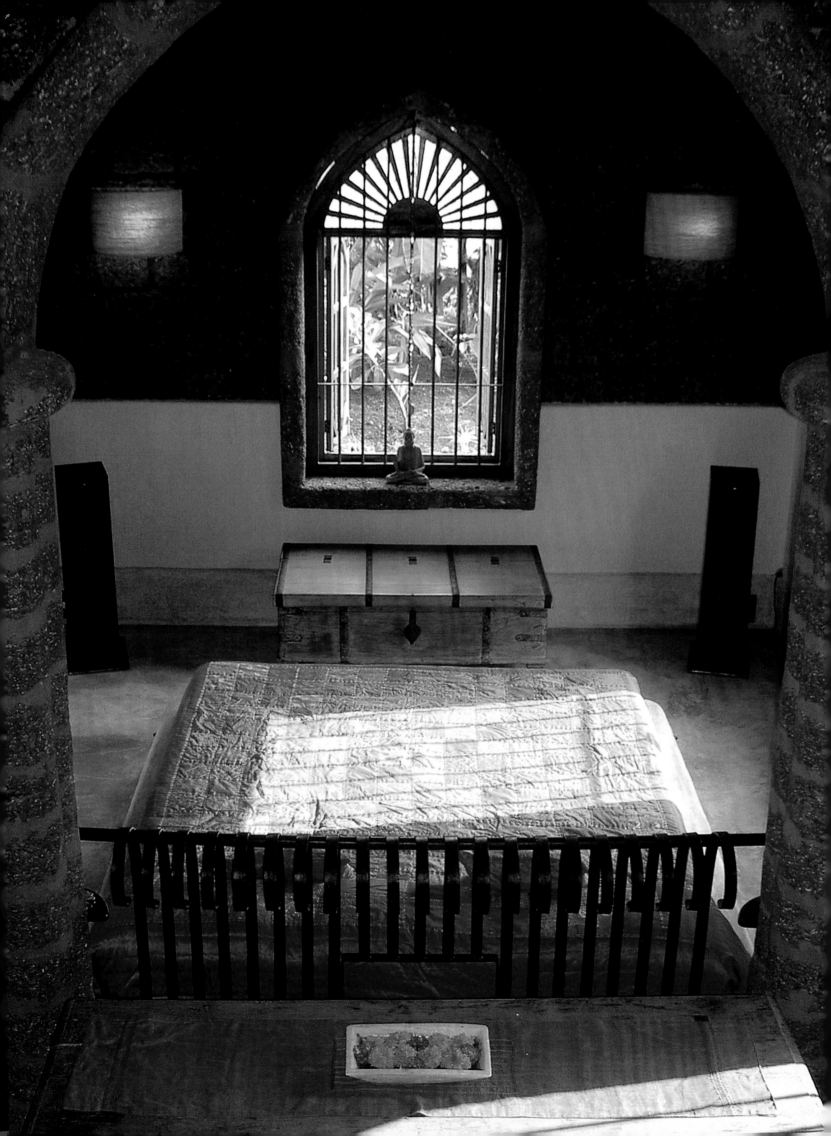

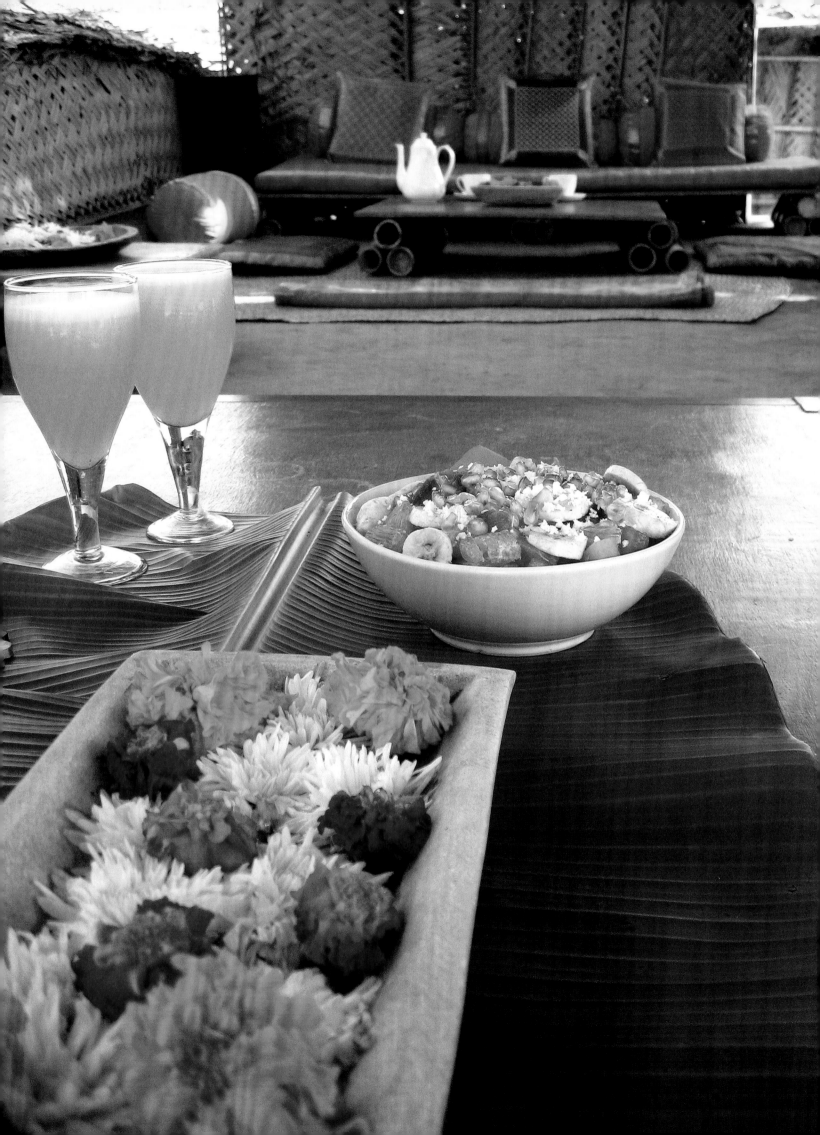

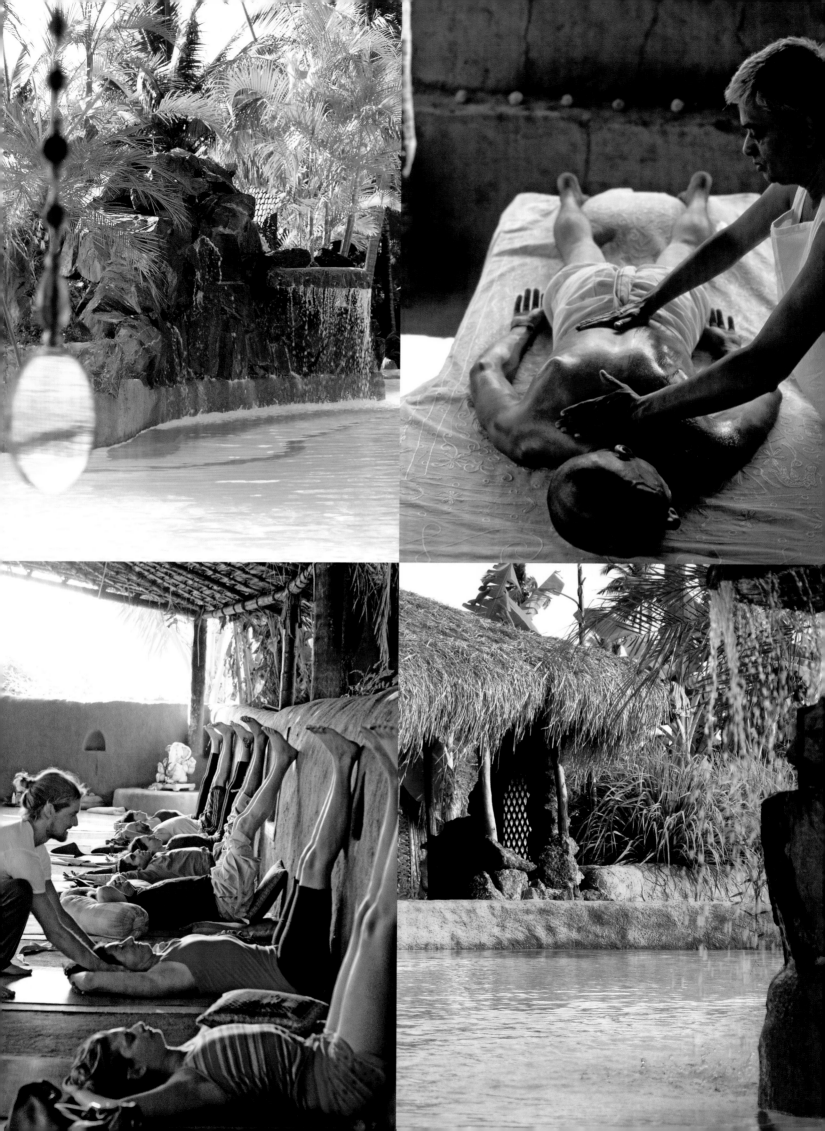

Peace in the Jungle of Thou

Ulpotha, Galgiriyawa Mountains

Ulpotha, Galgiriyawa Mountains

Peace in the Jungle of Thought

One of Asia's most extraordinary ecotourism projects came into being at the place where elephant paths crossed, Shiva's son had a shrine built and a prince fled with his legendarily beautiful but poor lover. Rebuilt as a traditional farming village, Ulpotha lies in the middle of former Ceylon's deepest jungle next to a small lake, surrounded by seven hills in which ascetics and shamans still meditate in their caves. But Ulpotha is by no means withdrawn. The Ayurveda treatments in the eco lodge, a treasure trove of centuries-old remedies, are considered an insiders' tip and are included in the price. With neither electricity nor mobile-phone reception, Ulpotha's luxury consists in making contact with nature: ambling between hibiscus plants along the sandy paths to the lake, observing how lizards stretch out in the sun, swimming among the water lilies or taking a stroll in the surrounding hills at sunset. A Yoga session with the legendary Tripsichore teacher Edward Clark even teaches the guest to feel like an ant. Typical British understatement in outstanding surroundings.

Books to pack: "Yoga and Ayurveda: Self-Healing and Self-Realization" by David Frawley and "Anil's Ghost" by Michael Ondaatje.

Ulpotha
Embogama Nr Galgamuwa
Kurunegala District
Sri Lanka
Tel. +44 208 123 3603
info@ulpotha.com
www.ulpotha.com

DIRECTIONS	Located in central Sri Lanka. Some 3 hrs away from Colombo Airport. Airport transfer by arrangement.
YOGA	Hatha, Ashtanga, Sivananda, Iyengar, Anusara.
TEACHERS	Edward Clark, Sam Cunningham, Mika, Anoushka Pletts, Jean Hall, Daniela Schmid. Each teacher gives instruction for a period of 14 days.
ROOMS	10 cottages, 2 rooms in the main building. Max. 19/20 people.
FOOD	Strictly organic vegetarian food with products grown on site, e.g. green mango curry with coconut milk.
TREATMENTS	Ayurveda therapy, Panchakarma, massages, sauna, herbal baths, detox and rejuvenation cures, Shiatsu.
RECREATION	Swimming, hiking.

Ruhe im Gedankendschungel

Wo sich Elefantenwege kreuzten, Shivas Sohn einen Schrein errichten ließ und wohin ein Prinz mit seiner legendär schönen, aber armen Geliebten floh, entstand eines der außergewöhnlichsten Ökotourismus-Projekte Asiens. Wieder aufgebaut als traditionelles Bauerndorf, liegt Ulpotha mitten im tiefsten Dschungel des ehemaligen Ceylon an einem kleinen See, umringt von sieben Hügeln, in denen noch immer Asketen und Schamanen in ihren Höhlen meditieren. Doch Ulpotha ist alles andere als weltabgewandt. Als Schatzkammer jahrhundertealter Heilmittel gelten die Ayurveda-Behandlungen in der Öko-Lodge als Geheimtipp und sind im Preis inbegriffen. Ohne Strom und Handyempfang besteht der Luxus von Ulpotha darin, Kontakt zur Natur aufzunehmen – auf den sandigen Wegen zwischen Hibiskuspflanzen zum See zu schlendern, zuzusehen, wie sich Eidechsen in der Sonne räkeln, zwischen den Wasserlilien zu schwimmen oder bei Sonnenuntergang eine Wanderung auf die umliegenden Hügel zu machen. Eine Yogastunde beim legendären Tripsichore-Lehrer Edward Clark lehrt den Gast sogar, sich wie eine Ameise zu fühlen. Typisch britisches Understatement in herausragender Umgebung.

Buchtipps: »Das große Handbuch des Yoga und Ayurveda« von David Frawley und »Anils Geist« von Michael Ondaatje.

Paix dans la jungle des pensées

Là où les routes des éléphants se croisaient, où le fils de Shiva fit ériger un sanctuaire et où un prince vint se réfugier avec sa bien-aimée, une très belle mais très pauvre jeune fille, a vu le jour un des projets les plus extraordinaires d'écotourisme en Asie. Ulpotha, reconstruit comme village de paysans traditionnel, est implanté au fin fond de la jungle, dans l'ancien territoire du Ceylan, au bord d'un petit lac entouré de sept collines, dans les grottes desquelles méditent, aujourd'hui encore, les ascètes et les chamans. Toutefois, Ulpotha est tout sauf isolé du monde. Trésors de remèdes séculaires, les traitements d'Ayurveda pratiqués dans l'écovillage sont une référence incontournable et sont inclus dans le prix. Sans électricité et sans réception portable, le luxe d'Ulpotha consiste à prendre contact avec la nature : sur les chemins sableux entre les plants d'hibiscus, flâner vers le lac, observer les lézards qui s'étirent au soleil, nager parmi les fleurs de lotus ou, au coucher du soleil, faire une promenade dans les collines environnantes. Une séance de yoga auprès d'Edward Clark, le fameux professeur de tripsichore, donne même au visiteur la sensation d'être une fourmi. Understatement typiquement britannique dans un cadre grandiose.

Livres à emporter : « Yoga et Ayurvéda : Autoguérison et Réalisation de Soi » de David Frawley et « Le fantôme d'Anil » de Michael Ondaatje.

ANREISE	Mitten in Sri Lanka gelegen. Etwa 3 Std. vom Colombo-Flughafen entfernt. Flughafentransfer nach Absprache.
YOGA	Hatha, Astanga, Sivananda, Iyengar, Anusara.
GASTLEHRER	Edward Clark, Sam Cunningham, Mika, Anoushka Pletts, Jean Hall, Daniela Schmid. Jeder Gastlehrer unterrichtet jeweils 14 Tage.
ZIMMER	10 Cottages, 2 Zimmer im Haupthaus. Max. 19/20 Personen.
KÜCHE	Streng organisch-vegetarisch.
ANWENDUNGEN	Ayurveda, Panchakarma, Massagen, Kräuterbad, Detox- und Verjüngungskuren, Shiatsu.
FREIZEIT	Schwimmen, Wandern.

ACCÈS	Situé au cœur du Sri Lanka à 3 h environ de l'aéroport de Colombo. Transfert de l'aéroport sur demande.
YOGA	Hatha, Ashtânga, Shivananda, Iyengar, Anusara.
PROFESSEURS	Edward Clark, Sam Cunningham, Mika, Anoushka Pletts, Jean Hall, Daniela Schmid. Chaque professeur invité enseigne pendant 14 jours.
CHAMBRES	10 cottages, 2 chambres dans la maison principale. 19–20 personnes max.
RESTAURATION	Cuisine organique et végétarienne stricte.
TRAITEMENTS	Panchakarma, massages, bains d'herbes, cures de désintoxication et de rajeunissement, shiatsu.
ACTIVITÉS	Natation, randonnées.

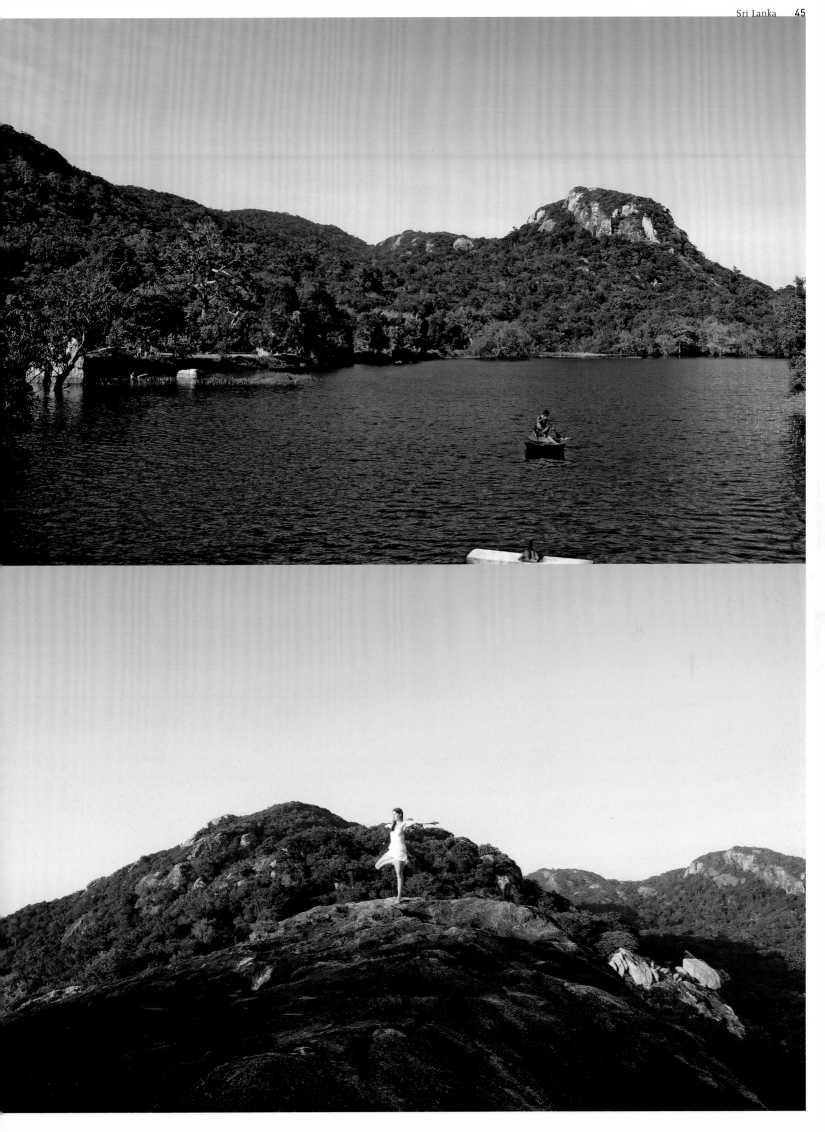

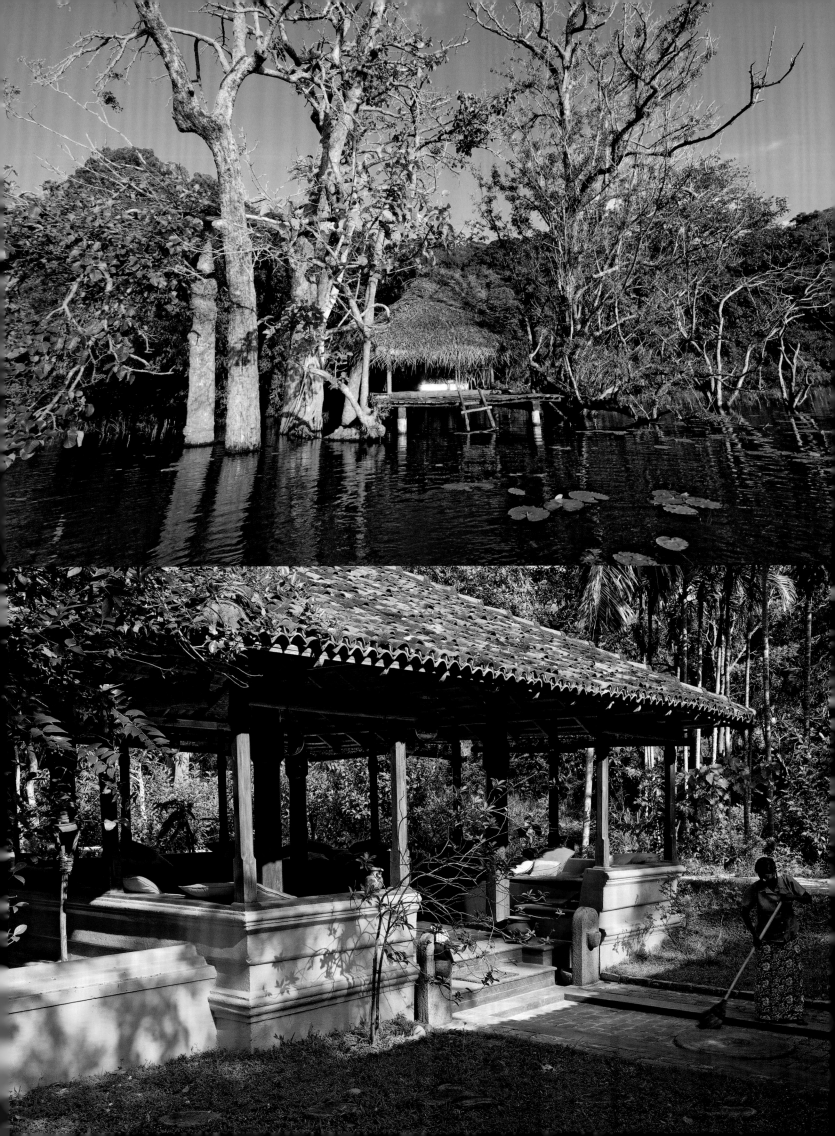

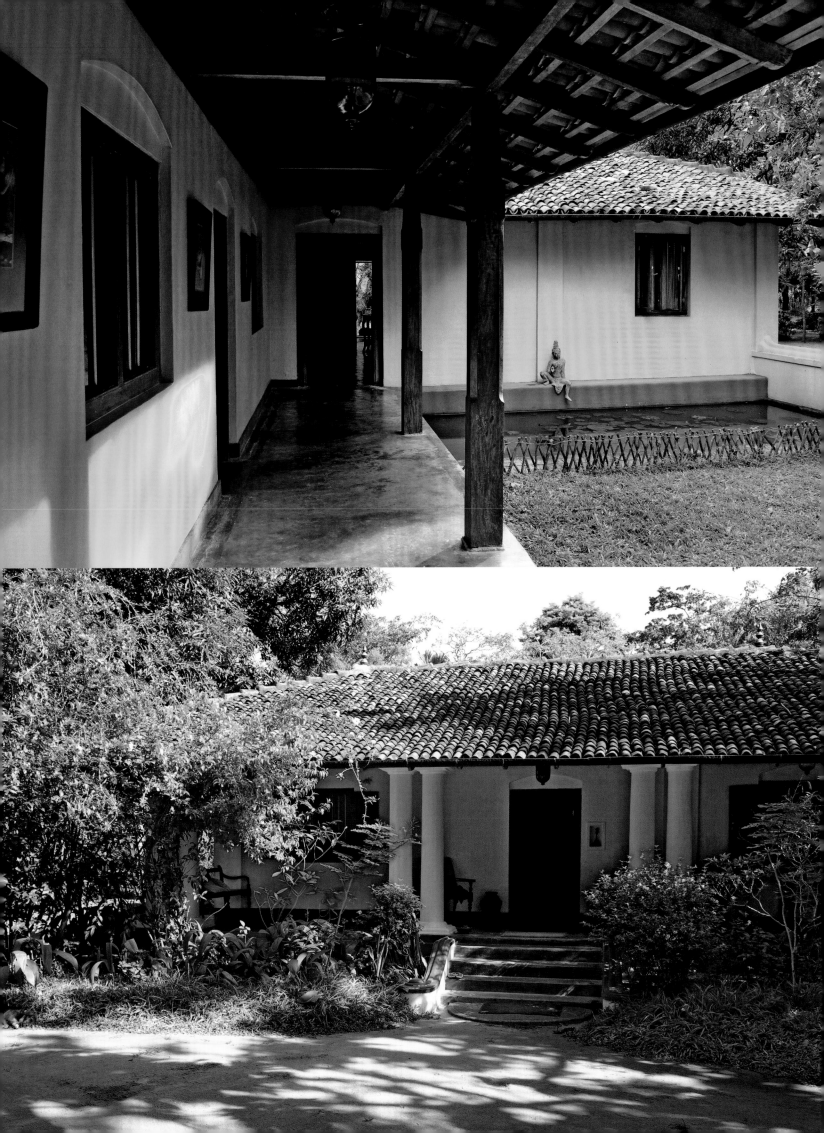

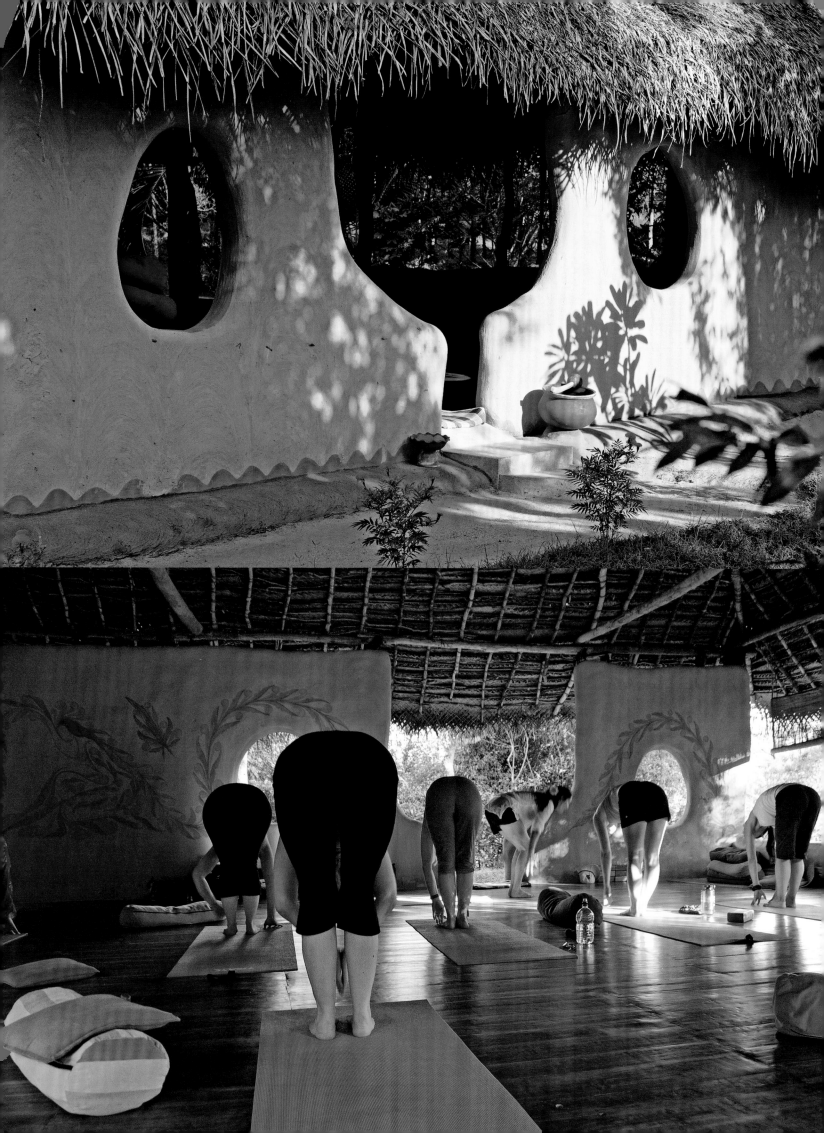

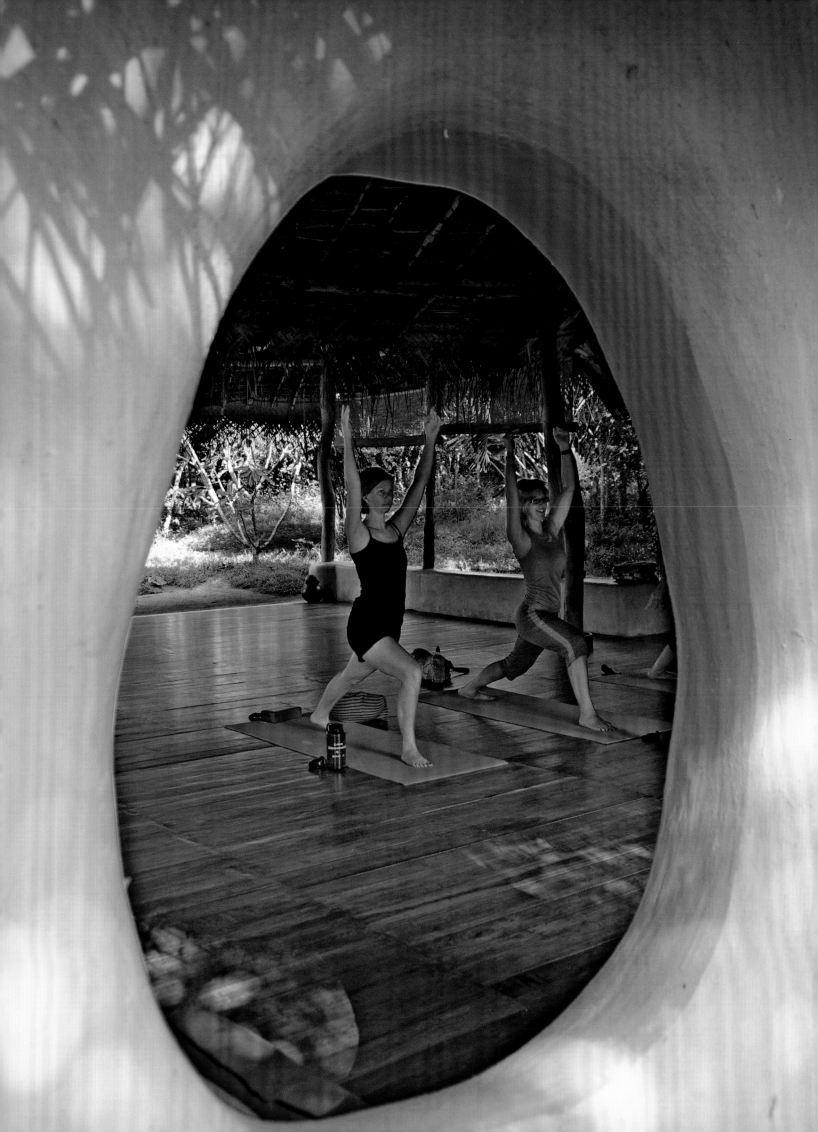

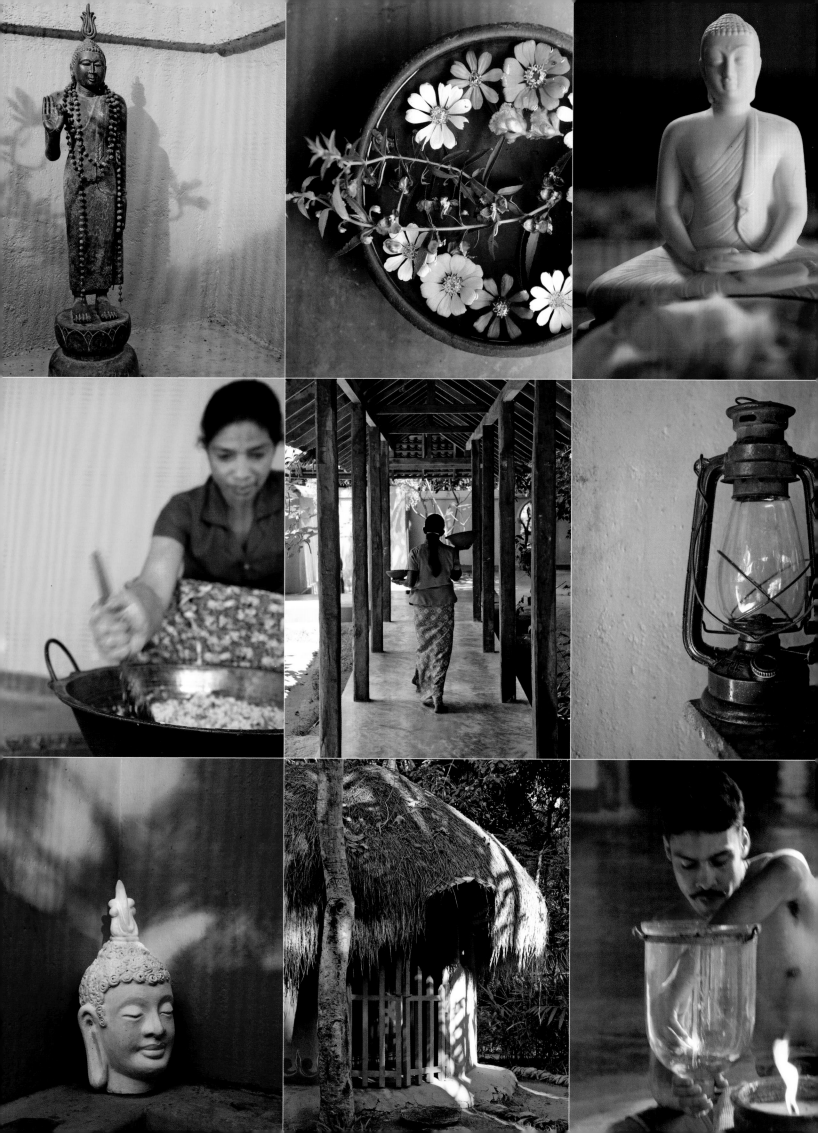

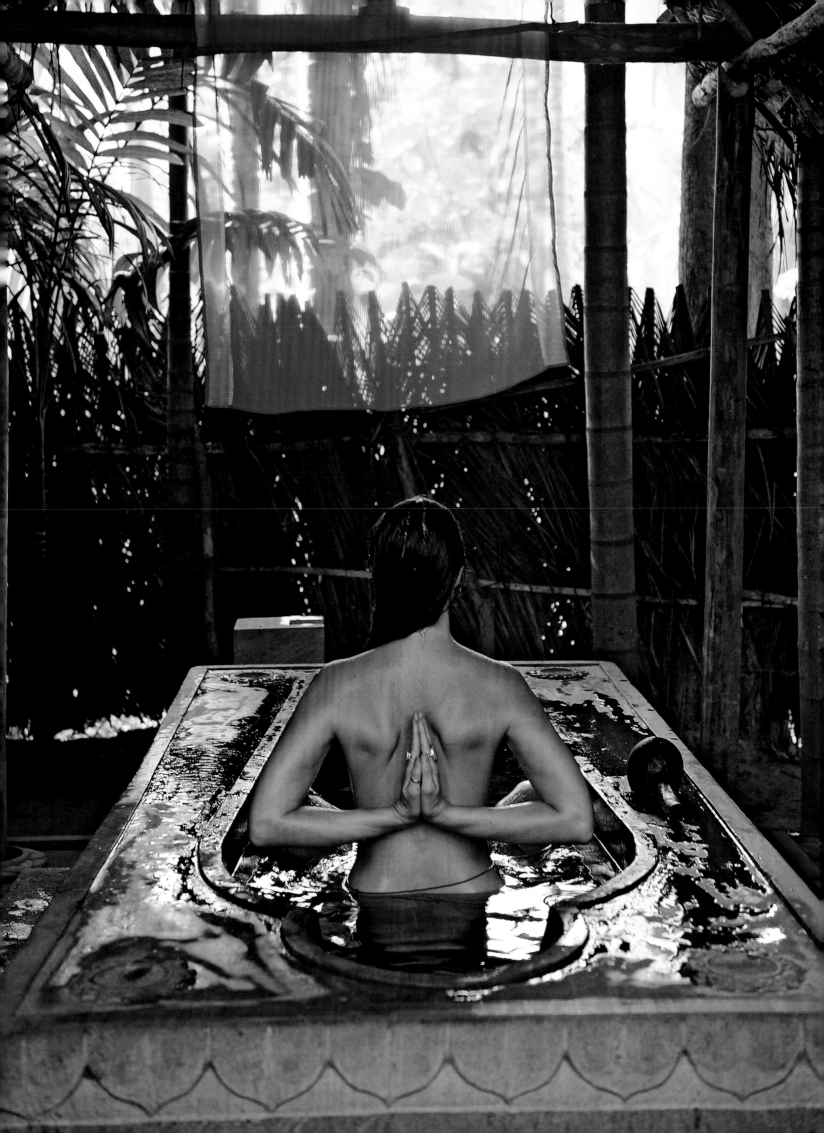

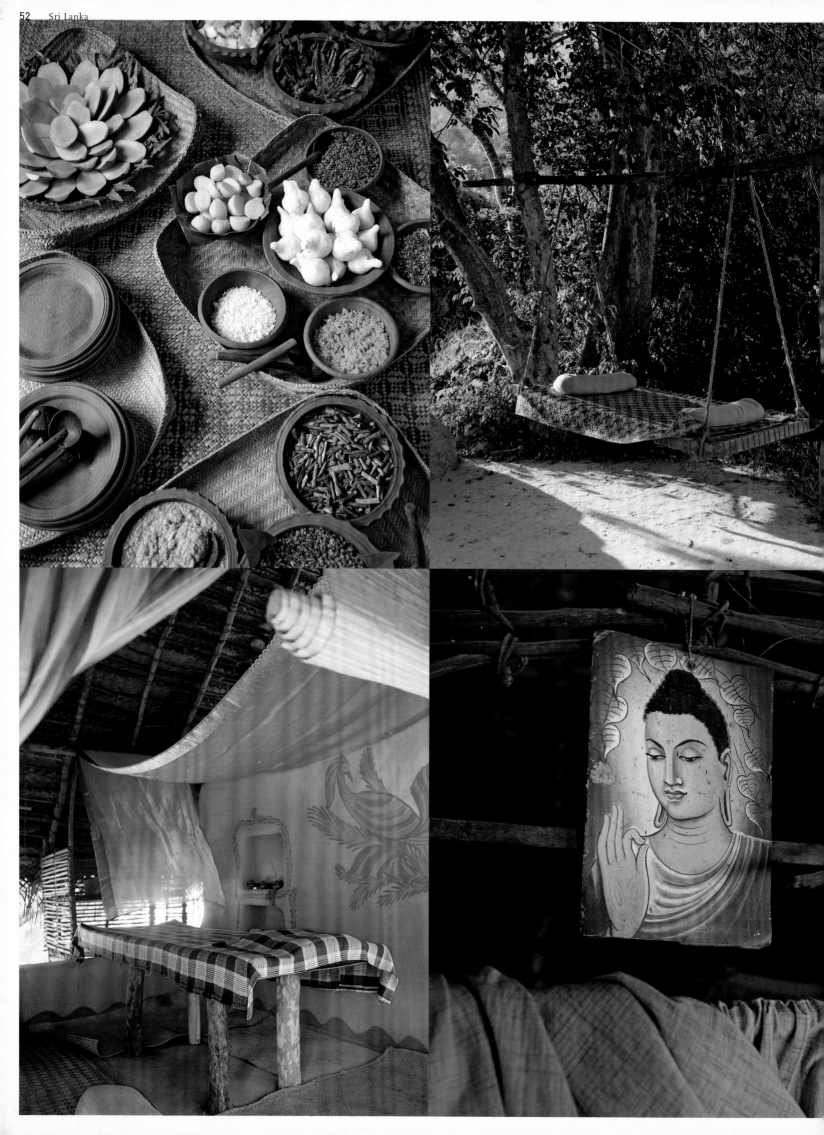

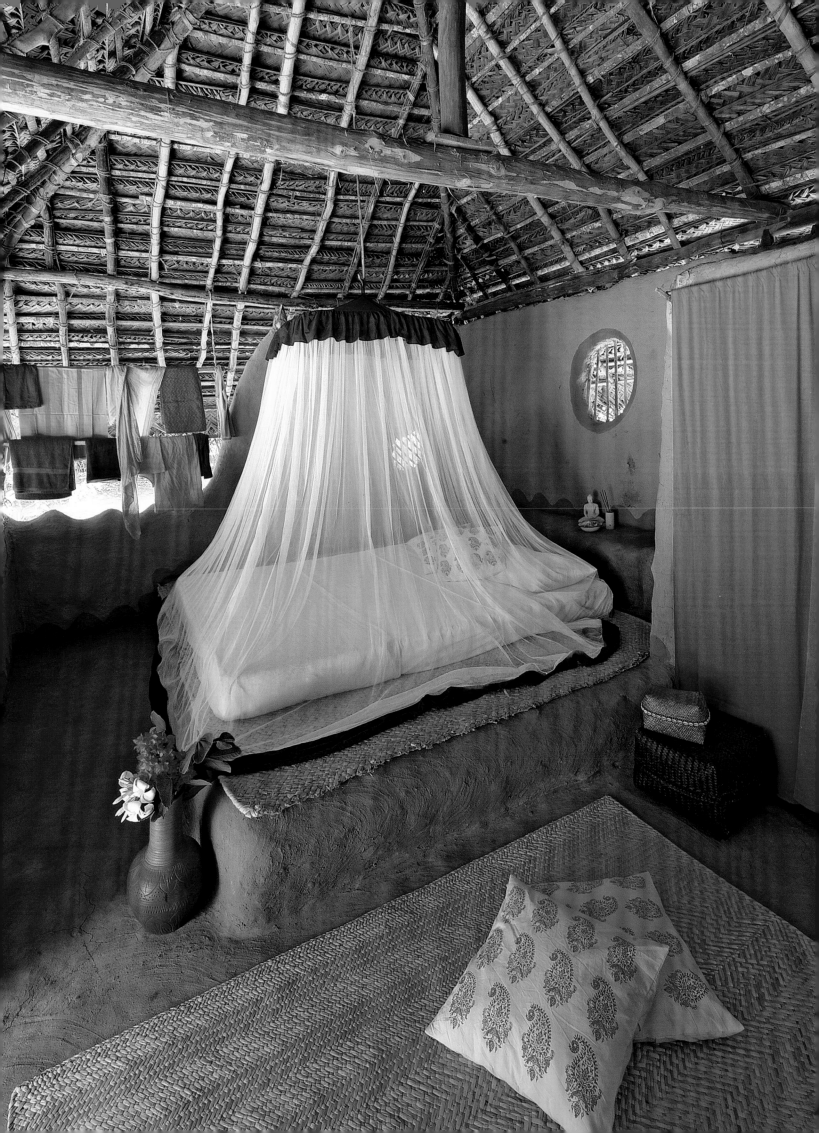

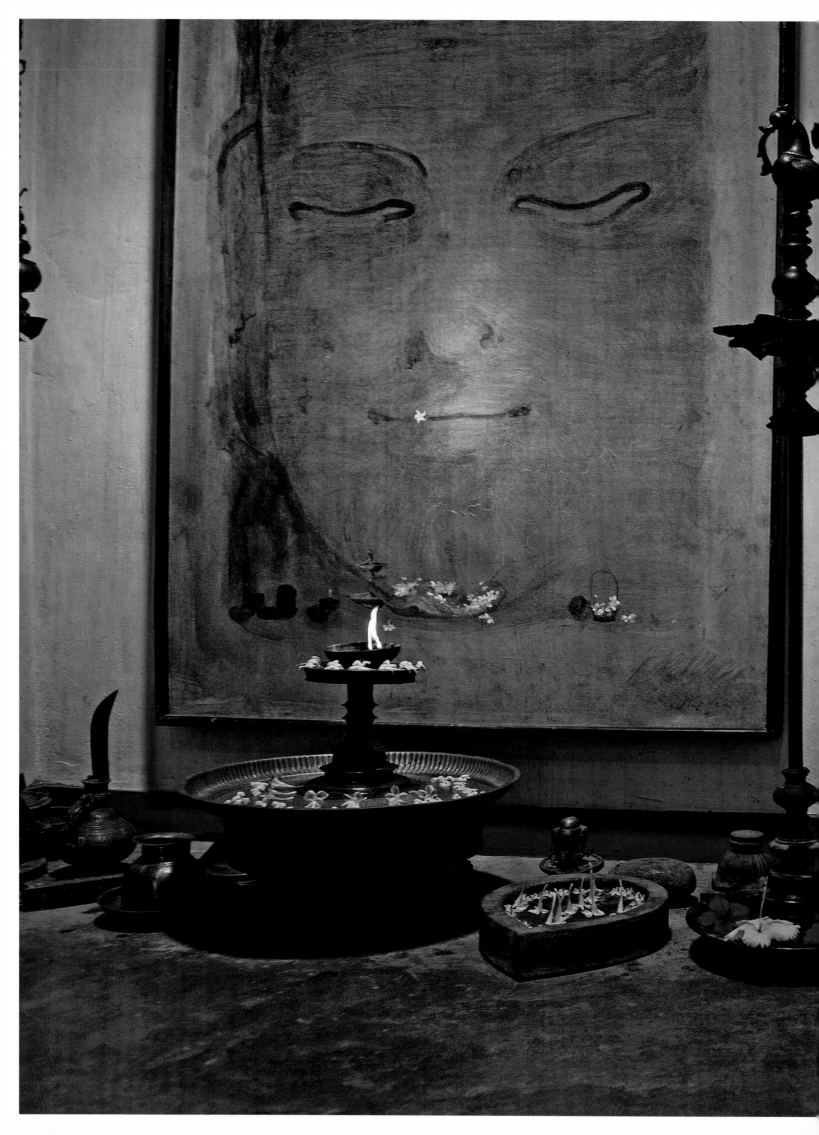

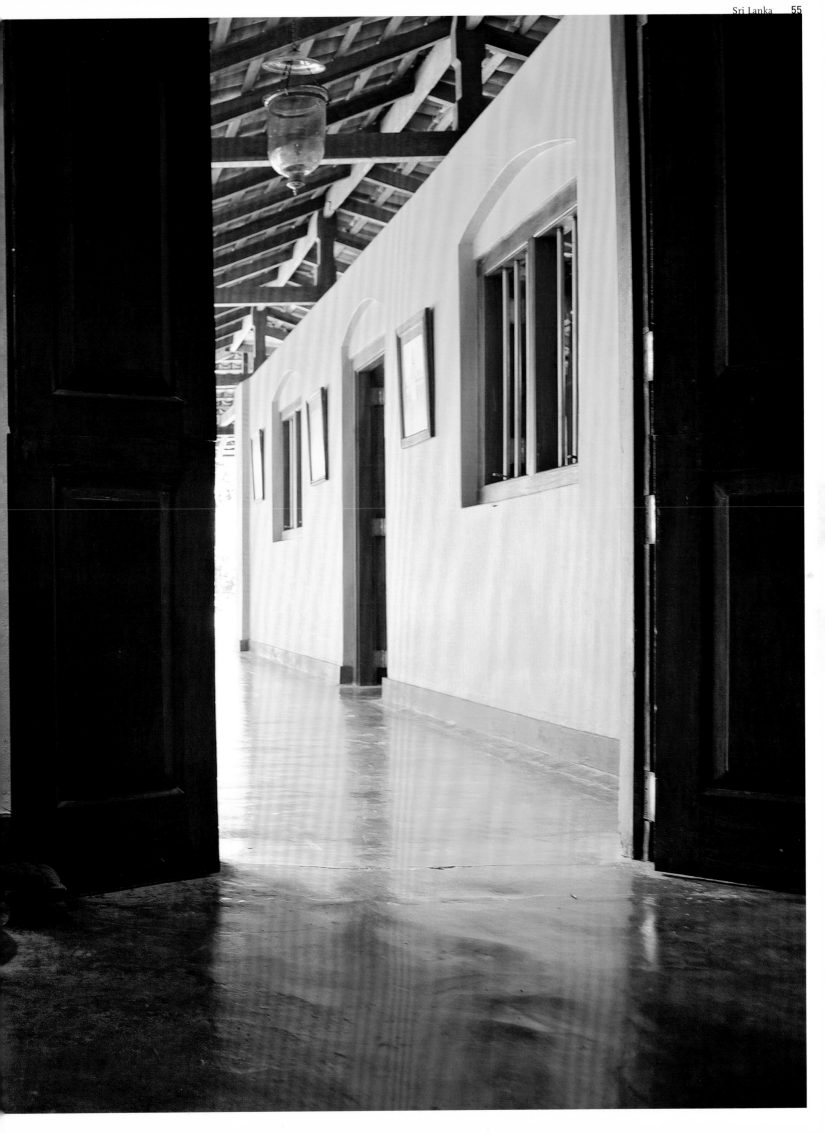

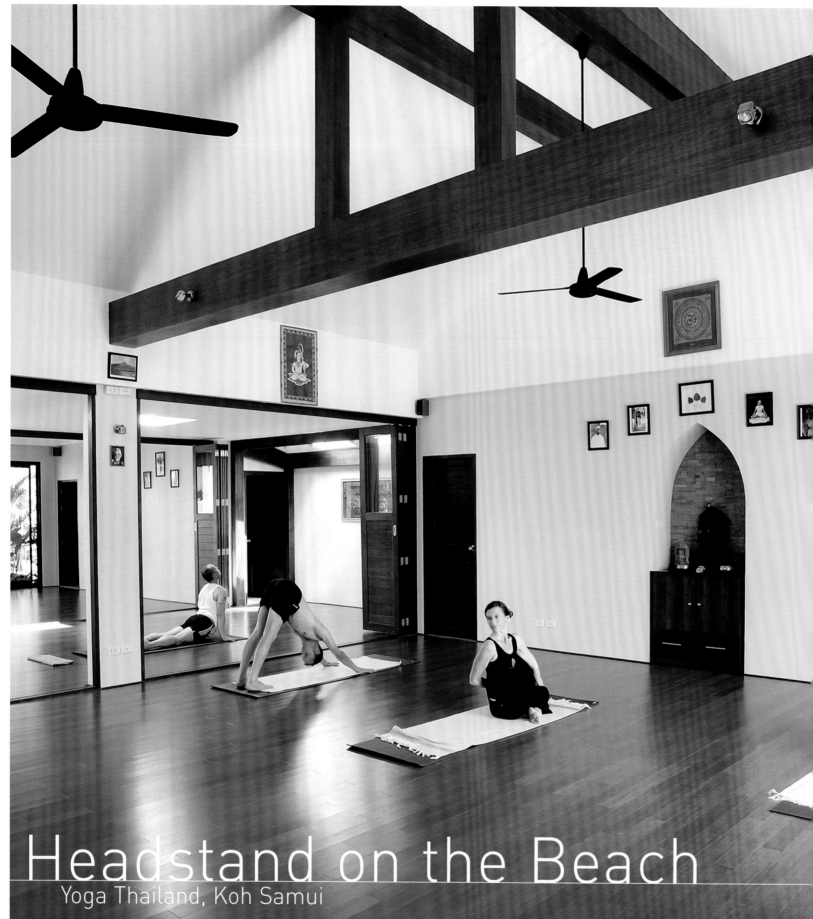

Headstand on the Beach
Yoga Thailand, Koh Samui

Yoga Thailand, Koh Samui

Headstand on the Beach

When in 2001, with modest savings, Paul and Jutima squinted at the light at the end of the Lincoln Tunnel, they were leaving not only New York but also their former years in training as yoga teachers behind them. Their destination was Los Angeles, their next stop Bangkok, Jutima's place of birth. Before they founded Yoga Thailand, they travelled to India in order to study in Mysore with their teacher Pattabhi Jois and his grandson Sharath. The respect and the seriousness that are the features of the constant practice of the couple are also present in every detail of this beautiful resort. From the light Yoga Shala – on whose bamboo floor sweating bodies raise themselves into a handstand, the excellent equipment including props such as Iyengar belts hanging from the ceiling and the wall – to the delightful meditation garden, the saltwater pool and on to the inviting lounge: lucidity and a cool head, obeisance to the masters and silent contentment are the goal. Yoga is everywhere. As Pattabhi Jois said: "Practise. And the rest will follow."

Books to pack: "The Yoga Sutras of Patanjali" by Sri Swami Satchidananda and "Shantaram" by Gregory David Roberts.

Yoga Thailand
55/20–24 Moo 4,
T. Namuang, Koh Samui
Suratthani 84140
Thailand
Tel. +66 77 920 090 and +66 77 920 091
info@yoga-thailand.com
www.yoga-thailand.com

DIRECTIONS	Located on the south coast of Koh Samui at Laem Sor Beach, 45 min from the airport.
YOGA	Ashtange, Vinyasa, Pranayama, Prenatal, Yoga Anatomy, teacher training.
TEACHERS	Richard Freeman, Sri O.P. Tiwari.
ROOMS	28 rooms.
FOOD	Asian-European freshly prepared using local produce, occasionally fish and eggs, juice bar.
TREATMENTS	Detox, bodywork, massages, infra-red sauna, steam bath, colon hydrotherapy.
RECREATION	Saltwater pool, walks along the beach.

Kopfstand am Strand

Als Paul und Jutima mit wenig Erspartem 2001 in das Licht
am Ende des Lincoln-Tunnels blinzelten, ließen sie nicht nur
New York, sondern auch ihre frühen Lehrjahre als Yogalehrer
hinter sich. Ihr Ziel war Los Angeles, nächster Halt Bangkok,
Jutimas Geburtsort. Bevor sie Yoga Thailand gründeten,
reisten sie nach Indien, um in Mysore bei ihrem Lehrer
Pattabhi Jois und dessen Enkel Sharath zu studieren. Der
Respekt und die Ernsthaftigkeit, die das beständige Üben
der beiden auszeichnen, steckt auch in jedem Detail dieses
wunderschönen Resorts. Von der lichten Yoga-Shala, auf
deren Bambusboden sich schwitzend die Körper in den
Handstand heben, und der ausgezeichneten Ausstattung mit
Hilfsmitteln inklusive Iyengar-Gurten, die von der Decke
und der Wand hängen, über den lieblichen Meditations-
garten, den Salzwasserpool, bis zur einladenden Lounge:
Transparenz und ein kühler Kopf, Verneigung vor den
Meistern und stille Fröhlichkeit sind das Ziel. Yoga ist
überall. Wie Pattabhi Jois sagte: »Übe. Der Rest ergibt sich.«
**Buchtipps: »The Yoga Sutras of Patanjali« von Sri Swami
Satchidananda und »Shantaram« von Gregory David Roberts.**

Faire le poirier sur la plage

Lorsqu'en 2001 Paul et Jutima, avec leurs quelques écono-
mies en poche, aperçurent une lueur au fond du tunnel
Lincoln, ils ne laissaient pas seulement New York derrière eux,
mais aussi leurs années de formation comme professeurs de
yoga. Leur but était Los Angeles, prochaine halte : Bangkok,
ville natale de Jutima. Avant de fonder le Yoga Thailand, ils
allèrent en Inde, à Mysore, pour s'instruire auprès de leur
professeur Pattabhi Jois et de son petit-fils Sharath. Le respect et le sérieux qui caractérisent l'entraînement constant
de ces deux-là sont également présents dans chaque détail
de ce merveilleux site. De la yoga-shala très aérienne au
plancher de bambou sur lequel les corps en sueur font le
poirier, à l'excellent équipement avec des accessoires comme
la ceinture Iyengar, accrochés au plafond et sur le mur, en
passant par l'exquis jardin de méditation, la piscine d'eau
salée jusqu'à l'attrayant salon : transparence et idées claires,
déférence pour les maîtres et joie sereine sont la finalité.
Le yoga est omniprésent. Comme Pattabhi Jois a dit :
« Entraînez-vous et le reste suivra. »
**Livres à emporter : « The Yoga Sutras of Patanjali » de Sri
Swami Satchidananda et « Shantaram » de Gregory David
Roberts.**

ANREISE	An der Südküste von Koh Samui am Laem Sor Beach gelegen, 45 min Fahrt vom Flughafen.
YOGA	Astanga, Vinyasa, Pranayama, Prenatal, Yoga Anatomie, Teacher Training.
GASTLEHRER	Richard Freeman, Sri O.P. Tiwari.
ZIMMER	28 Zimmer.
KÜCHE	Asiatisch-europäisch, frisch zubereitet mit Produkten der Region, gelegentlich Fisch und Eier, Saftbar.
ANWENDUNGEN	Detox, Bodywork, Massagen, Infrarotsauna, Dampf-bad, Darmspülung durch Colon-Hydro-Therapie.
FREIZEIT	Salzwasserpool, Strandspaziergänge.

ACCÈS	Situé sur la côte sud de Koh Samui sur la Laem Sor Beach, à 45 min de l'aéroport.
YOGA	Ashtânga, Vinyasa, Pranayama, Prénatal, Yoga Anatomie, Teacher Training.
PROFESSEURS	Richard Freeman, Sri O.P. Tiwari.
CHAMBRES	28 chambres.
RESTAURATION	Asiatique et européenne à base de produits bio de la région, occasionnellement poisson et œufs, jus de fruits et de légumes.
TRAITEMENTS	Detox, bodywork, massages, sauna infrarouge, bains de vapeur, hydrothérapie du côlon.
ACTIVITÉS	Piscine d'eau salée, promenades sur la plage.

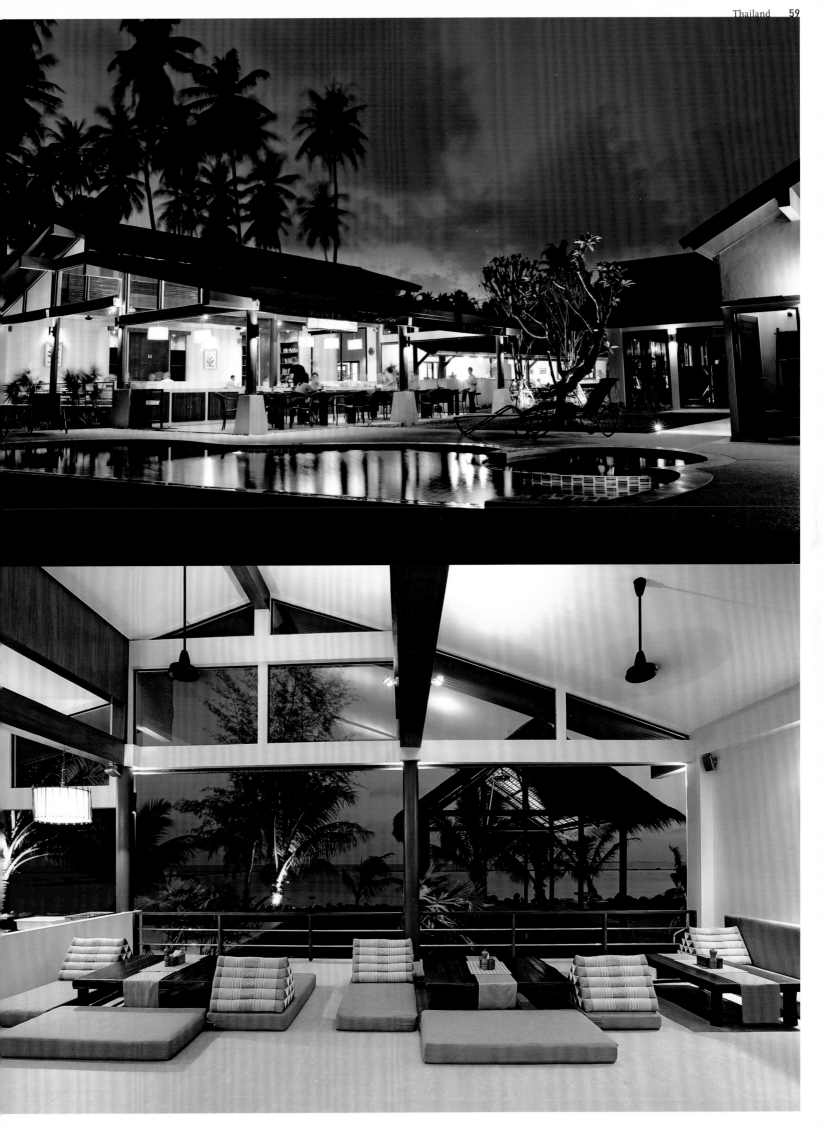

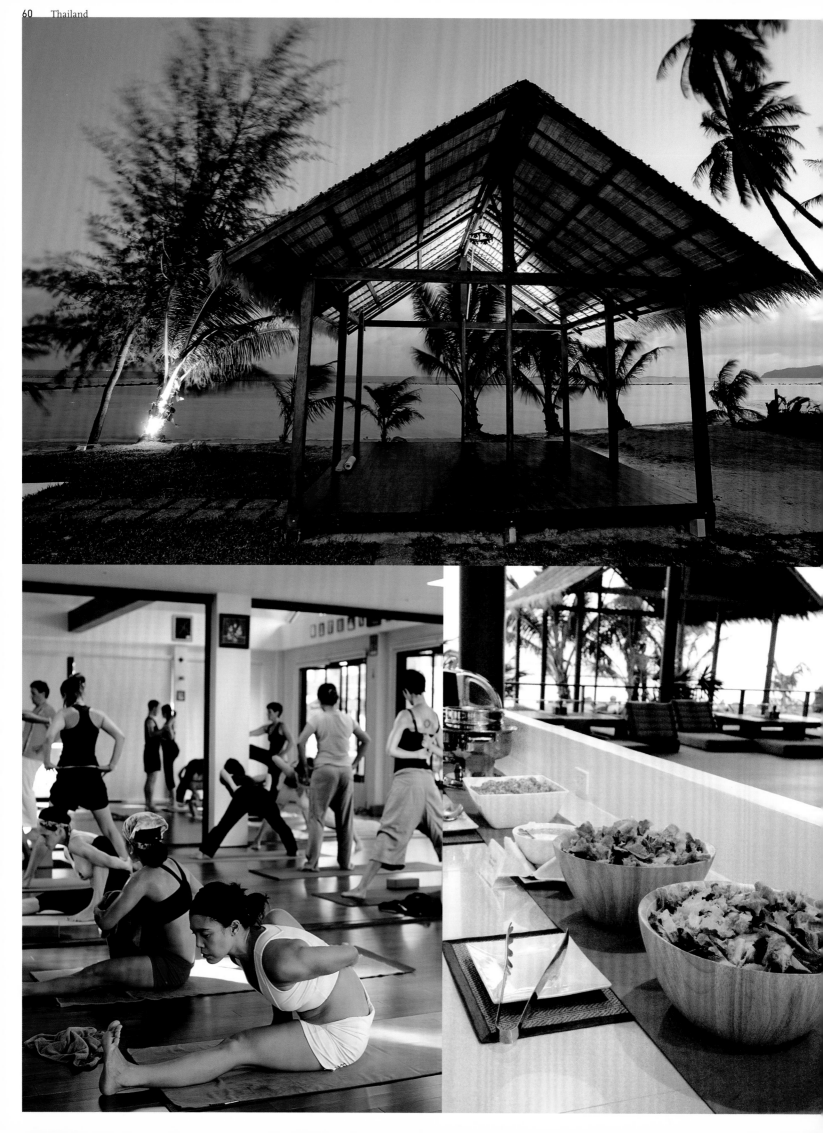

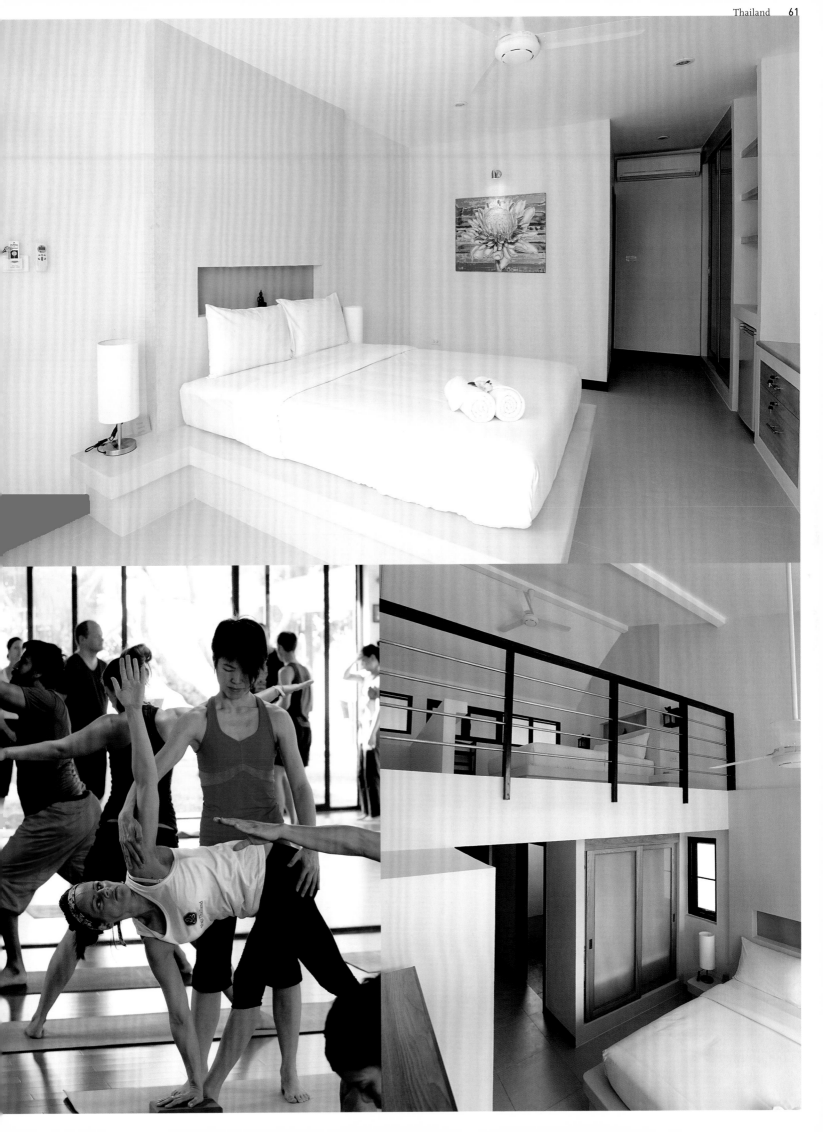

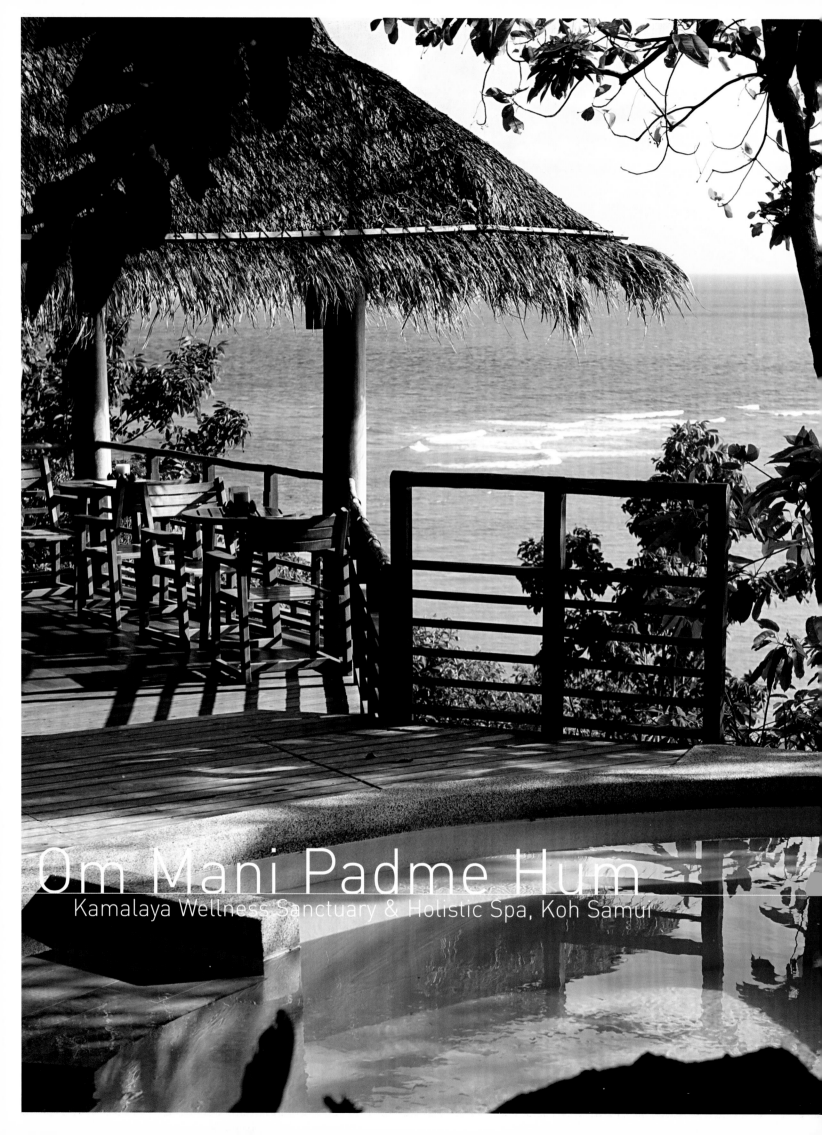

Om Mani Padme Hum

Kamalaya Wellness Sanctuary & Holistic Spa, Koh Samui

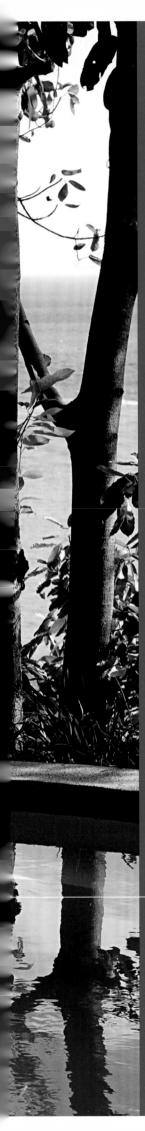

Kamalaya Wellness Sanctuary & Holistic Spa, Koh Samui

Om Mani Padme Hum

Lotus flowers grow best in a muddy subsoil; their beauty is first revealed at the surface. Translated, Kamalaya means "lotus realm", and this is no exaggeration: they bloom here everywhere in bright pink, well known to the Yogis as a symbol for change. In contrast to other spa resorts the quality of the multiple prize-winning Kamalaya doesn't come from bathrobes that you are allowed to take home along with a light holiday tan. In the middle of the resort between honeysuckle bushes and plunge pools under coconut palms lies the cave in which Buddhist monks have meditated for several hundred years. Located on a steep slope, the site compels you to walk everywhere on shady paths, an activity that leads to its own form of meditation and keeps you from descending into apathy. On the way the quite breathtaking view changes constantly: the Thai coastal landscape, the turquoise-coloured small bay of the resort's own private beach and, in the end, even your perspective on your own significance. And that, finally, is what the Yoga taught in a beautiful pavilion up on a cliff is all about. Here, you can create space on all levels, and that includes making room for the outstanding breakfast. **Books to pack: "Autobiography of a Yogi" by Paramahansa Yogananda and "The Beach" by Alex Garland.**

Kamalaya Wellness Sanctuary & Holistic Spa	
102/9 Moo 3, Laem Set Road	
Na-Muang, Koh Samui	
Suratthani 84140	
Thailand	
Tel. +66 77 429 800	
Fax +66 77 429 899	
info@kamalaya.com	
www.kamalaya.com	

DIRECTIONS	Located on the southeastern side of Koh Samui. About 45 min from Koh Samui Airport.
YOGA	Hatha, Vinyasa, Kundalini, Ashtanga.
TEACHERS	Lieve Powell, Lara Baumann, Danny Paradise, Jessie Chapman.
ROOMS	59 hillside rooms, suites and villas for max. 120 guests.
FOOD	Vegetarian dishes, fish, poultry, lamb.
TREATMENTS	Chi Nei Tsang (Taoist belly massage), lymph drainage, Reiki, colon hydrotherapy, infra-red sauna, trad. Chin. medicine, detox, Ayurveda, naturopathy.
RECREATION	Lap pool, painting, kayaking, snorkelling, diving, fitness centre, healthy cooking classes.

Om Mani Padme Hum

Lotosblüten wachsen am besten in schlammigem Untergrund und entfalten ihre Schönheit erst an der Oberfläche. Reich des Lotos heißt Kamalaya übersetzt, was nicht übertrieben ist, denn er blüht hier überall in hellem Rosa, den Yogis wohlbekannt als Symbol für Veränderung. Anders als gewöhnliche Spa-Resorts bezieht das mehrfach preisgekrönte Kamalaya seine Qualität nicht aus Bademänteln, die man mit nach Hause nehmen darf, und einer leichten Urlaubsbräune. In der Mitte des Resorts zwischen Geißblattbüschen und Badekuhlen unter Kokosnusspalmen liegt die Höhle, in der jahrhundertelang buddhistische Mönche meditierten. An einem steilen Hang gelegen, nötigt die Anlage dazu, auf schattigen Wegen überall hinzuwandern, was zu einer eigenen Art von Meditation führt und davor bewahrt, in Apathie zu verfallen. Ständig wechselt dabei die atemberaubende Aussicht auf die thailändische Küstenlandschaft, die türkisfarbene kleine Bucht des eigenen Privatstrands und am Ende sogar die Perspektive auf die eigenen Belange. Darum geht es schließlich im Yoga, das in einem wunderschönen Pavillon oben auf einem Fels unterrichtet wird. Platz schaffen auf allen Ebenen, unter anderem für das hervorragende Frühstück.

Buchtipps: »Autobiographie eines Yogi« von Paramahansa Yogananda und »Der Strand« von Alex Garland.

Om Mani Padme Hum

Les fleurs de lotus poussent de préférence dans un sous-sol vaseux et ne dévoilent toute leur beauté qu'à la surface. Kamalaya signifie littéralement empire du lotus, à juste titre, car partout ils fleurissent ici en une couleur rose pâle, symbole de la métamorphose, bien connu des yogis. A l'inverse des spas habituels, la qualité du Kamalaya, qui a été plusieurs fois récompensé, ne lui vient pas des manteaux de bain que l'on peut emporter chez soi, ni d'un léger bronzage de vacances. Au centre du domaine, entre les buissons de chèvrefeuille et les cuves de bains sous les cocotiers, se trouve la caverne où, tout au long des siècles, des moines bouddhistes vinrent méditer. Situé sur une pente escarpée, ce lieu appelle à sillonner tous les chemins ombragés, ce qui génère une forme particulière de méditation et empêche de céder à la léthargie. Ce faisant, la vue époustouflante sur les côtes thaïlandaises évolue en permanence, la petite crique couleur turquoise de la plage privée et, enfin, même le regard que l'on porte sur soi. Car c'est bien de cela qu'il s'agit dans le yoga enseigné dans un magnifique pavillon ou tout en haut d'un rocher. Créer de l'espace à tous les niveaux, entre autres pour le succulent petit-déjeuner.

Livres à emporter : « Autobiographie d'un yogi » de Paramahansa Yogananda et « La Plage » d'Alex Garland.

ANREISE	Auf der südöstlichen Seite von Koh Samui gelegen. Etwa 45 min vom Koh-Samui-Flughafen entfernt.
YOGA	Hatha, Vinyasa, Kundalini, Astanga.
GASTLEHRER	Lieve Powell, Lara Baumann, Danny Paradise, Jessie Chapman.
ZIMMER	59 Zimmer, Suiten und Villen für max. 120 Gäste.
KÜCHE	Rohkost, vegetarisch, Fisch, Geflügel und Lamm.
ANWENDUNGEN	Chi Nei Tsang (taoistische Bauchmassage), Lymphdrainage, Reiki, Colon-Hydro-Therapie, Infrarotsauna, Trad. chin. Medizin, Detox, Ayurveda, Naturheilkunde.
FREIZEIT	Lap Pool, Strandspaziergänge, Malen, Ausflüge, Kajak, Schnorcheln, Tauchen, Fitnesscenter, Kochkurse.

ACCÈS	À environ 45 min de l'aéroport de Koh Samui.
YOGA	Hatha, Vinyasa, Kundalini, Ashtânga.
PROFESSEURS	Lieve Powell, Lara Baumann, Danny Paradise, Jessie Chapman.
CHAMBRES	59 chambres, suites et villas pour 120 personnes max.
RESTAURATION	Cuisine végétarienne, poisson, volaille, agneau.
TRAITEMENTS	Chi Nei Tsang (massage du ventre), drainage lymphatique, reiki, hydrothérapie du côlon, sauna infrarouge, médecine chinoise traditionnelle, Detox, Ayurveda.
ACTIVITÉS	Lap pool, peinture, kayak, plongée libre, plongée sous-marine, centre de mise en forme, cours de cuisine.

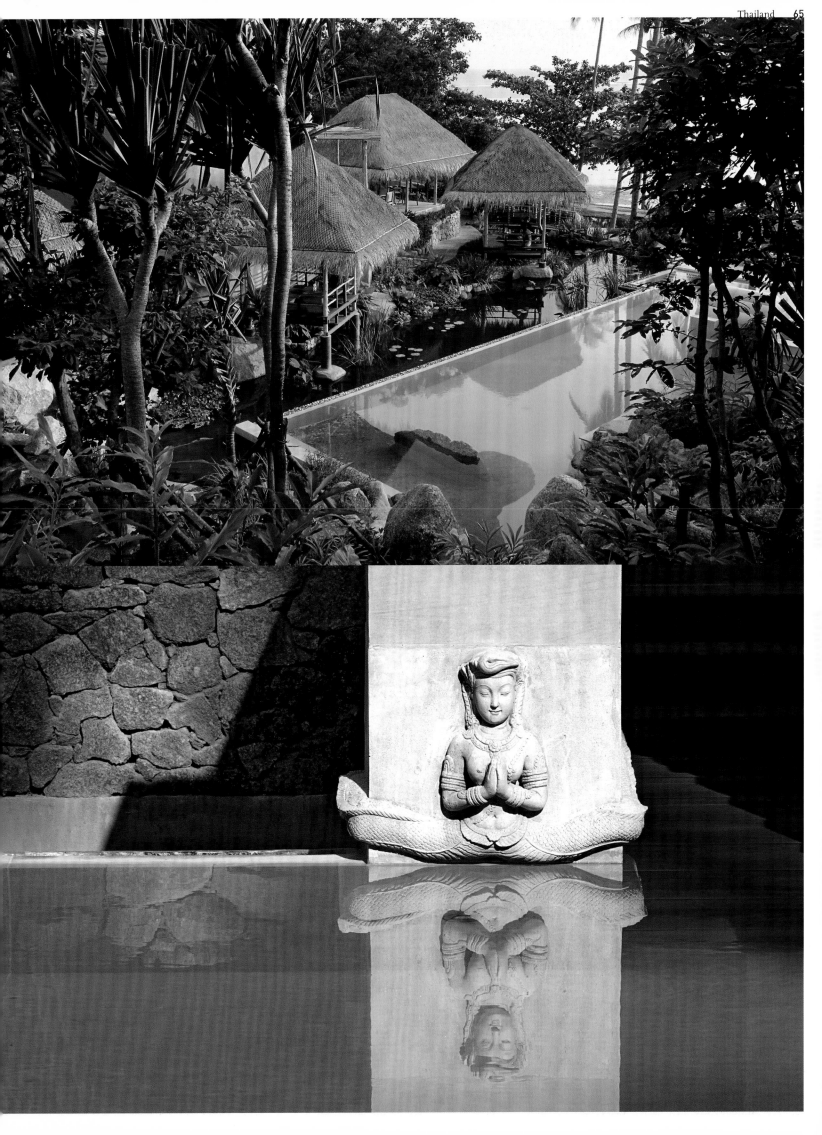

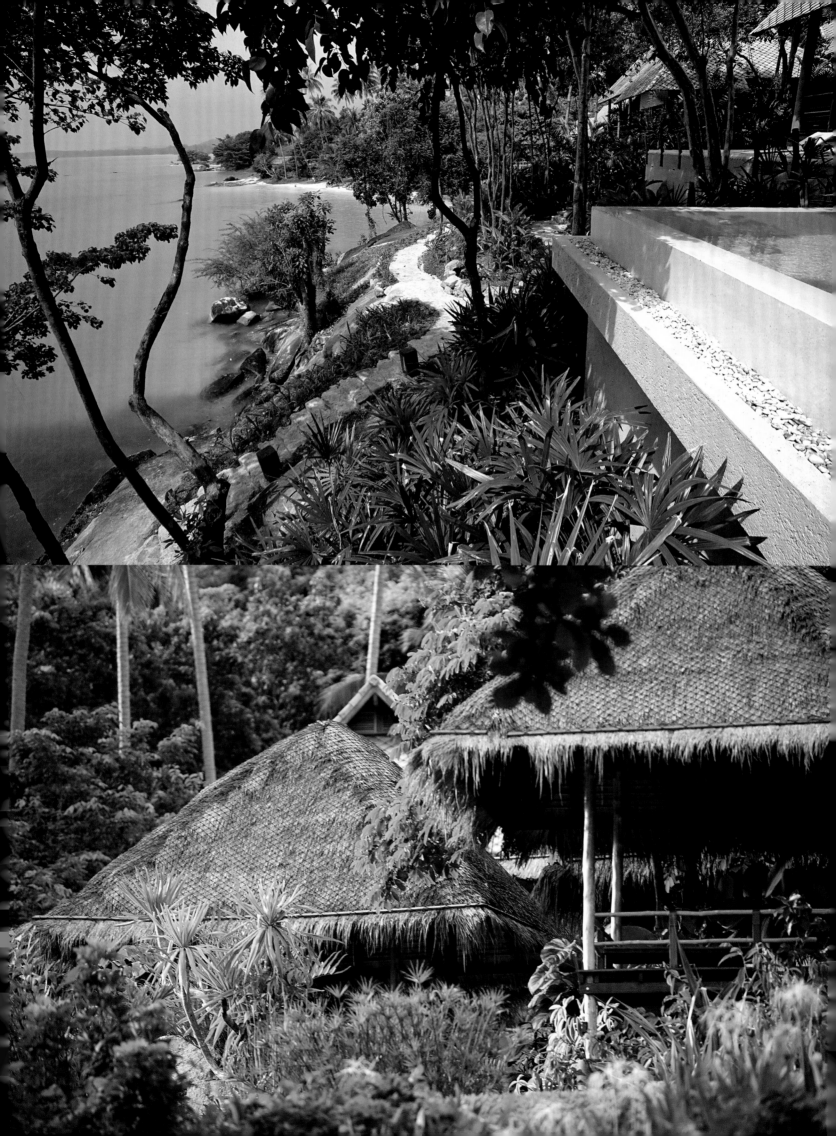

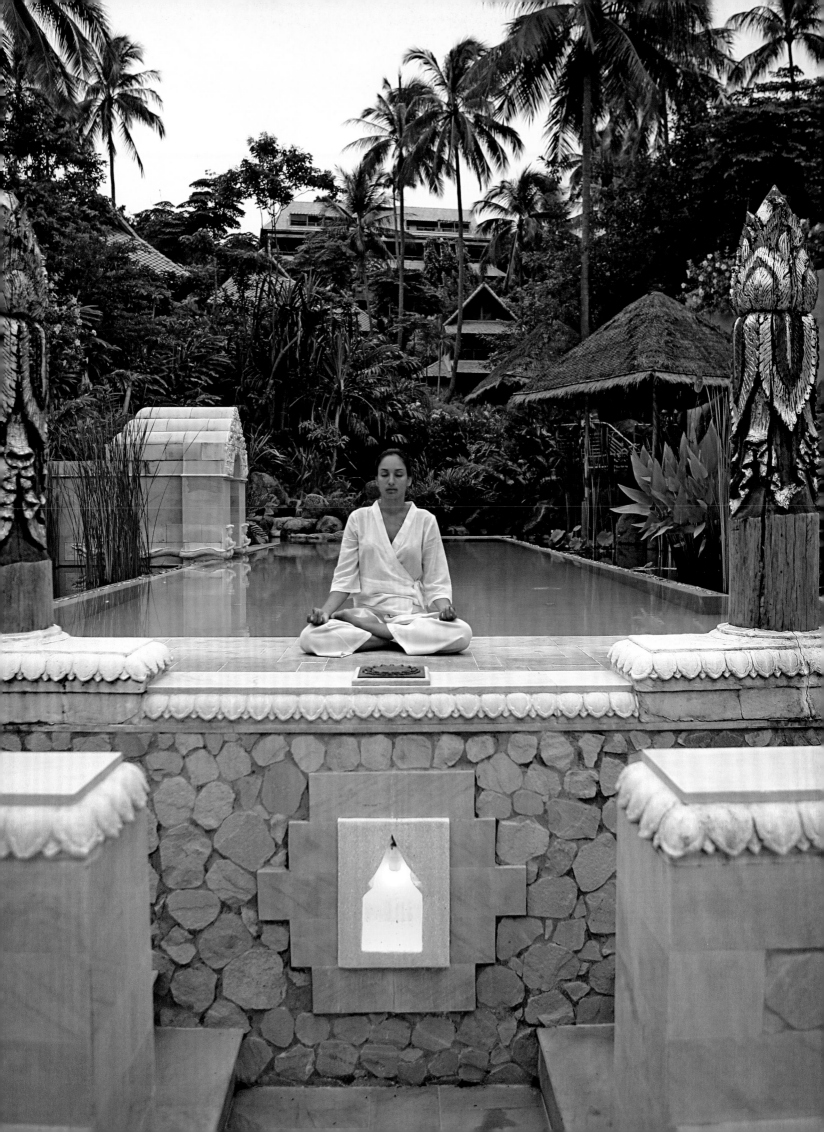

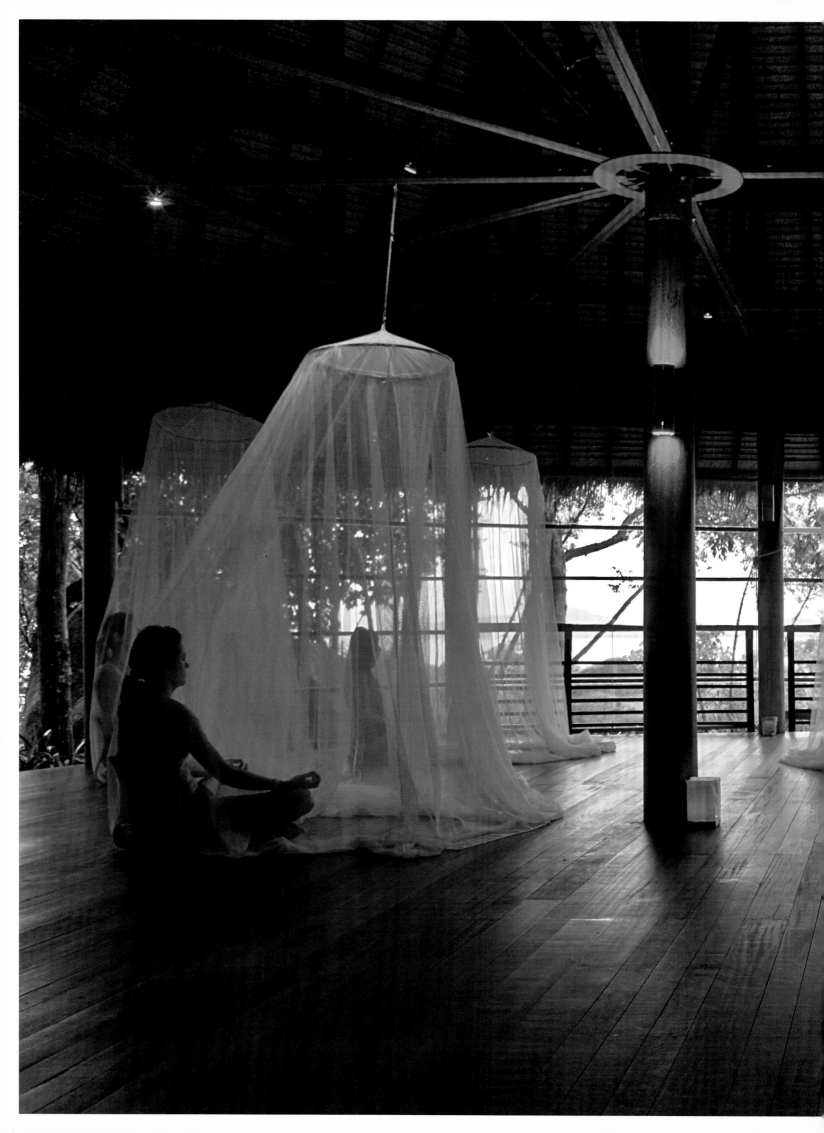

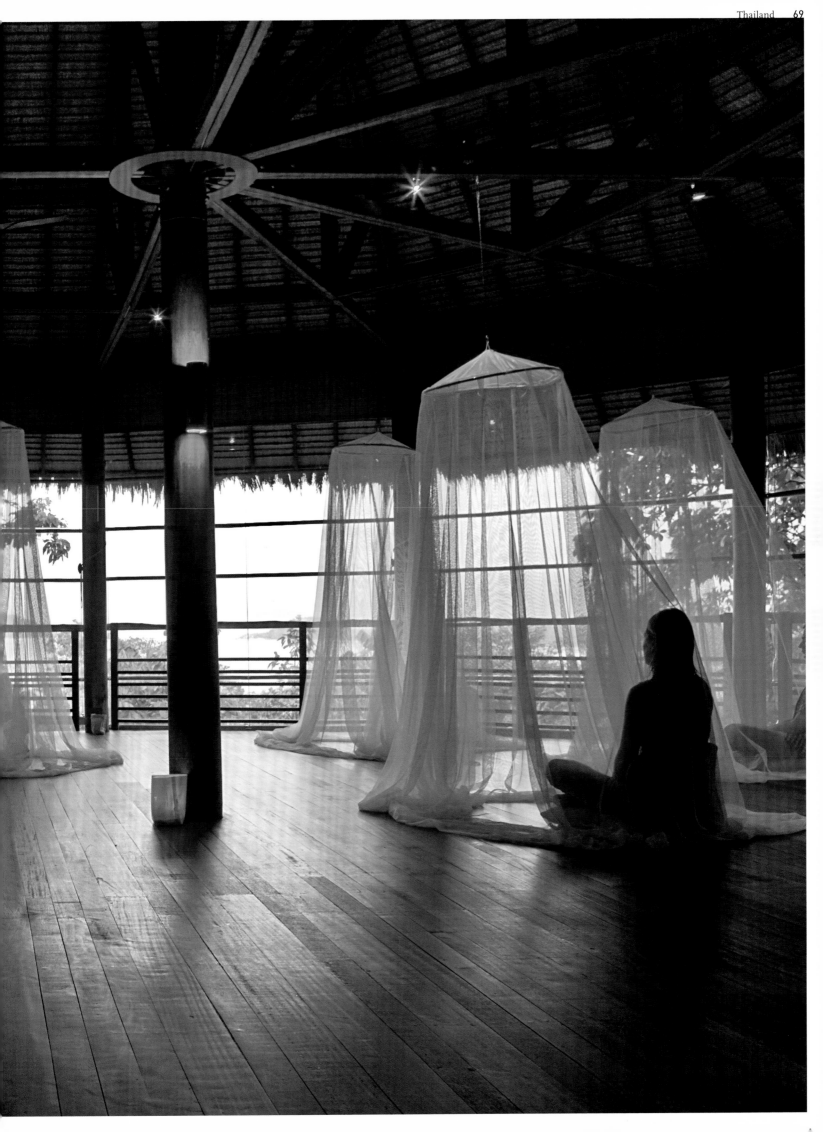

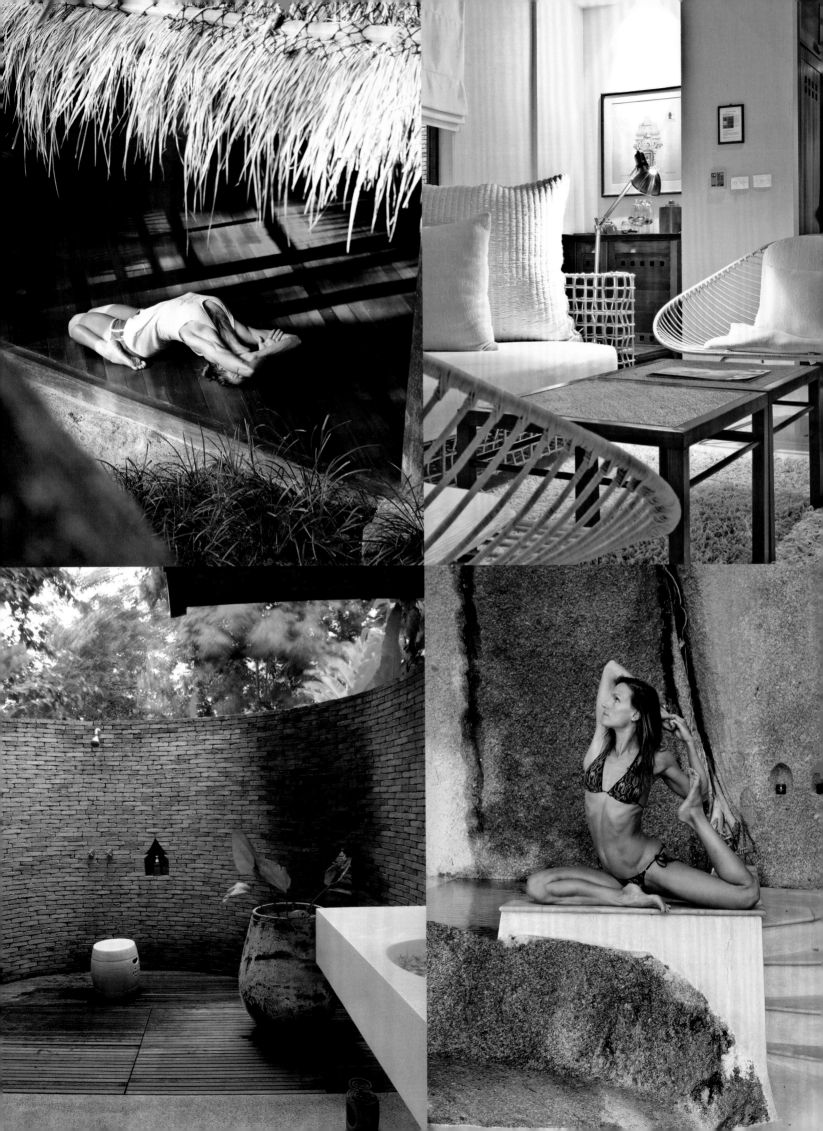

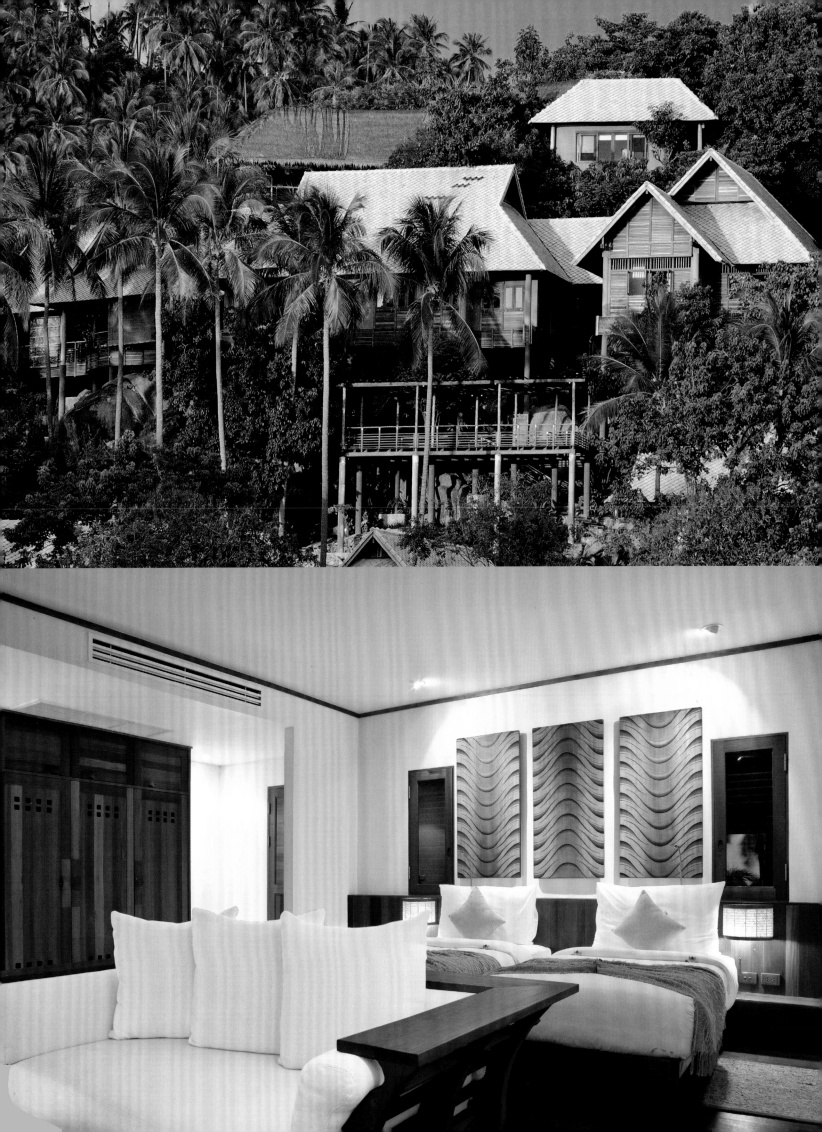

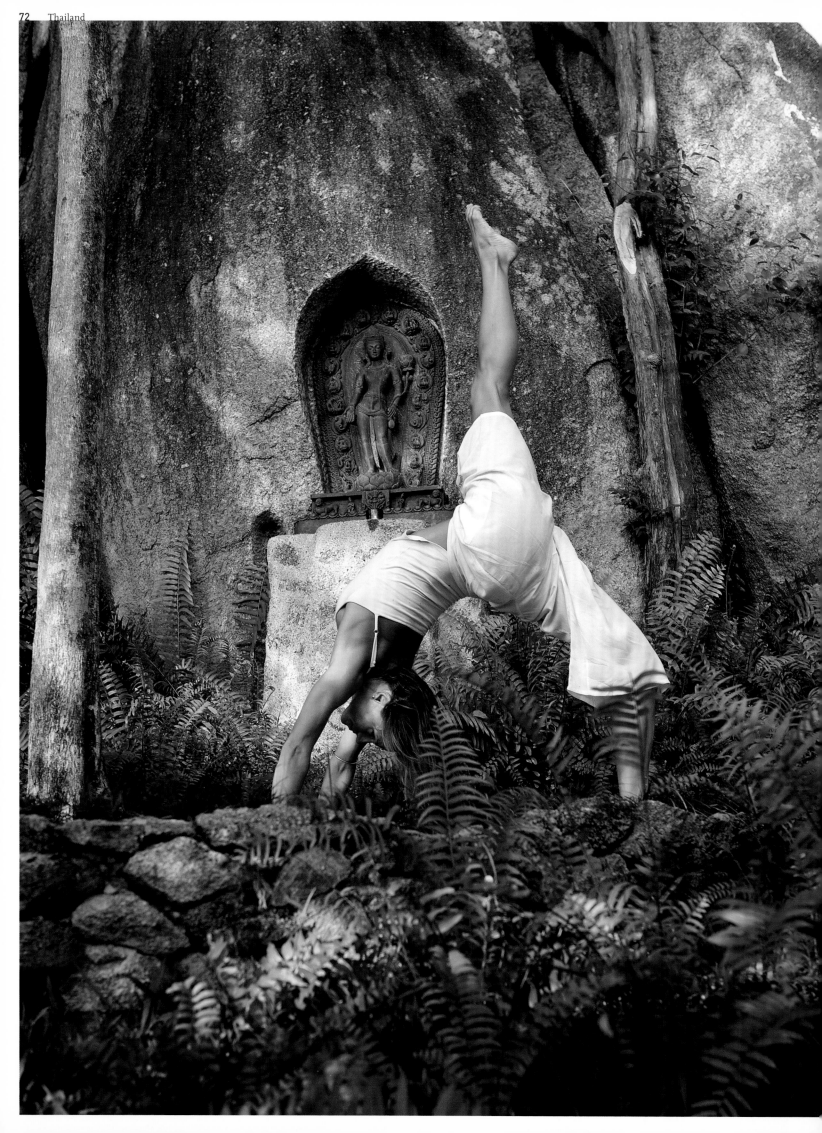

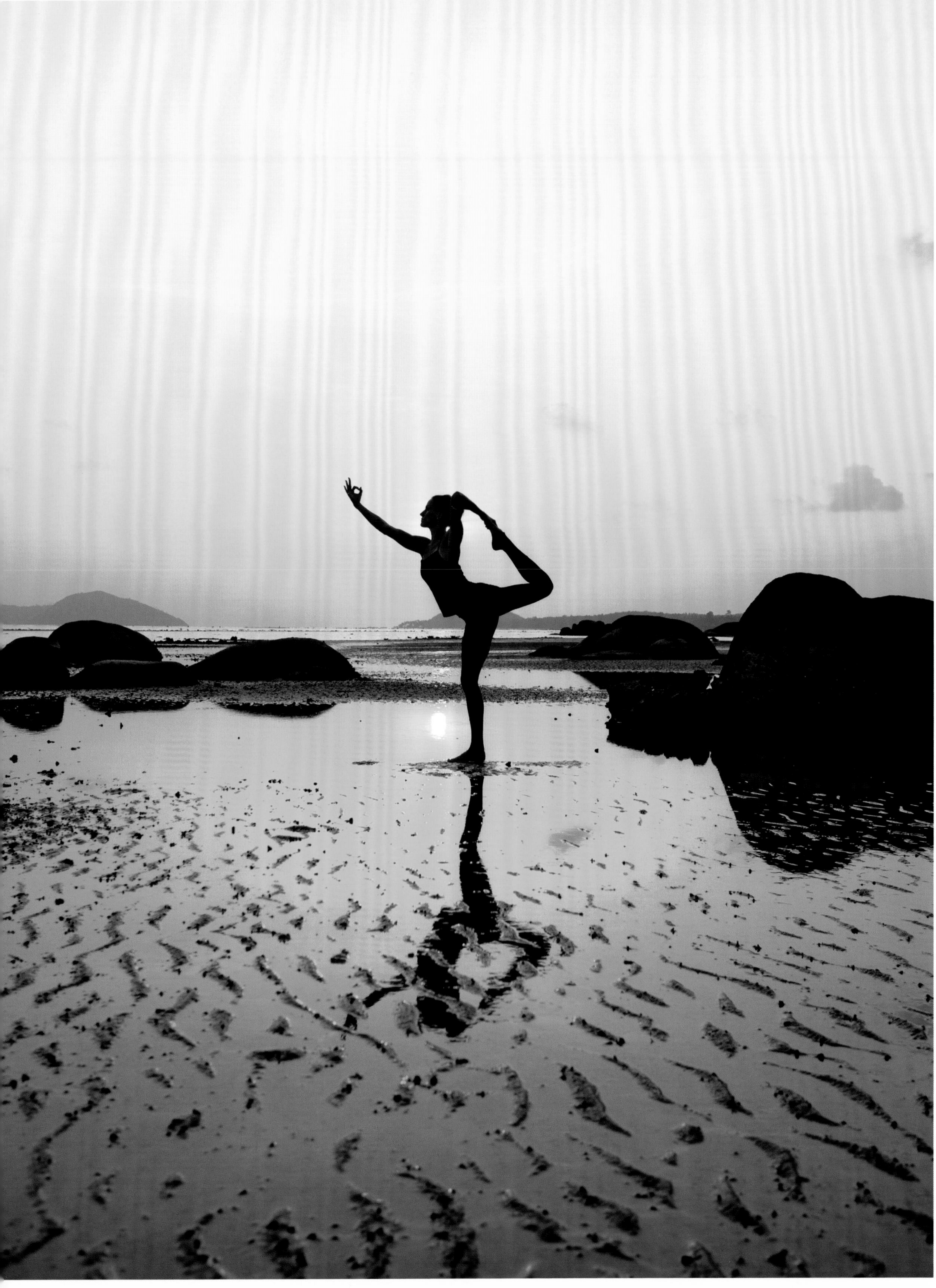

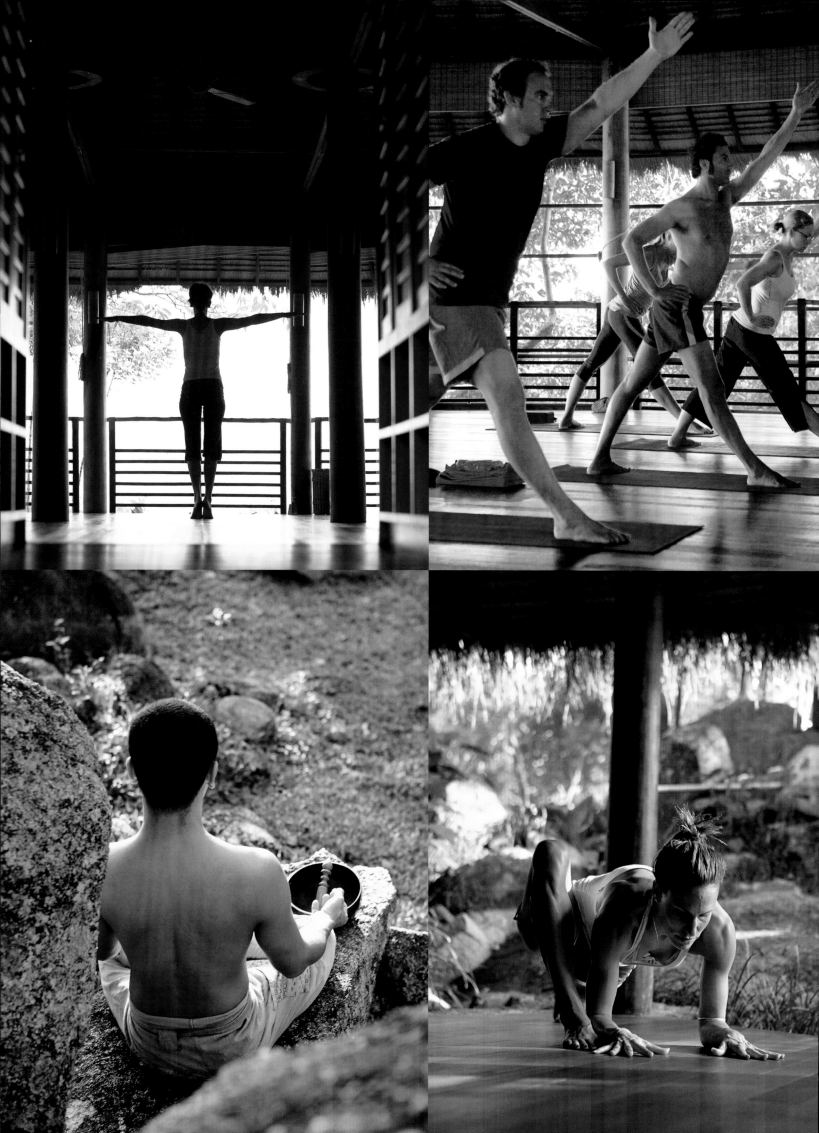

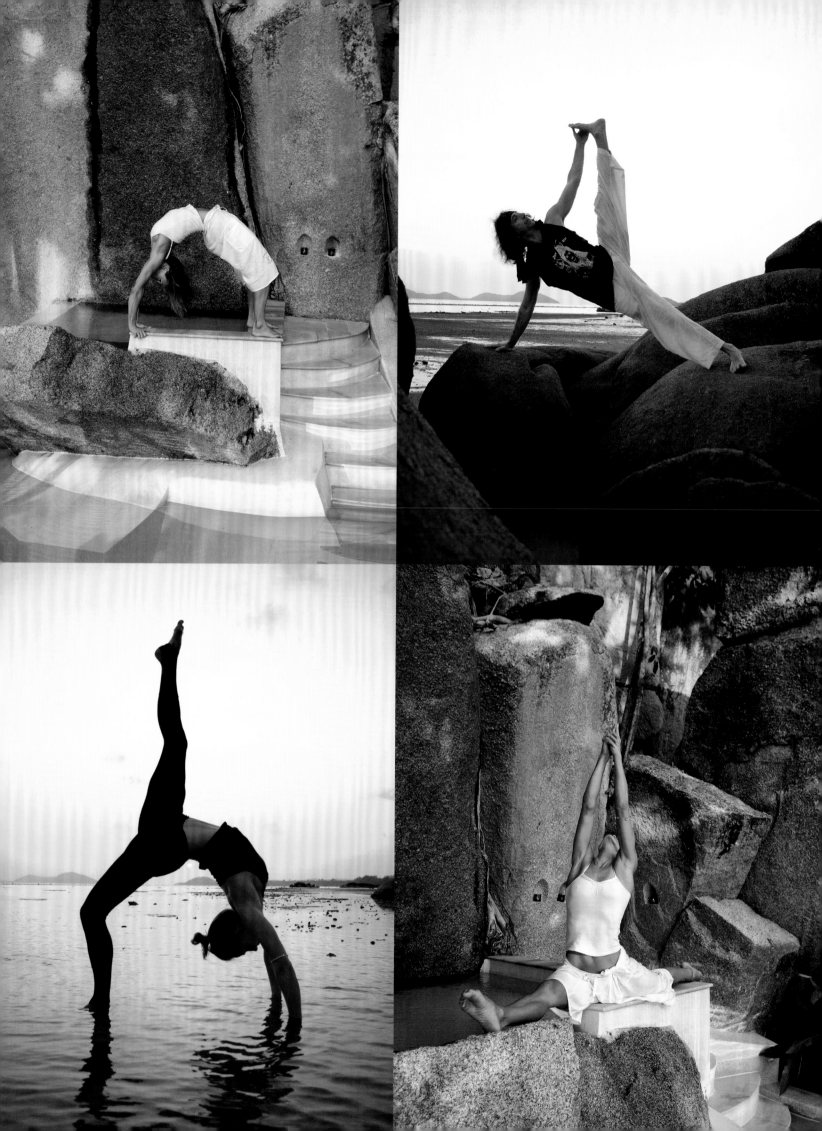

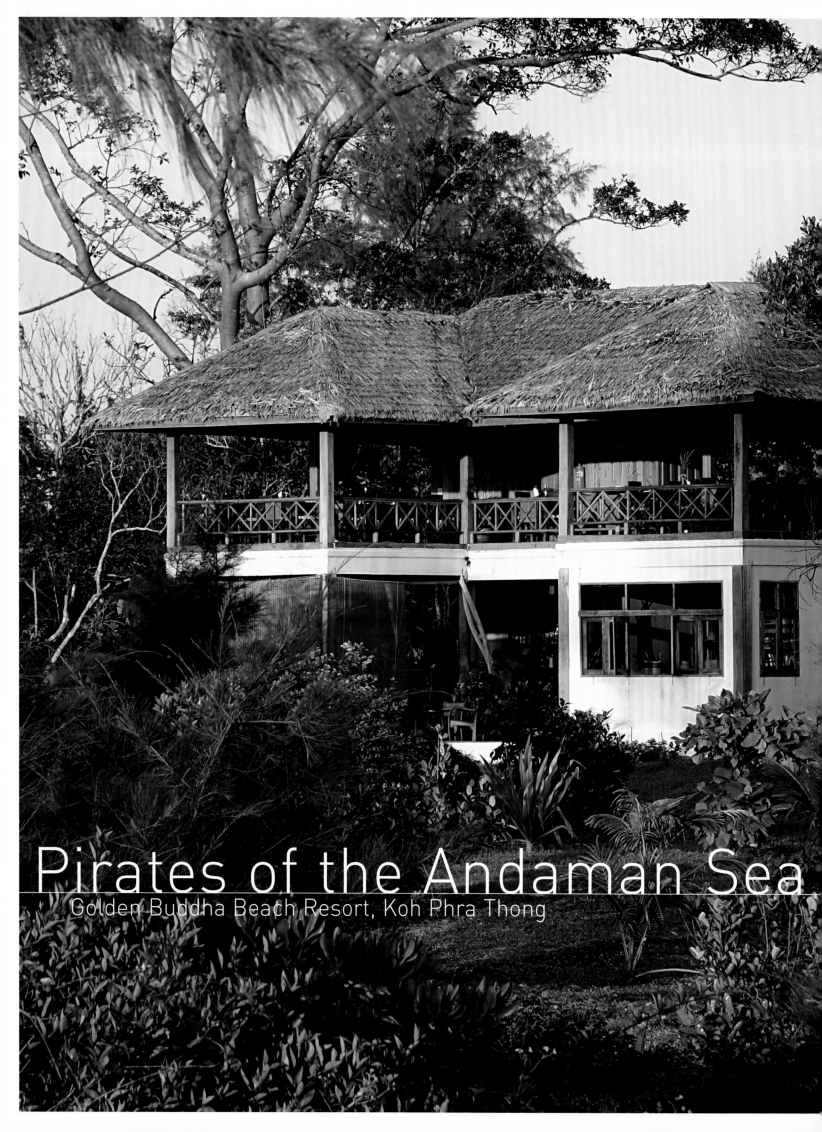

Pirates of the Andaman Sea
Golden Buddha Beach Resort, Koh Phra Thong

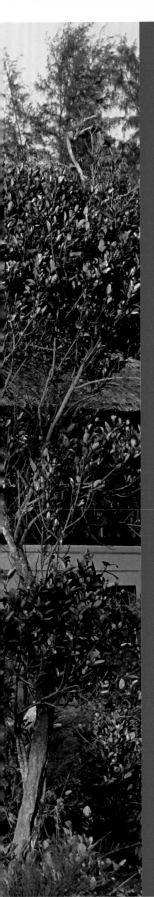

Golden Buddha Beach Resort,
Koh Phra Thong

Pirates of the Andaman Sea

What a wise decision the pirates made in hiding a golden Buddha statue precisely here, on the lonely island of Koh Phra Thong. It lies a couple of hours north of Phuket; enough of a distance away, indeed, to have the feeling of touching down on another planet. Monkeys inhabit their own cliffs here, and water buffaloes doze in the sun. The Golden Buddha Beach Resort, an eco lodge that seems as if it was made for dynamic Yoga on the beach, lies between green rice fields and dense forest. From the spacious veranda of the wooden stilt houses you look either onto the steep lime-stone cliffs in the turquoise Andaman Sea or into a small, shady wood, where the monkeys romp in the trees. Siddhartha Gautama, the young man from a wealthy background who left his family to seek enlightenment, could well have stopped off here. Or Roger Moore maybe, "the man with the golden gun". One reason to get shipwrecked on the island is without doubt the turtles, threatened with extinction, that bury their eggs in the white sand of the ten-mile-long beach in absolute peace and quiet.

Books to pack: "Buddha" by Karen Armstrong and "The Glass Palace" by Amitav Ghosh.

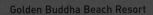

Golden Buddha Beach Resort		
131 Moo 2, T. Koh Phra Thong		
A. Kuraburi, Phang-nga 82150		
Thailand		
Tel. +66 818 922 208 and +66 818 925 228		
info@goldenbuddharesort.com		
www.goldenbuddharesort.com		

DIRECTIONS	Some 93 miles away from Phuket Airport, transfer on request.
YOGA	Hatha, Vinyasa, Anusara.
TEACHERS	Danny Paradise, Carolina Smilas, Susan Desmarais.
ROOMS	25 small houses for 2–6 people.
FOOD	Thai, green papaya salad, pancakes with hibiscus jam, sea bass with coriander and chilli.
TREATMENTS	Thai Ayurveda massage, aromatherapy massage, Swedish massage, Chakra head massage, foot reflexology massage.
RECREATION	Hiking, safaris, bird-watching, diving, snorkelling, kayaking.

Piraten der Andamanensee

Was für eine weise Entscheidung die Piraten getroffen haben, genau auf dieser einsamen Insel eine goldene Buddha-Statue zu verstecken. Koh Phra Thong liegt ein paar Stunden nördlich von Phuket, weit genug, um das Gefühl zu haben, einen anderen Planeten zu betreten. Affen bewohnen hier ihren eigenen Felsen, Wasserbüffel dösen in der Sonne, zwischen grünen Reisfeldern und dichten Wäldern liegt das Golden Buddha Beach Resort, eine Öko-Lodge wie geschaffen für dynamisches Yoga am Strand. Von der großzügigen Veranda der auf Stelzen gebauten Holzhäuser sieht man entweder auf die steilen Kalksteinfelsen in der türkisfarbenen Andamanensee oder in ein schattiges Wäldchen, wo die Affen auf den Bäumen turnen. Siddhartha Gautama, der junge Mann aus gutem Haus, der seine Familie verließ, um Erleuchtung zu suchen, könnte hier gut Station gemacht haben. Oder war es Roger Moore, »der Mann mit dem goldenen Colt«? Ein Grund, hier vor Anker zu gehen, sind in jedem Fall die vom Aussterben bedrohten Meeresschildkröten, die in aller Ruhe ihre Eier im weißen Sand des 16 Kilometer langen Strandes vergraben.
Buchtipps: »Buddha« von Karen Armstrong und »Der Glaspalast« von Amitav Ghosh.

Les pirates de la mer d'Andaman

Quelle sage décision prirent les pirates qui cachèrent une statue dorée de Bouddha précisément sur cette île déserte. Koh Phra Thong se trouve à quelques heures au nord de Phuket, assez loin pour qu'on ait l'impression d'accéder à une autre planète. Ici, les singes sont chez eux dans leurs roches, les buffles d'eau somnolent au soleil, entre les rizières vertes et les forêts touffues s'étend le Golden Buddha Beach Resort, station écologique idéale pour l'exercice dynamique du yoga sur la plage. Depuis la vaste véranda des maisons de bois construites sur pilotis, le regard se pose sur les rochers de calcaire escarpés dans une mer d'Andaman aux reflets turquoise ou sur un bosquet ombragé où les singes virevoltent dans les arbres. Siddhartha Gautama, le jeune homme de bonne famille qui quitta sa famille pour trouver l'Eveil, pourrait bien avoir fait halte ici. Ou était-ce Roger Moore, « l'homme au pistolet d'or » ? En tout cas, les tortues marines menacées d'extinction, qui viennent, en toute quiétude sur la plage longue de 16 kilomètres enfouir leurs œufs dans le sable blanc vous donneraient bien envie de faire naufrage ici.
Livres à emporter : « Bouddha » de Karen Armstrong et « Le Palais des miroirs » d'Amitav Ghosh.

ANREISE	150 km südlich vom Phuket Airport entfernt, Transfer auf Wunsch.
YOGA	Hatha, Vinyasa, Anusara.
GASTLEHRER	Danny Paradise, Carolina Smilas, Susan Desmarais.
ZIMMER	25 Häuschen für 2–6 Personen.
KÜCHE	Thai, grüner Papayasalat, Pfannkuchen mit Hibiskusmarmelade, Loup de mer mit Koriander und Chili.
ANWENDUNGEN	Thai-Ayurveda-Massage, Aromatherapie-Massage, Schwedische Massage, Kopf-Chakra-Massage, Fußreflexzonen-Massage.
FREIZEIT	Wandern, Safari, Vogelbeobachtung, Tauchen, Schnorcheln, Kajak.

ACCÈS	À 150 km de l'aéroport de Phuket, transport sur demande.
YOGA	Hatha, Vinyasa, Anusara.
PROFESSEURS	Danny Paradise, Carolina Smilas, Susan Desmarais.
CHAMBRES	25 maisonnettes pour 2 à 6 personnes.
RESTAURATION	Thaïlandaise, salade verte de papayes, crêpes à la confiture d'hibiscus, loup de mer au coriandre et au chili.
TRAITEMENTS	Massage ayurvédique thaïlandais, aromathérapie, massage suédois, massage crânien et des chakras, massage réflexe des pieds.
ACTIVITÉS	Promenades, safaris, observations des oiseaux, plongée sous-marine, plongée libre, kayak.

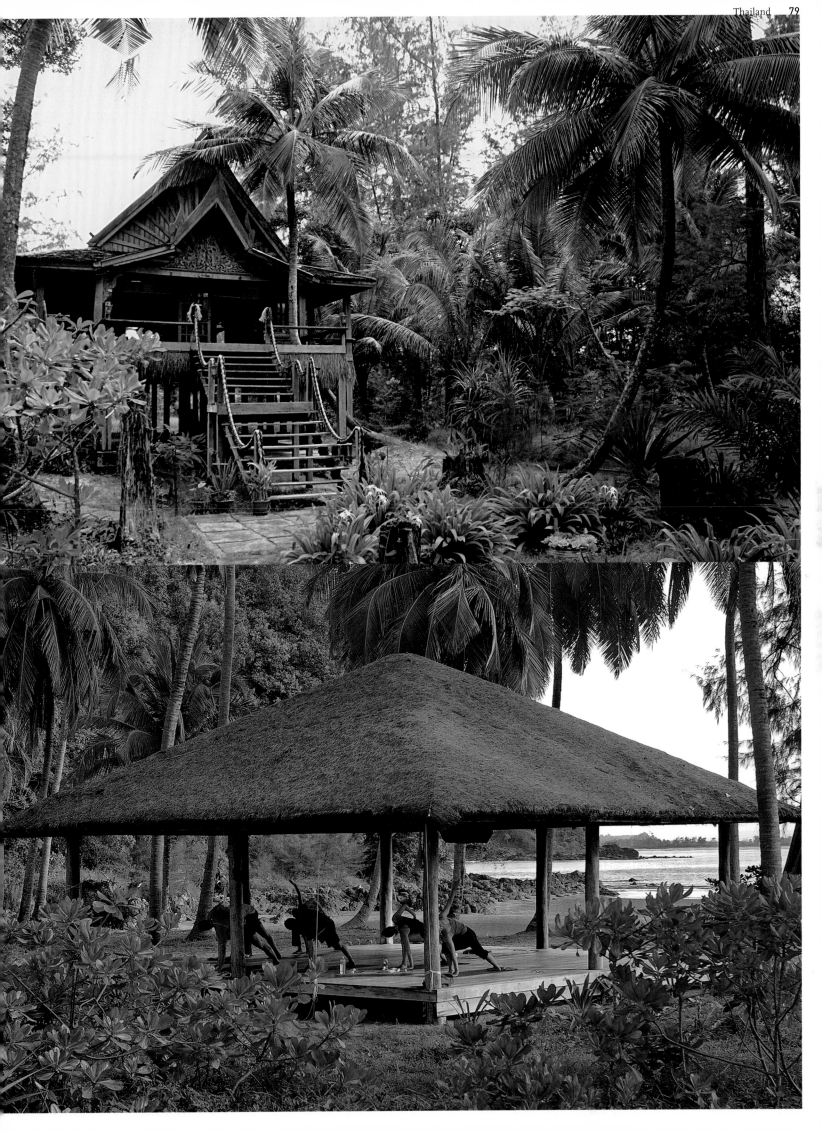

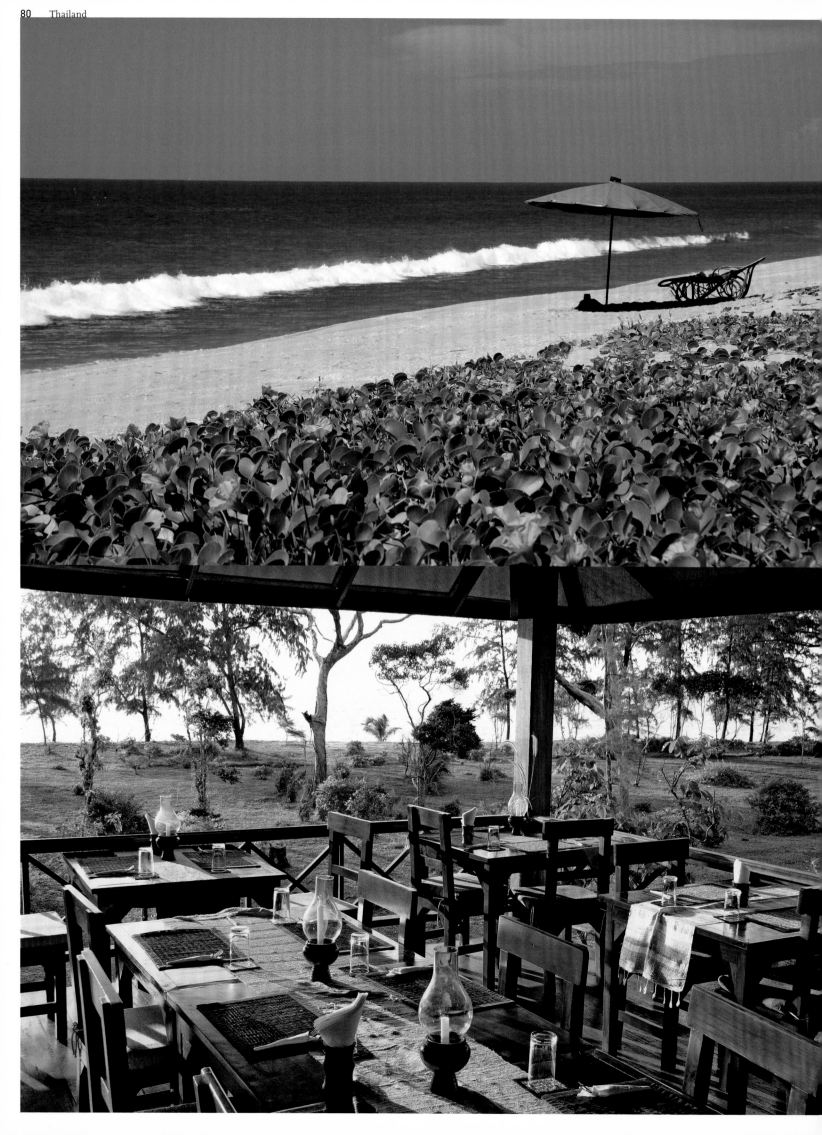

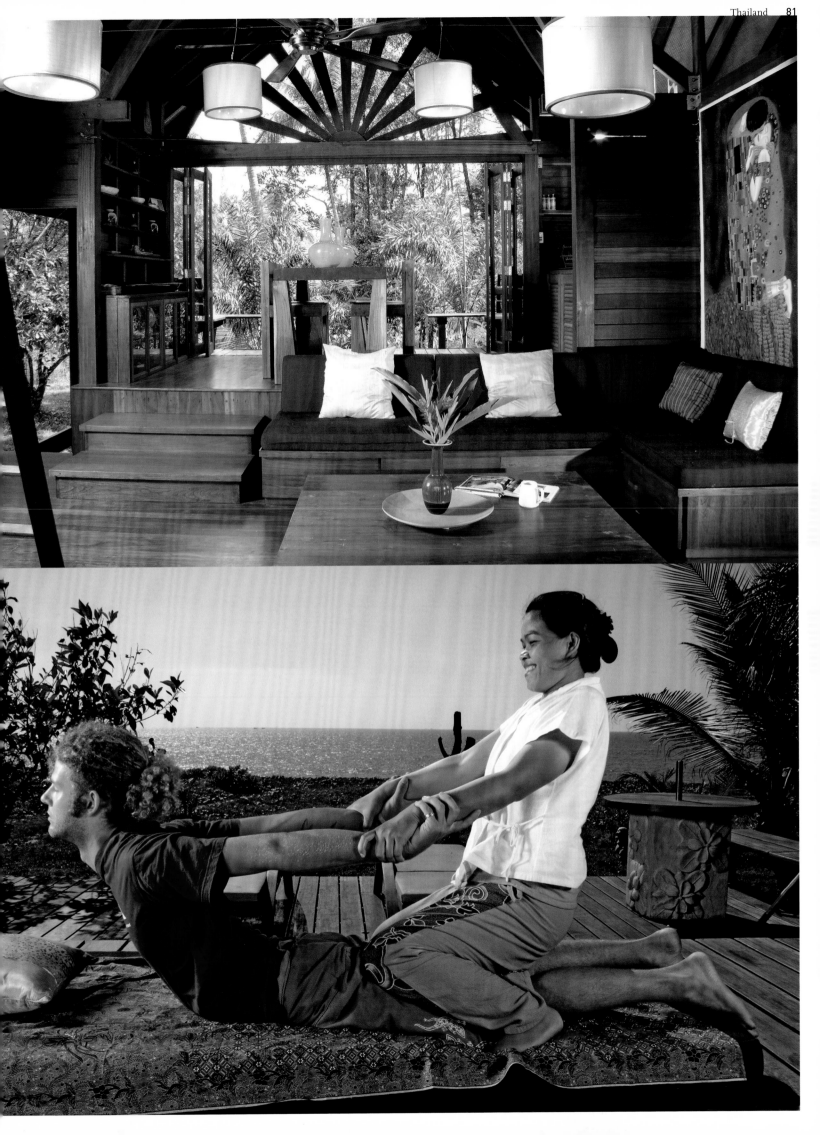

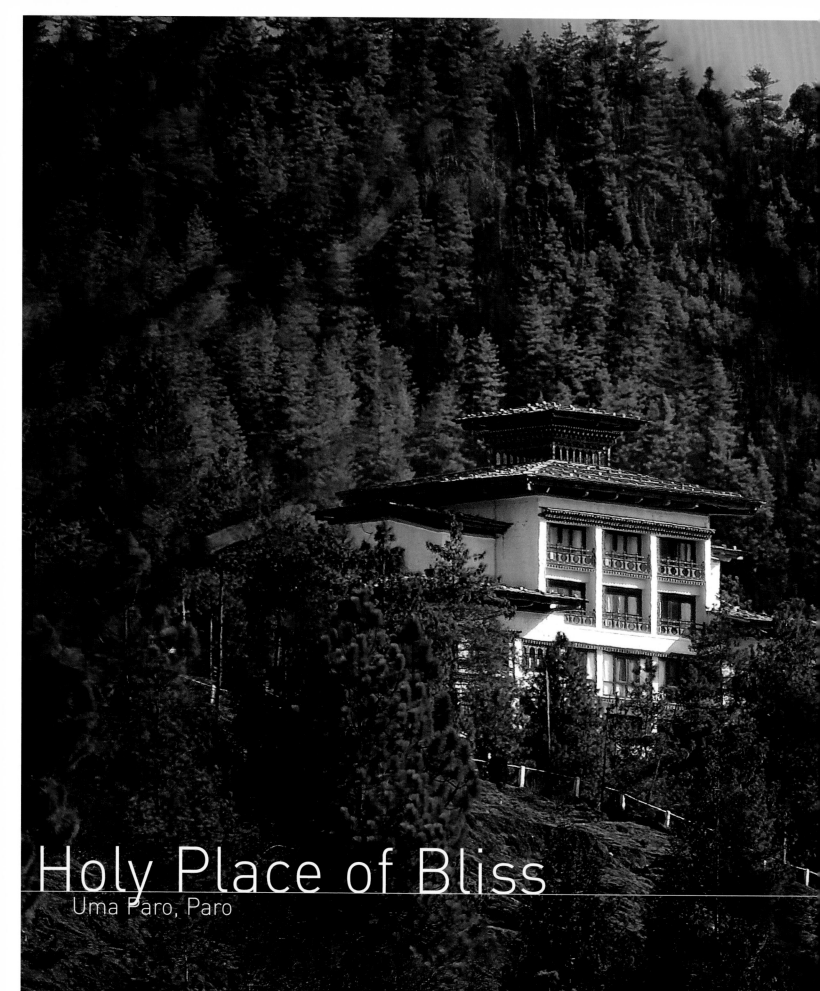

Holy Place of Bliss
Uma Paro, Paro

Uma Paro, Paro

Holy Place of Bliss

The heart violently pumps oxygen into all the body's cells. Slowly the pulse steadies, and the muscles breathe a sigh of relief. The Australian Judy Krupp teaches five hours of Yoga a day here on the polished sprung parquet of the open-air pavilion, from which the eyes are gently drawn towards nature. The star-shaped magnolia flowers sparkle white between Bhutan pines and Himalayan cypresses in the garden, brightly coloured flags flutter in the wind and the sky over the Paro valley is a cobalt blue. The ringing of the prayer wheel, turned by the monks to cleanse their Karma, is audible from far off. Is there a better place than this to meditate? In the 8th century the religion's founder, Guru Rinpoche, after his flight over the Himalayas on the back of a tigress, is said to have landed here in order to free the people from the curse of the outraged spirits of nature and to convert them to Buddhism. Today, the white walls of the Taktsang monastery cling to the steep rock face at this spot. After a day trip to one of the many monasteries, drinking a green tea martini or a chai-spiced hot chocolate, the saffron and burgundy coloured robes of the monks still in your mind's eye, or being treated in the spa on hot stones with herbs from Bhutan, it is easy to live in the here and now.

Books to pack: "Tibetan Book of the Dead" by Sogyal Rinpoche and "Seven Years in Tibet" by Heinrich Harrer.

Uma Paro	
P.O. Box 222	
Paro	
Bhutan	
Tel. +975 827 1597	
Fax +975 827 1513	
info.paro@uma.como.bz	
www.uma.paro.como.bz	

DIRECTIONS	Via Bangkok to Paro; 10 min away from the airport there.
YOGA	Hatha, Vinyasa Flow.
TEACHERS	Judy Krupp, Eileen Hall, Ming Lee.
ROOMS	29 guest rooms and suites, incl. 9 bungalows.
FOOD	Holistic Bhutanese-Indian and Western cuisine.
TREATMENTS	Holistic therapies, including reflex zone massage, Ayurveda, facial treatments. Bhutanese hot-stone bath with hot boulders and massage.
RECREATION	Hot-stone bath house, indoor pool, camping and trekking tours, mountain biking, temple visits.

Heiliger Ort der Glückseligkeit

Heftig pumpt das Herz Sauerstoff in alle Körperzellen, langsam beruhigt sich der Puls, und die Muskeln atmen auf. Fünf Stunden Yoga täglich unterrichtet die Australierin Judy Krupp hier auf dem federnden, polierten Parkett des Open-Air-Pavillons, von dem der Blick sanft in die Natur schweift. Weiß blitzen die sternförmigen Blüten der Magnolien im Garten zwischen Tränenkiefern und Himalaja-Zypressen, knallbunt wehen kleine Fahnen im Wind, und kobaltblau strahlt der Himmel über dem Paro-Tal. Von Weitem ist das helle Klingeln der Gebetsmühlen zu hören, die die Mönche drehen, um ihr Karma zu reinigen. Gibt es einen besseren Platz, um zu meditieren? Im 8. Jahrhundert soll der Religionsstifter Guru Rinpoche nach seinem Flug über den Himalaja auf dem Rücken einer Tigerin gelandet sein, um die Menschen vom Fluch der aufgebrachten Naturgeister zu befreien und sie zum Buddhismus zu bekehren. Heute kleben an dieser Stelle die weißen Mauern des Taktsang-Klosters in der steilen Felswand. Nach einem Ausflug zu einem der vielen Klöster am Kaminfeuer im Salon einen Green Tea Martini oder eine Chai-gewürzte heiße Schokolade zu trinken, die safran- und burgunderfarbenen Roben der Mönche noch vor Augen, oder im Spa auf heißen Steinen mit Kräutern aus Bhutan behandelt zu werden, macht es einem leicht, im Hier und Jetzt zu leben.

Buchtipps: »Das tibetische Buch vom Leben und vom Sterben« von Sogyal Rinpoche und »Sieben Jahre in Tibet« von Heinrich Harrer.

Lieu sacré de la félicité

Avec ardeur le cœur pompe l'oxygène dans toutes les cellules du corps, le pouls ralentit peu à peu et les muscles se détendent. Cinq heures par jour, l'Australienne Judy Krupp enseigne le yoga ici sur le parquet souple et luisant du pavillon en plein air, d'où le regard s'élève doucement vers la nature environnante. Dans le jardin, entre pins pleureurs et cyprès de l'Himalaya, les fleurs des magnolias brillent comme des étoiles blanches, les petits drapeaux colorés flottent dans le vent et le ciel bleu de cobalt resplendit au-dessus de la vallée de Paro. Au loin retentit le son clair des moulins à prières que les moines font tourner pour purifier leur karma. Existe-t-il un meilleur endroit pour méditer ? Au 8e siècle, dit-on, le fondateur de la religion connu sous le nom de Guru Rinpoché aurait atterri sur le dos d'une tigresse après avoir survolé l'Himalaya pour libérer les hommes de la malédiction des esprits de la nature alors furieux, et les convertir au bouddhisme. Aujourd'hui, à cet endroit, les murs blancs du monastère de Taktshang s'accrochent à la paroi rocheuse s'élevant à pic. Après une excursion dans l'un des nombreux cloîtres, boire un martini au thé vert ou un chocolat chaud aromatisé au chai devant le feu de cheminée du salon, les robes couleur safran ou bordeaux des moines encore en mémoire, ou dans le spa sur les pierres chaudes s'adonner à un traitement aux herbes de Bhoutan, rien de tel pour vivre l'ici et maintenant.

Livres à emporter : « Le livre tibétain de la vie et de la mort » de Sogyal Rinpoché et « Sept ans d'aventures au Tibet » de Heinrich Harrer.

ANREISE	Über Bangkok nach Paro, dort 10 min vom Flughafen entfernt.	ACCÈS	Par Bangkok pour aller à Paro, situé à 10 min de l'aéroport.
YOGA	Hatha, Vinyasa Flow.	YOGA	Hatha, Vinyasa Flow.
GASTLEHRER	Judy Krupp, Eileen Hall, Ming Lee.	PROFESSEURS	Judy Krupp, Eileen Hall, Ming Lee.
ZIMMER	29 Gästezimmer und Suiten inkl. 9 Bungalows.	CHAMBRES	29 chambres d'hôtes et suites, y compris 9 bungalows.
KÜCHE	Ganzheitlich bhutanisch-indisch und westlich.	RESTAURATION	Cuisine intégrale indo-bhoutanaise et occidentale.
ANWENDUNGEN	Ganzheitliche Therapien inklusive Reflexzonenmassage, Ayurveda, Gesichtsbehandlungen. Bhutanisches Hot-Stone-Bad mit heißen Flusssteinen und Massage.	TRAITEMENTS	Thérapies intégrales comprenant massage des zones de réflexe, Ayurveda, soins du visage, bain bhoutanais sur galets chaud et massages.
FREIZEIT	Hot-Stone-Badehaus, Indoor-Pool, Camping- und Trekkingtouren, Mountainbiking, Tempelbesuche.	ACTIVITÉS	Pavillon de bains aux pierres chaudes, piscine couverte, camping et trekking, VTT, visites de temples.

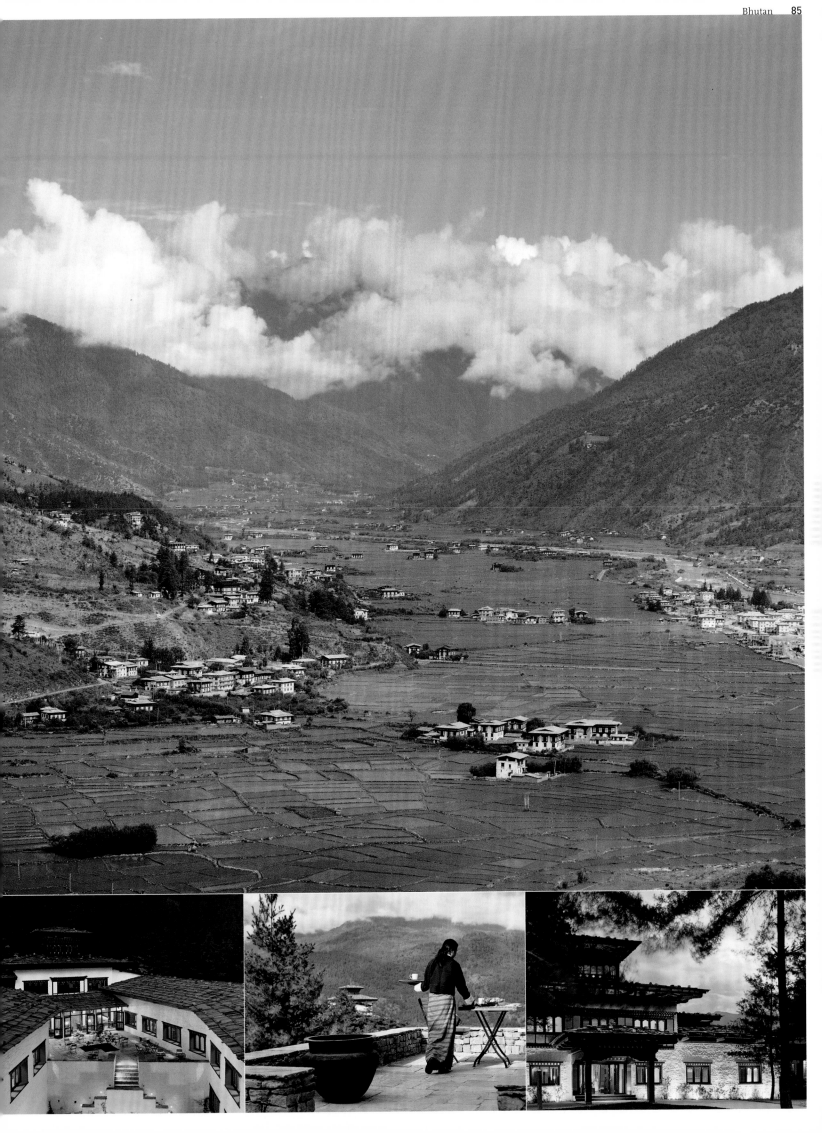

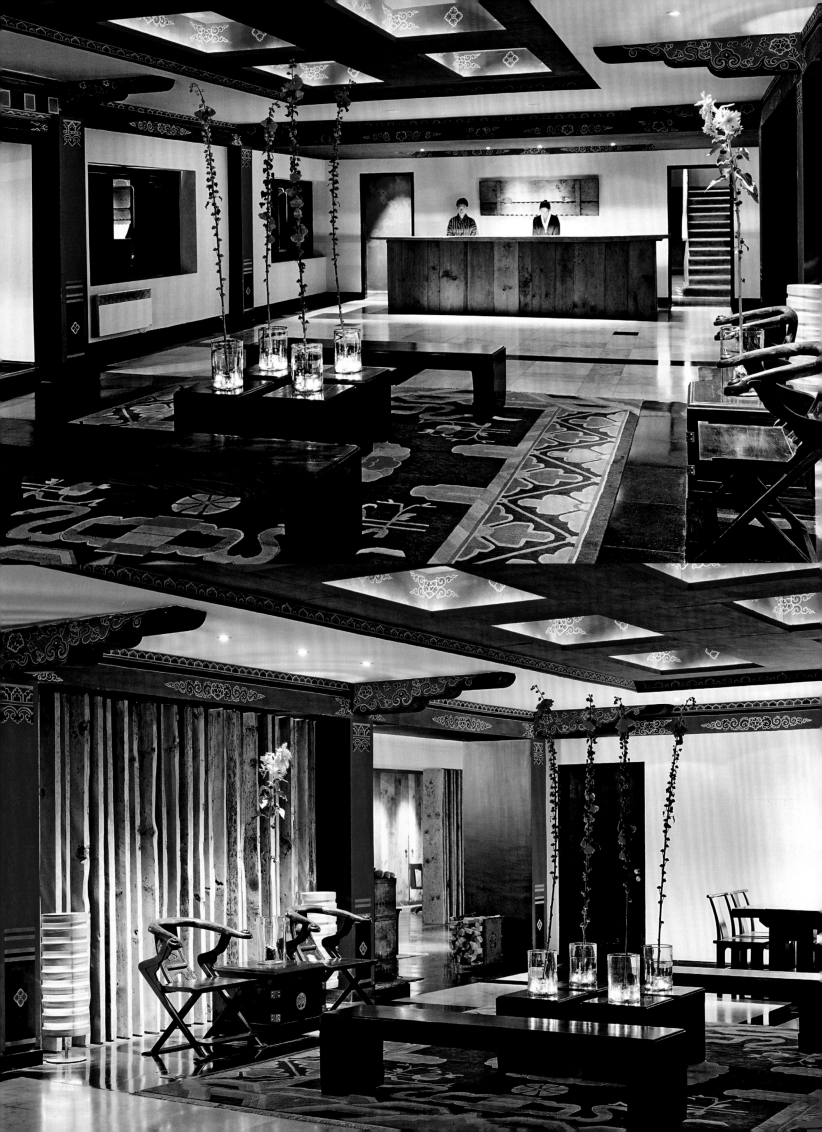

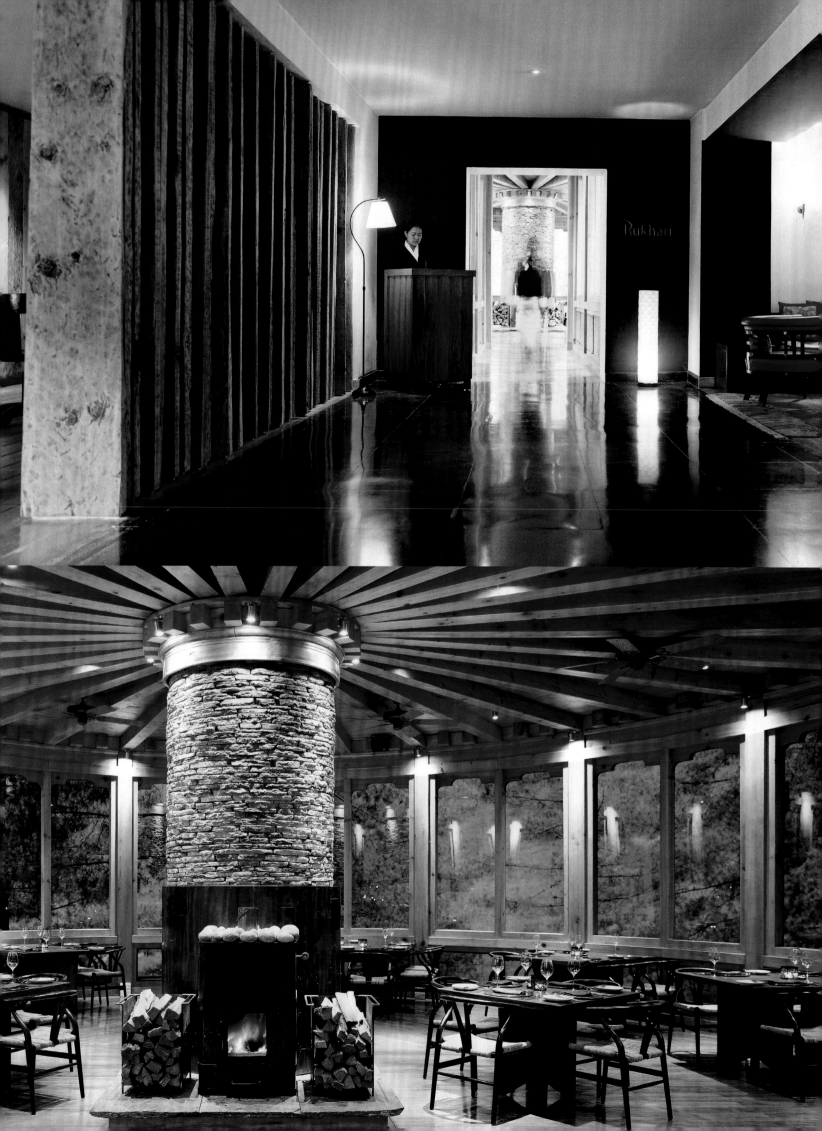

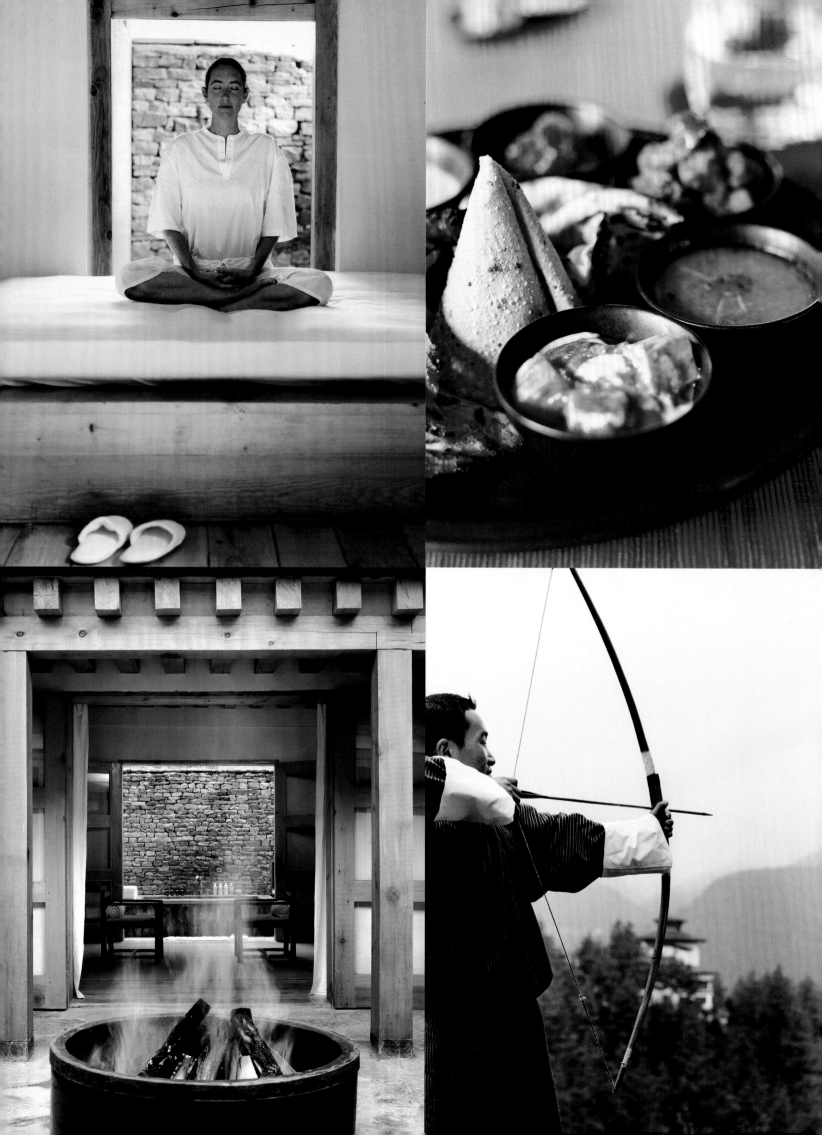

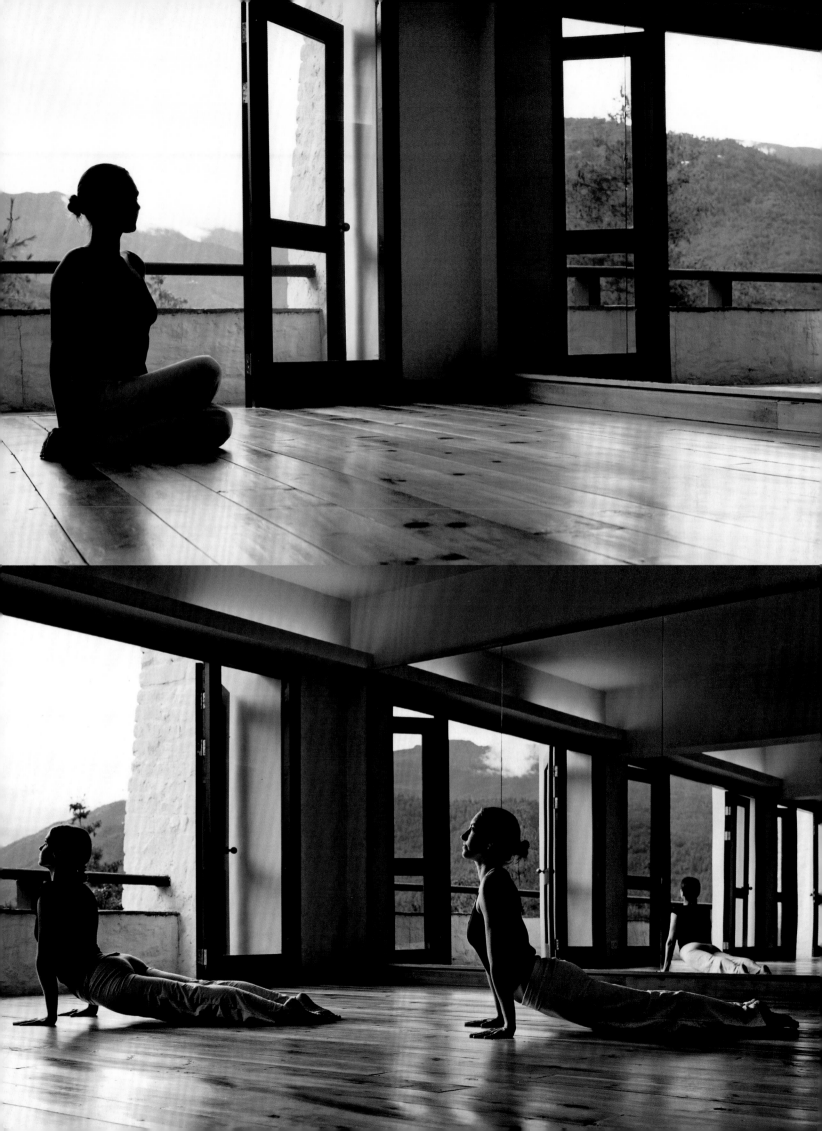

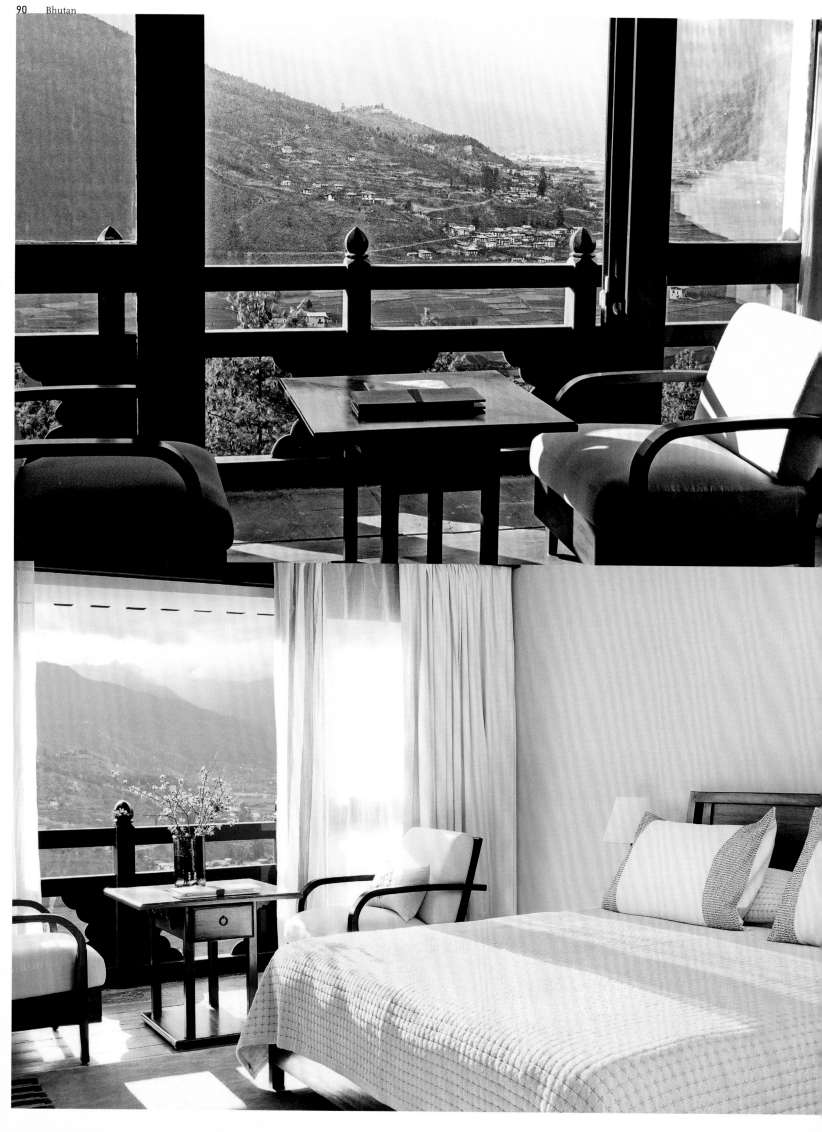

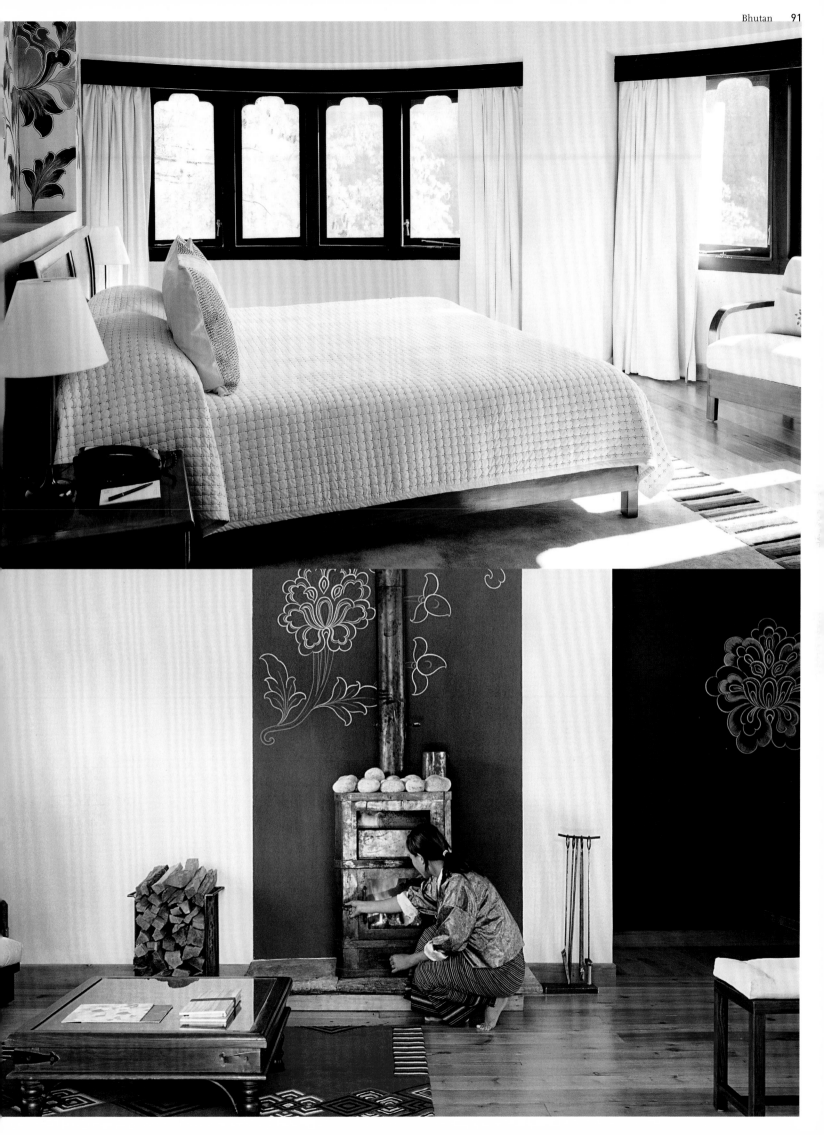

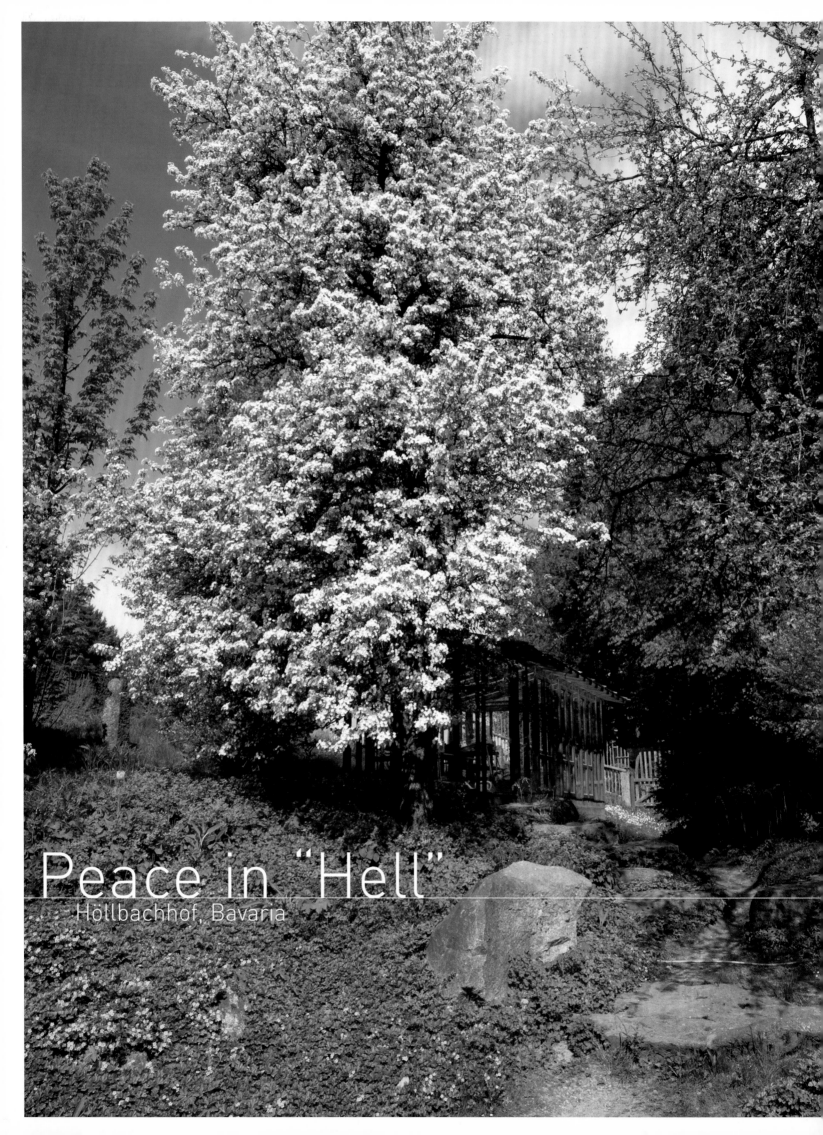

Peace in "Hell"
Höllbachhof, Bavaria

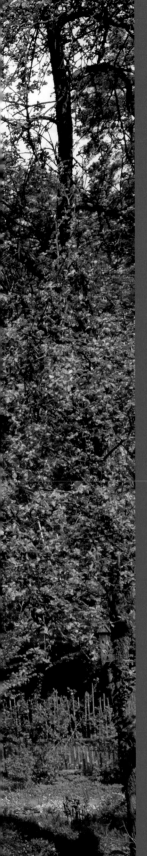

Höllbachhof, Bavaria

Peace in "Hell"

Einstein said: "Strive not to be a success, but rather to be of value." If the Nazis hadn't driven him out, it is easy to imagine him here in the spring sunshine reading with interest about what Chiara J. Greber, Vivian Dittmar and Oryon Load have planned. They want to create a place of learning, of searching and of finding oneself; also, in these times of social isolation, a place where people communicate with each other without Facebook and text messaging. It may sound a lot like a church meeting, but it is founded on solid science. The love of nature here goes much further than raked park paths and floral wallpaper in the hall. There is the Wilderness School, a goat shed, a greenhouse built out of wood and glass, an ecological vegetable garden and marvellous fields intended for the cultivation of organic cereals in future. Take a long walk through the "Hölle" ("hell") conservation area after one of the intensive Yoga sessions, courageously leaping over the Höll brook or hiding behind the moss-covered rocks, and then relax beside the fire in this 16th-century farmstead – and you could almost forget just how much you learn here.

Books to pack: "Jivamukti Yoga" by Sharon Gannon & David Life and "Measuring the World" by Daniel Kehlmann.

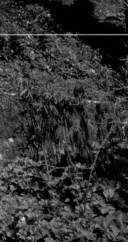

Höllbachhof
Postfelden 20
93131 Rettenbach
Germany
Tel. +49 948 4743
Fax +49 948 495 2883
info@hoellbachhof.net
www.hoellbachhof.net

DIRECTIONS	Located 22 miles east of Regensburg, 1 1/2 hrs drive from Munich Airport, in the middle of the Bavarian Forest.
YOGA	Jivamukti, Hatha.
TEACHERS	Patrick Broome, Gabriela Bozic, Antje Schäfer, Petros Haffenrichter.
ROOMS	7 1–2-bed rooms, 2 rooms with several beds, 2 dormitories for max. 38 guests.
FOOD	Predominantly organic regional vegetarian food. Aubergines in fenugreek wild herbs, millet with steamed apricots, rapadura and cream.
RECREATION	Swimming, hiking, Wilderness School, music.

Frieden in der Hölle

Einstein sagt: »Versuche nicht, ein erfolgreicher, sondern ein wertvoller Mensch zu werden.« Hätten ihn die Nazis nicht vertrieben, kann man sich gut vorstellen, wie er hier in der Frühlingssonne im Hof interessiert lesen würde, was Chiara J. Greber, Vivian Dittmar und Oryon Load sich vorgenommen haben. Einen Ort des Lernens, des Forschens und der Selbstfindung wollen sie schaffen, auch einen Platz, wo Menschen in Zeiten sozialer Isolierung ohne Facebook und SMS zusammentreffen. Was sehr nach Kirchengruppe klingt, steht wissenschaftlich auf festem Boden. Die Liebe zur Natur erschöpft sich hier nicht in geharkten Parkwegen und einer Blumentapete im Flur. Es gibt eine Wildnisschule, einen Ziegenstall, ein Gewächshaus aus Holz und Glas, einen ökologischen Gemüsegarten und herrliche Wiesen, auf denen in Zukunft Biogetreide wachsen soll. Nach einer der intensiven Yogastunden einen langen Spaziergang durch das Naturschutzgebiet »Hölle« zu machen, mutig über den Höllbach zu springen oder sich hinter mit Moos bewachsenen Felsbrocken zu verstecken, sich dann in diesem Gehöft aus dem 16. Jahrhundert vor dem Kamin auszuruhen, lässt einen fast vergessen, wie viel man dabei lernt.

Buchtipps: »Jivamukti Yoga« von Sharon Gannon & David Life und »Die Vermessung der Welt« von Daniel Kehlmann.

La paix en enfer

Einstein a dit : « Ne cherche pas à être quelqu'un, mais plutôt un homme de valeur. » Si les nazis ne l'avaient pas forcé à l'exil, on l'imagine aisément ici, dans la cour, plongé dans un livre sous un soleil printanier, comme Chiara J. Greber, Vivian Dittmar et Oryon Load se sont promis de faire. C'est un lieu d'étude, de recherche et de méditation qu'ils veulent créer, mais aussi, en ces temps d'isolement social, un endroit où les hommes se rencontrent sans Facebook et sans SMS. Ce qui sent le cercle religieux est en fait fondé scientifiquement sur des bases solides. Ici, l'amour de la nature ne se limite pas à des allées bien entretenues et à un papier peint fleuri dans l'entrée. On trouve une école en milieu sauvage, une étable pour les chèvres, une serre en bois et en verre et de magnifiques prairies où, il est prévu de cultiver des céréales bio. Après l'une des séances intensives de yoga, une longue promenade à travers la réserve naturelle de « Hölle – l'enfer », un saut téméraire pour enjamber le ruisseau Höllbach ou encore une partie de cache-cache derrière les grands rochers recouverts de mousse, puis, dans cette ferme du 16e siècle, la détente devant la cheminée, tout ceci vous fait presque oublier combien vous avez appris entre-temps.

Livres à emporter : « Jivamukti Yoga » de Sharon Gannon & David Life et « Les Arpenteurs du monde » de Daniel Kehlmann.

ANREISE	35 km östlich von Regensburg, 1,5 Std. Fahrtzeit vom Flughafen München, mitten im Bayerischen Wald.
YOGA	Jivamukti, Hatha.
GASTLEHRER	Patrick Broome, Gabriela Bozic, Antje Schäfer, Petros Haffenrichter.
ZIMMER	Sieben 1–2-Bettzimmer, 2 Mehrbettzimmer, 2 Schlafsäle für max. 38 Gäste.
KÜCHE	Überwiegend biologisch-regional vegetarisch. Auberginen in Bockshornklee mit Wildkräutern, Hirse mit gedämpften Aprikosen, Rapadura und Sahne.
FREIZEIT	Schwimmen, Wandern, Wildnisschule, Musik.

ACCÈS	A 35 km de Ratisbonne, 1 h 30 de l'aéroport de Munich, au cœur de la Forêt de Bavière.
YOGA	Jivamukti, Hatha.
PROFESSEURS	Patrick Broome, Gabriela Bozic, Antje Schäfer, Petros Haffenrichter.
CHAMBRES	7 chambres simples et doubles, 2 chambres à plusieurs lits, 2 dortoirs pour 38 personnes max.
RESTAURATION	Essentiellement végétarienne, produits bio de la région. Aubergines au fenugrec et aux herbes sauvages, millet aux abricots vapeur, au rapadura et à la crème.
ACTIVITÉS	Natation, randonnées, musique.

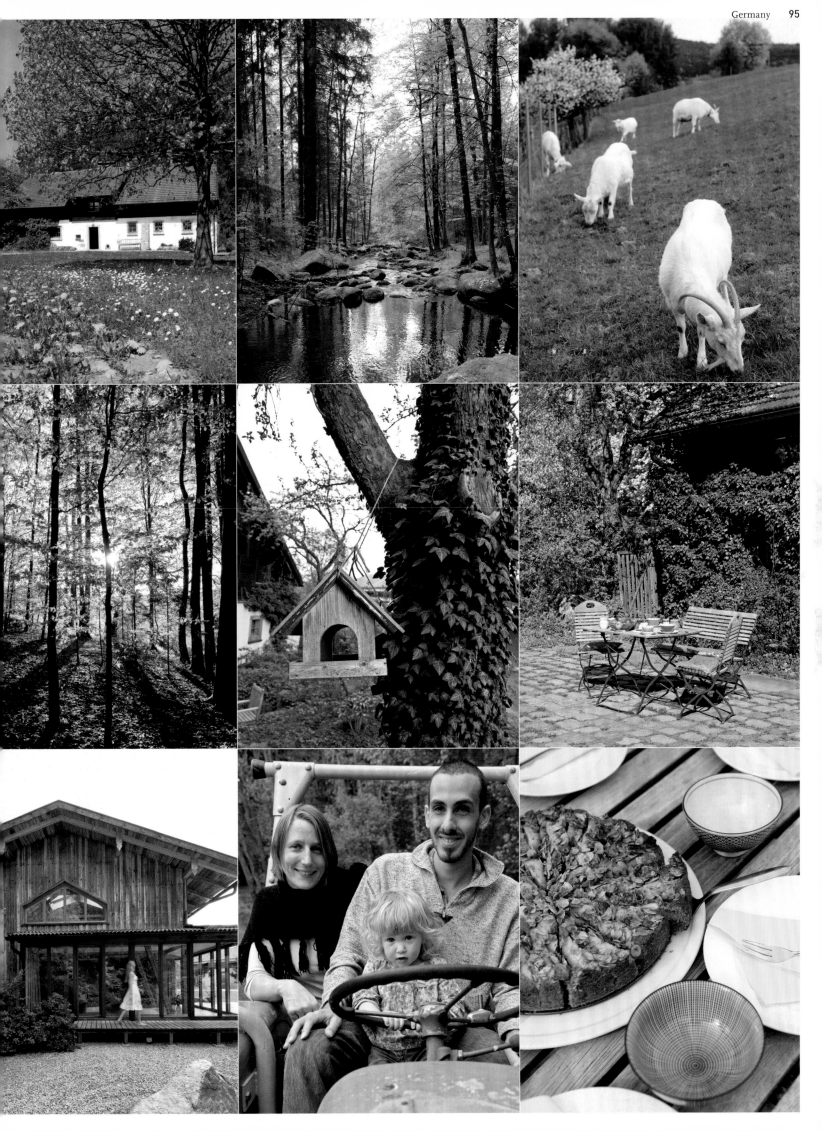

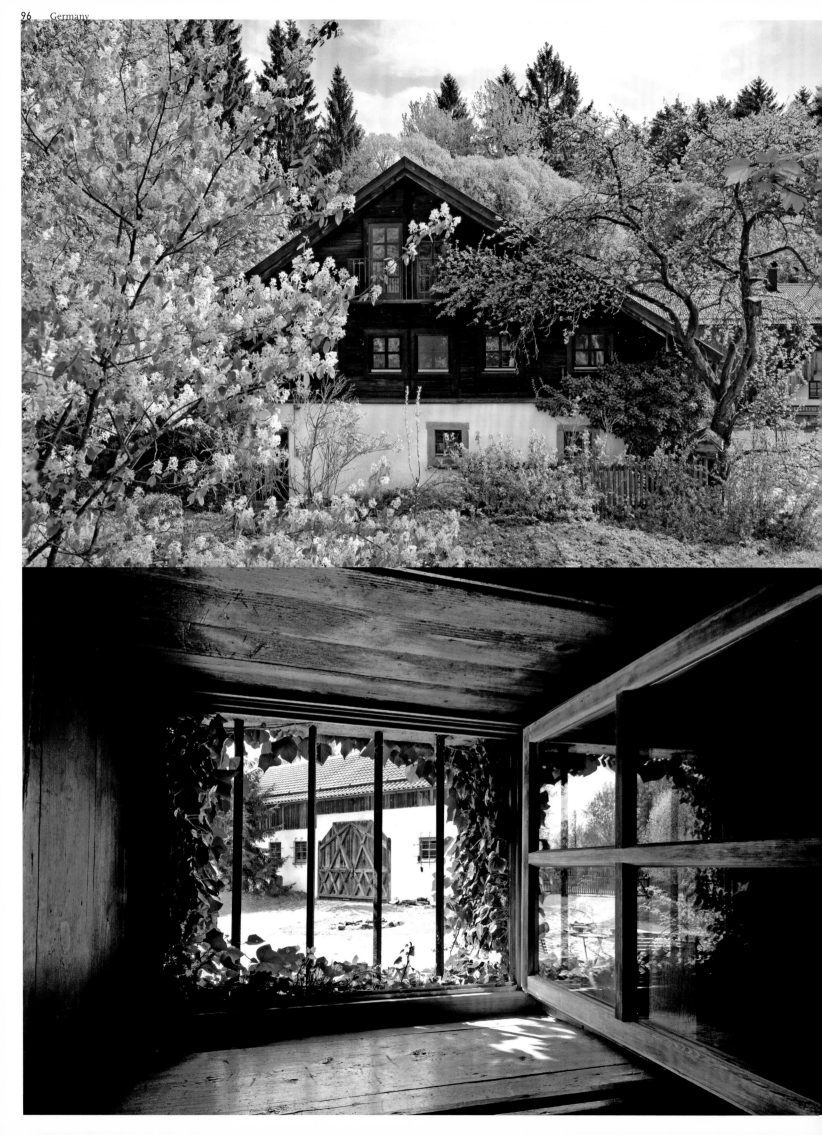

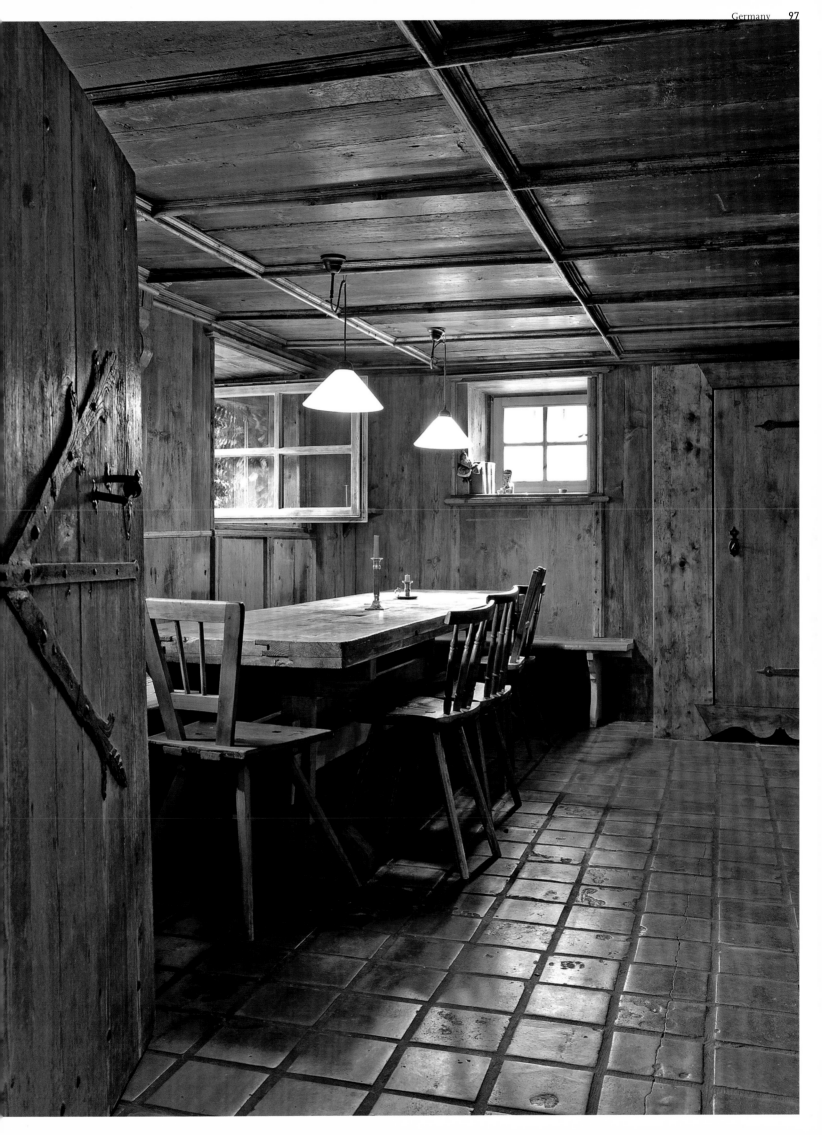

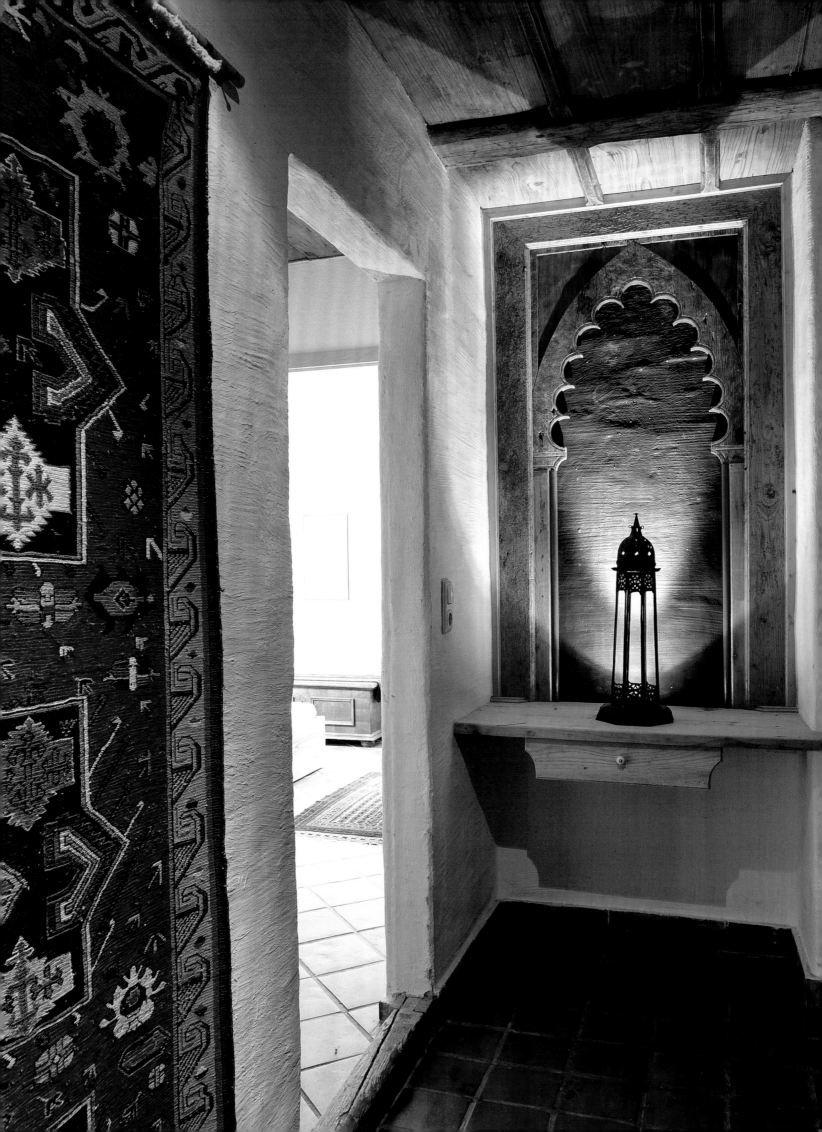

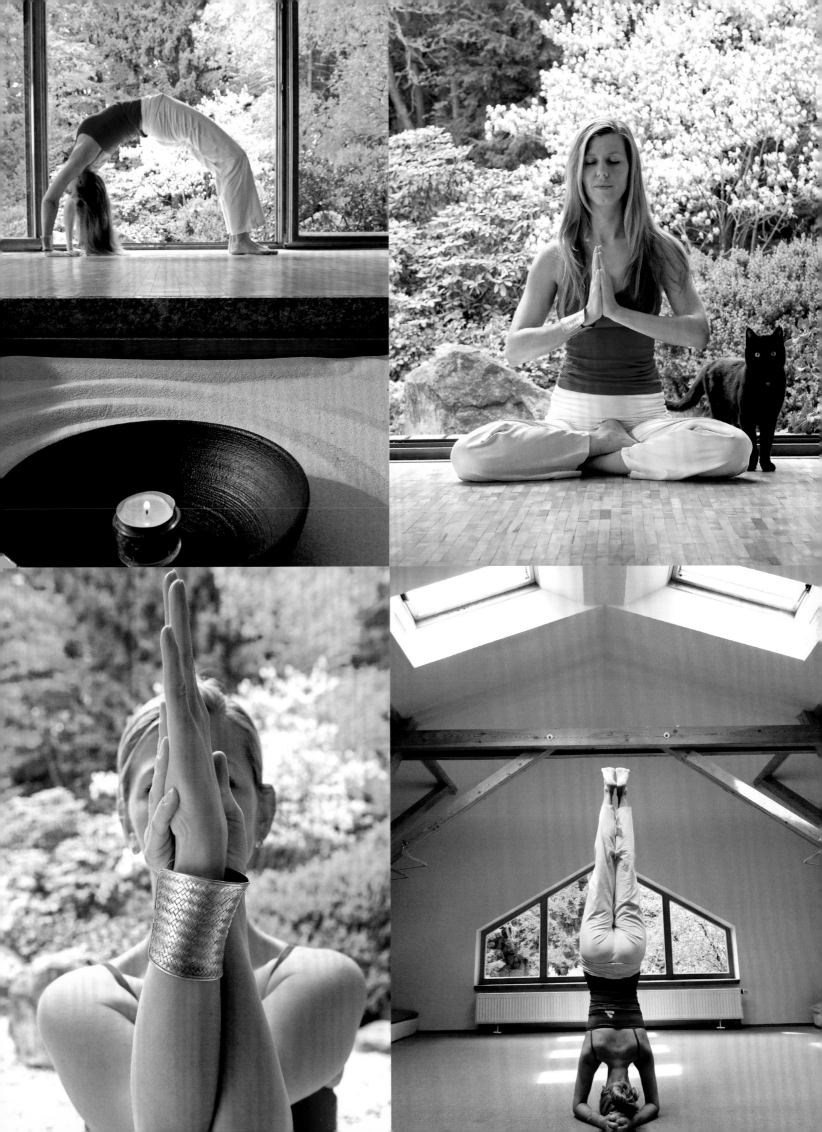

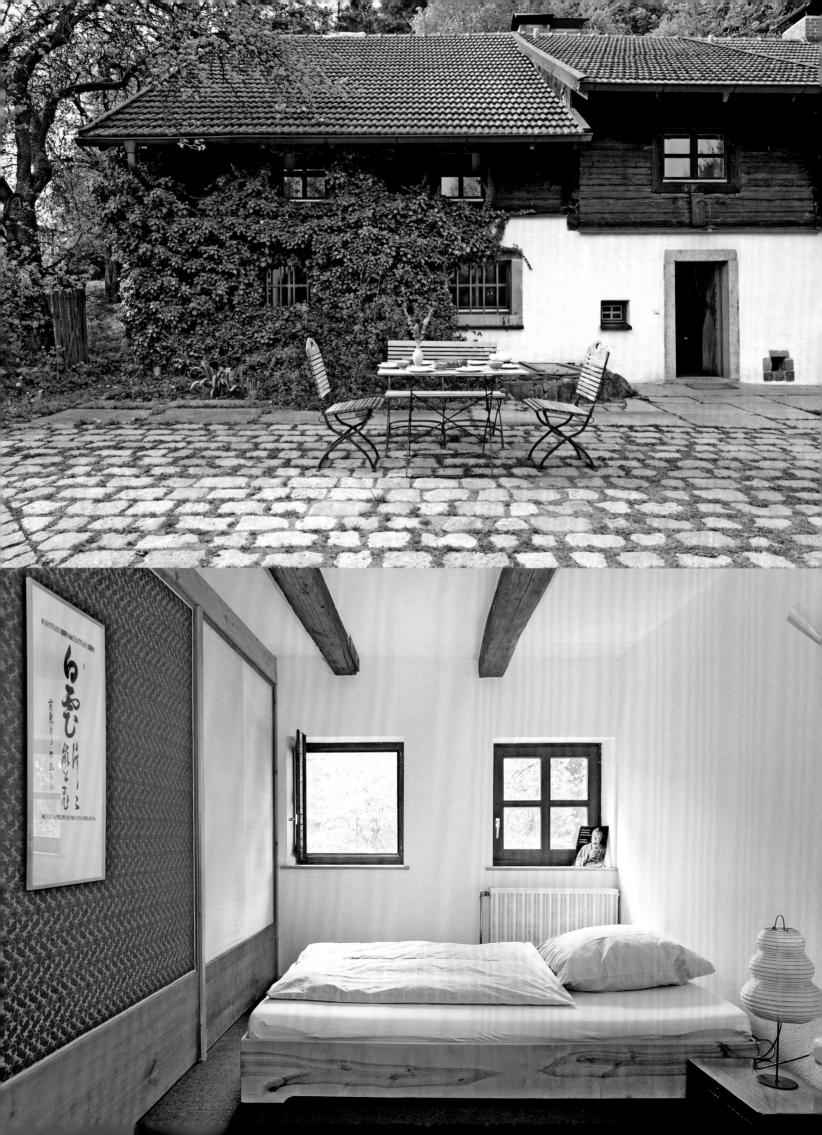

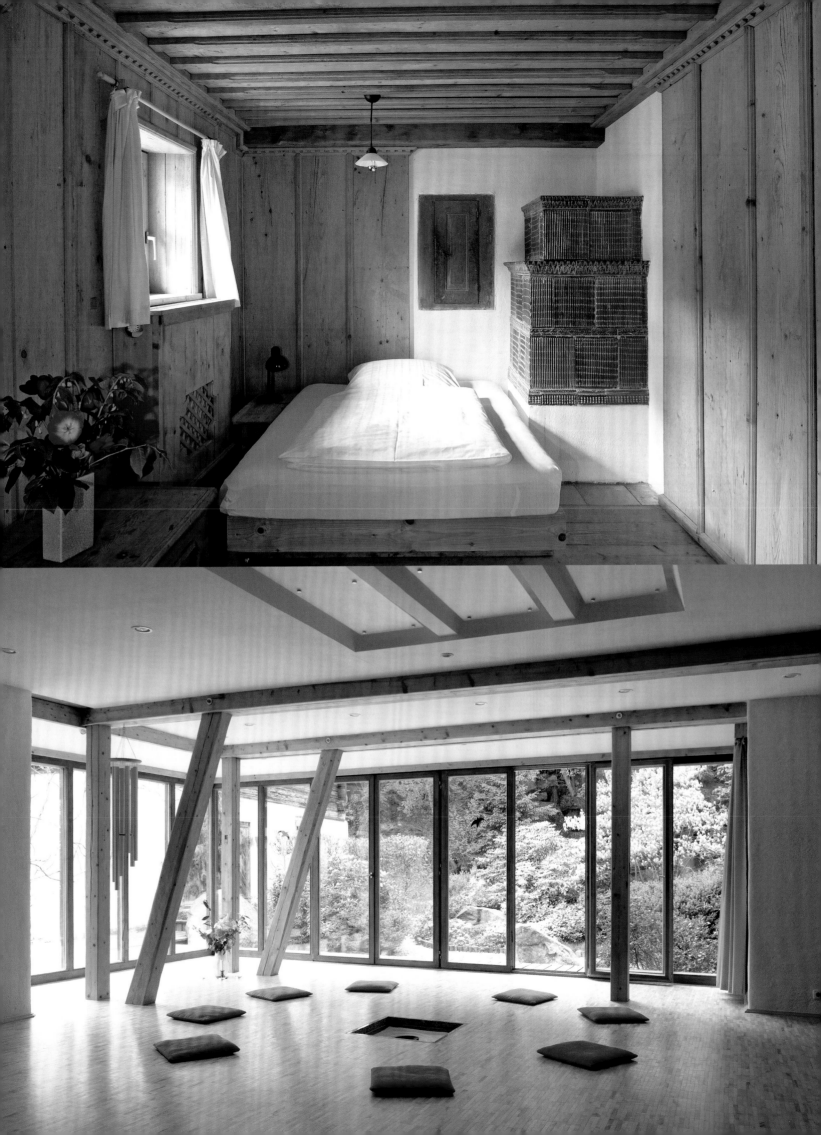

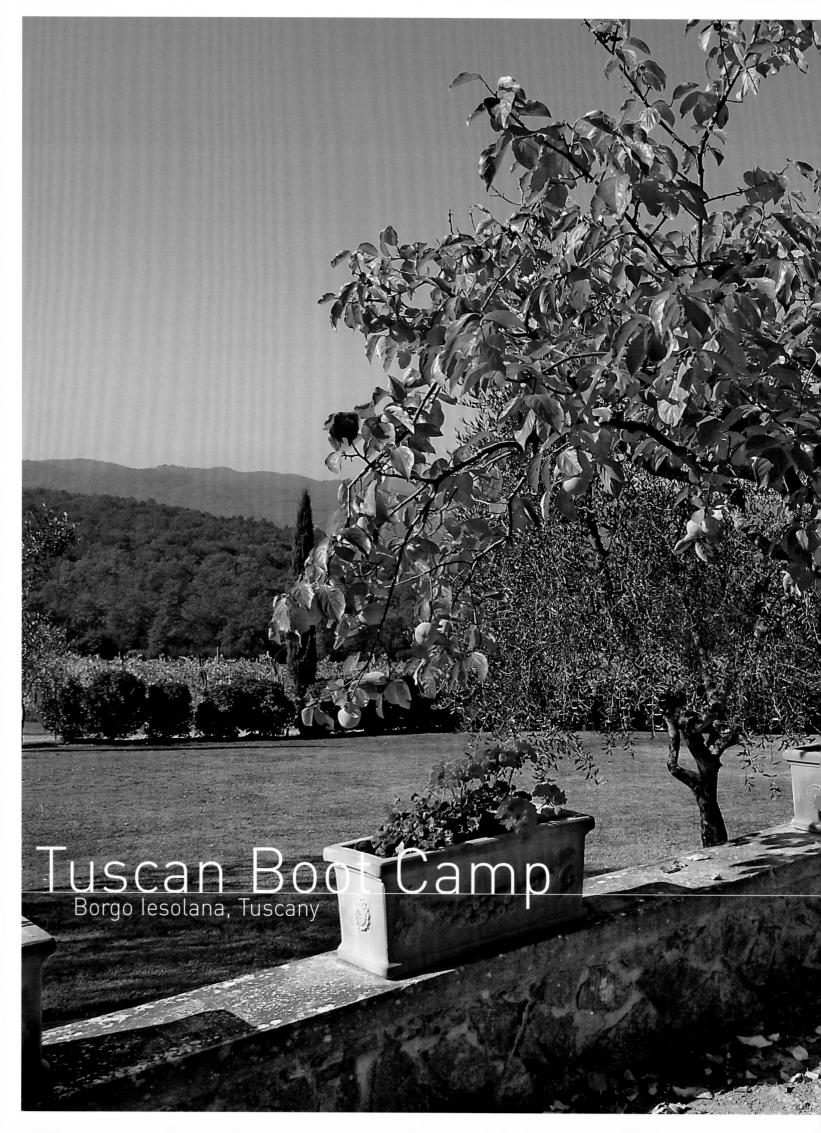

Tuscan Boot Camp

Borgo Iesolana, Tuscany

Borgo Iesolana, Tuscany

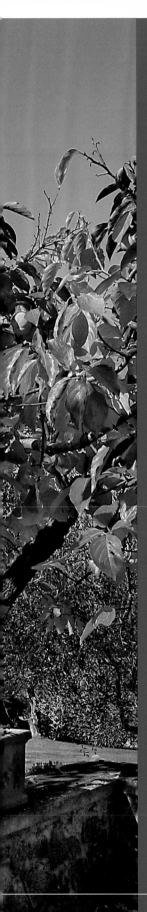

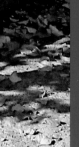

Tuscan Boot Camp

A last look across the vineyards, gently sloping down into the valley in the first light of dawn, and then the eyes are closed for meditation, until the aromas of toast and fresh orange juice announce the end of the extended Yoga session. A brisk march lasting several hours, undertaken in silence, through dried-out river beds and hip-high grasses, gorse, myrtle and rose hip bushes, past gnarled shrubs and shady pine forests, in the hills between Arezzo, Siena and Florence further clears the thoughts and sharpens the senses. How intense suddenly is the scent of the rosemary and the wild thyme, the oleander and the lemon trees. Frogs, butterflies, geckos and deer cross the path. At lunch the rescinded vow of silence and a delicious zucchini quiche provide for a lively cheerfulness. Contrary to the example set by "The Ashram" in Malibu, the organiser of Yogahikes, British film producer and Yoga fan Ian Flooks, sets great store by good food. A lazy afternoon by the pool, with the silvery olive trees around you and the wide azure sky above, is also tolerated. We are in Italy after all, Madonna!

Books to pack: "An Enigma by the Sea" by Carlo Fruttero & Franco Lucentini and "The English Patient" by Michael Ondaatje.

Borgo Iesolana
Loc. Iesolana
52021 Bucine, Tuscany
Italy
Tel. +44 7796 671 549 and +39 055 992 988
Fax +39 055 992 879
info@iesolana.it
mail@yogahikes.com
www.yogahikes.com and www.iesolana.it

DIRECTIONS	From Florence, Pisa or Milan, exit Valdarno on the A1 Florence-Rome in the direction of Montevarchi. At the next intersection continue in the direction of Levane, Bucine and Borgo Iesolana.
YOGA	Workshops only through www.yogahikes.com.
TEACHERS	Alexa Harris.
ROOMS	1 single room, 17 double rooms.
FOOD	Predominantly vegetarian; specialities: sautéed mushrooms, aubergine parmigiana, fennel bake.
TREATMENTS	Massages.
RECREATION	Mountain trekking, pool, Prada outlet.

Toskana Boot Camp

Noch ein letzter Blick über die im Morgengrauen sanft ab-
fallenden Weinberge hinunter ins Tal – und schon schließen
sich die Augen zur Meditation, bis der Geruch nach Toast
und frischem Orangensaft das Ende der ausgedehnten Yogastunde ankündigt. Ein mehrstündiger strammer Marsch,
schweigend unternommen, durch ausgetrocknete Flussbetten
und hüfthohe Gräser, Ginster, Myrte und Hagebuttensträucher
an knorrigen Büschen und schattigen Pinienwäldern vorbei,
in den Hügeln zwischen Arezzo, Siena und Florenz klärt
weiter die Gedanken und schärft die Sinne. Wie stark auf
einmal Rosmarin und wilder Thymian duften, der Oleander
und die Zitronenbäume. Frösche, Schmetterlinge, Geckos,
Rehe kreuzen den Weg. Beim Mittagessen sorgen das aufge-
hobene Schweigegebot und eine köstliche Zucchini-Quiche
für ausgelassene Fröhlichkeit. Anders als beim Vorbild
»The Ashram« in Malibu legt der Veranstalter von Yogahikes,
der britische Filmproduzent und Yogafan Ian Flooks, größten
Wert auf gute Küche. Ein fauler Nachmittag am Pool, die
silbrigen Olivenbäume vor sich und darüber der weite azur-
farbene Himmel, ist ebenfalls geduldet. Wir sind schließlich
in Italien, Madonna!
**Buchtipps: »Das Geheimnis der Pineta« von Carlo Fruttero &
Franco Lucentini und »Der englische Patient« von Michael
Ondaatje.**

Camp d'entraînement en Toscane

Un dernier regard, à l'aube naissante, sur les vignobles
glissant en pente douce vers la vallée, et déjà les yeux se
ferment pour la méditation jusqu'à ce que l'odeur de toast et
de jus d'orange frais annonce la fin de la longue séance de
yoga. Une marche soutenue de plusieurs heures, effectuée
en silence à travers lits de fleuve desséchés et hautes herbes,
genêts, myrtes et buissons de cynorhodon, devant les arbustes
noueux et les forêts de pins ombragées des collines ondulant
entre Arezzo, Sienne et Florence finit d'éclaircir l'esprit en
aiguisant les sens. Avec quelle intensité soudaine le romarin
et le thym sauvage, les lauriers roses et les citronniers n'em-
baument-ils pas ! Grenouilles, papillons, geckos et biches
croisent le chemin. Pendant le déjeuner, la consigne de silence
levée et une délicieuse quiche aux courgettes permettent à
une joyeuse convivialité de s'installer. Se démarquant du
modèle « The Ashram » à Malibu, l'organisateur de Yogahikes
Ian Flooks, producteur de films britannique et adepte du
yoga, attache la plus grande importance à une cuisine raffinée.
De même, un après-midi à se prélasser au bord de la piscine,
les oliviers argentés devant soi et l'immense ciel bleu azur
au-dessus, peut être envisagé. Après tout, nous sommes
dans la « bella Italia » !
**Livres à emporter : « Place de Sienne, coté ombre » de Carlo
Fruttero & Franco Lucentini et « Le Patient anglais » de Michael
Ondaatje.**

ANREISE	Von Florenz, Pisa oder Mailand, Ausfahrt Valdarno auf der A1 Florenz–Rom, Richtung Montevarchi. An der nächsten Kreuzung Richtung Levane, Bucine und Borgo Iesolana.
YOGA	Nur Workshops über www.yogahikes.com.
GASTLEHRER	Alexa Harris.
ZIMMER	1 Einzelzimmer, 17 Doppelzimmer.
KÜCHE	Überwiegend vegetarisch, Spezialitäten: sautierte Pilze, Auberginen parmigiana, Fenchelauflauf.
ANWENDUNGEN	Massagen.
FREIZEIT	Bergwandern, Pool, Prada-Outlet.

ACCÈS	Venant de Florence, Pise ou Milan, sortie Valdarno sur l'A1 Florence-Rome, direction Montevarchi. Au prochain carrefour, direction Levane, Bucine und Borgo Iesolana.
YOGA	Stages uniquement via www.yogahikes.com.
PROFESSEURS	Alexa Harris.
CHAMBRES	1 chambre individuelle, 17 chambres doubles.
RESTAURATION	Essentiellement végétarienne, spécialités : champignons sautés à la poêle, aubergines au parmesan, gratin de fenouil.
TRAITEMENTS	Massages.
ACTIVITÉS	Randonnées en montagne, piscine, espace Prada.

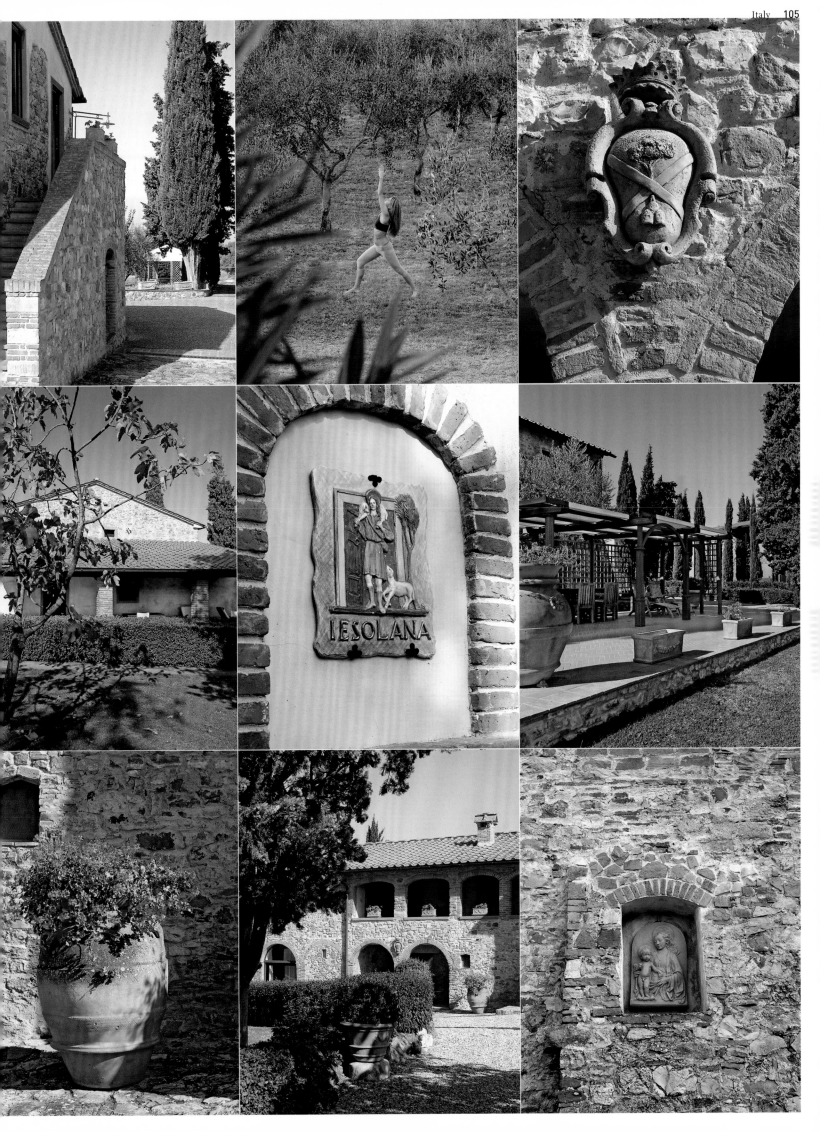

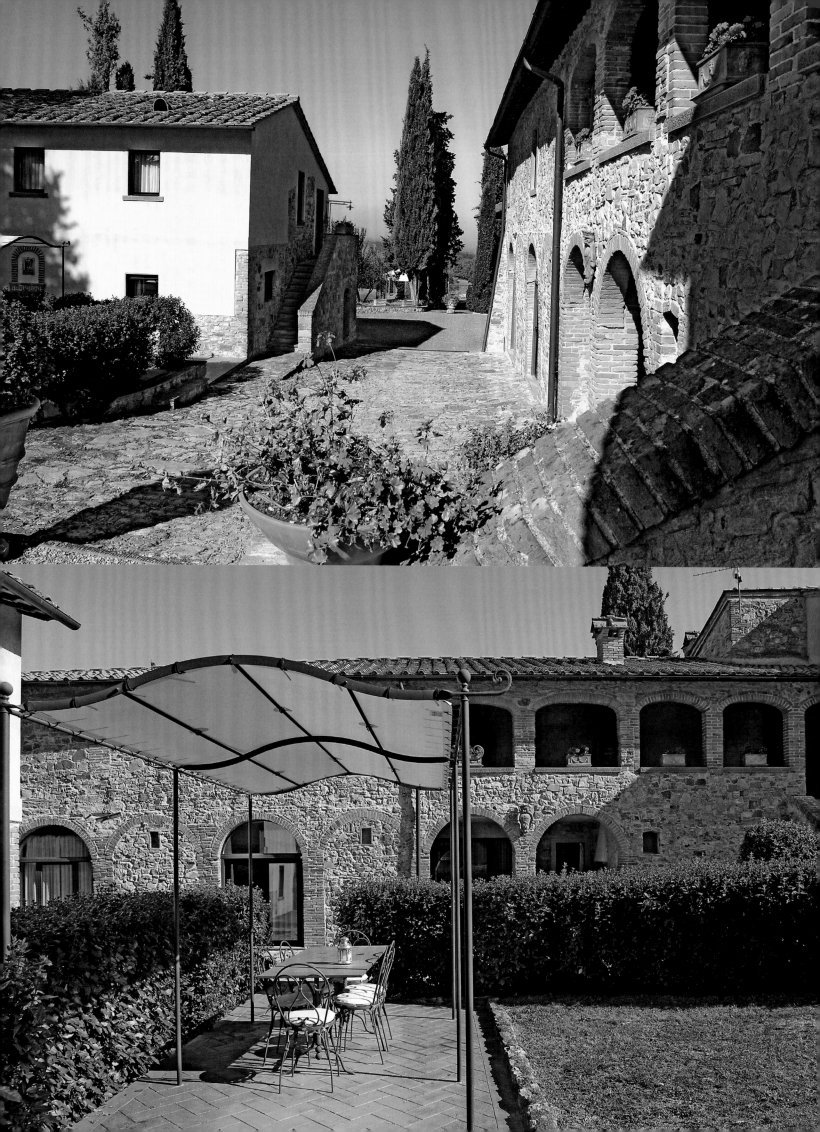

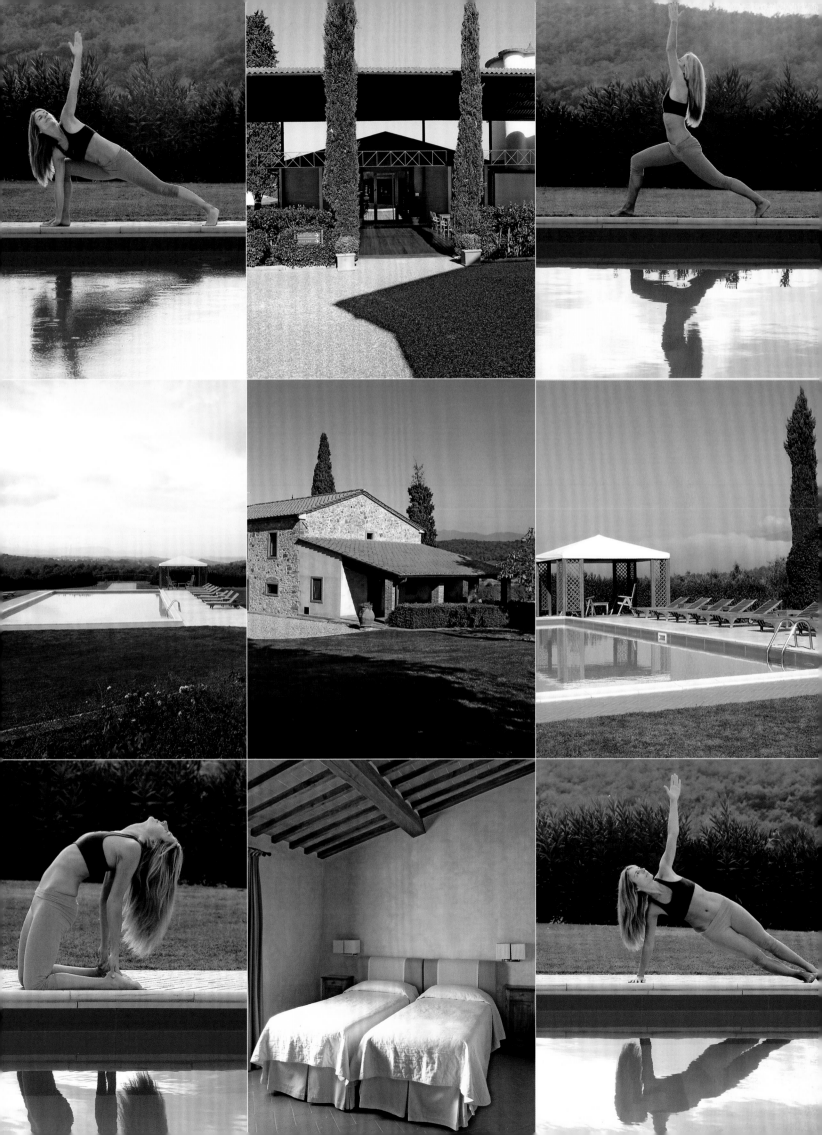

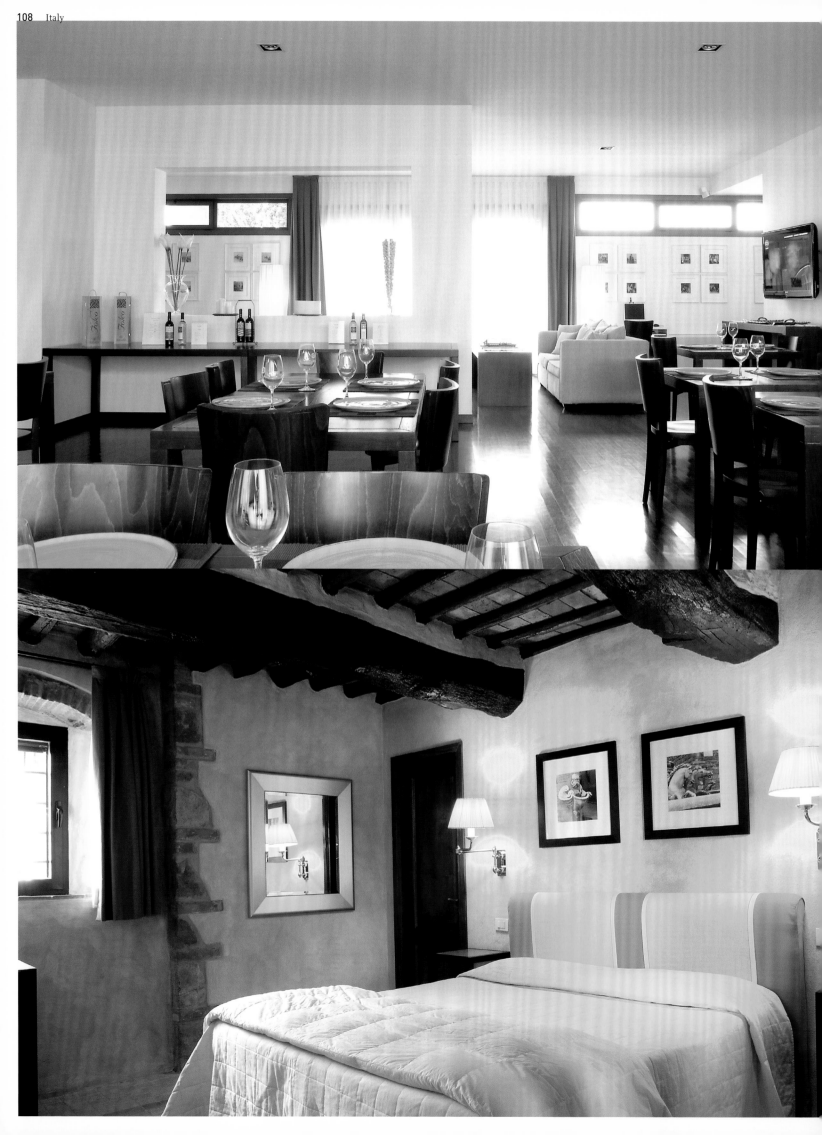

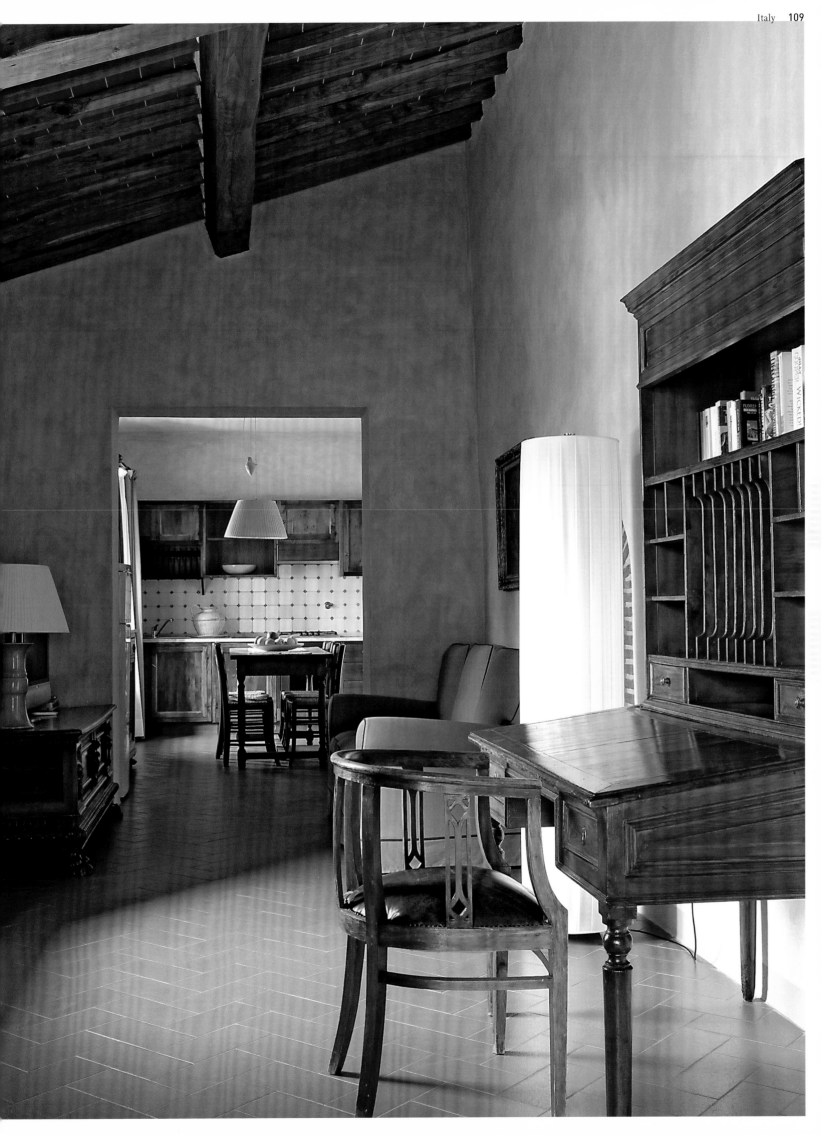

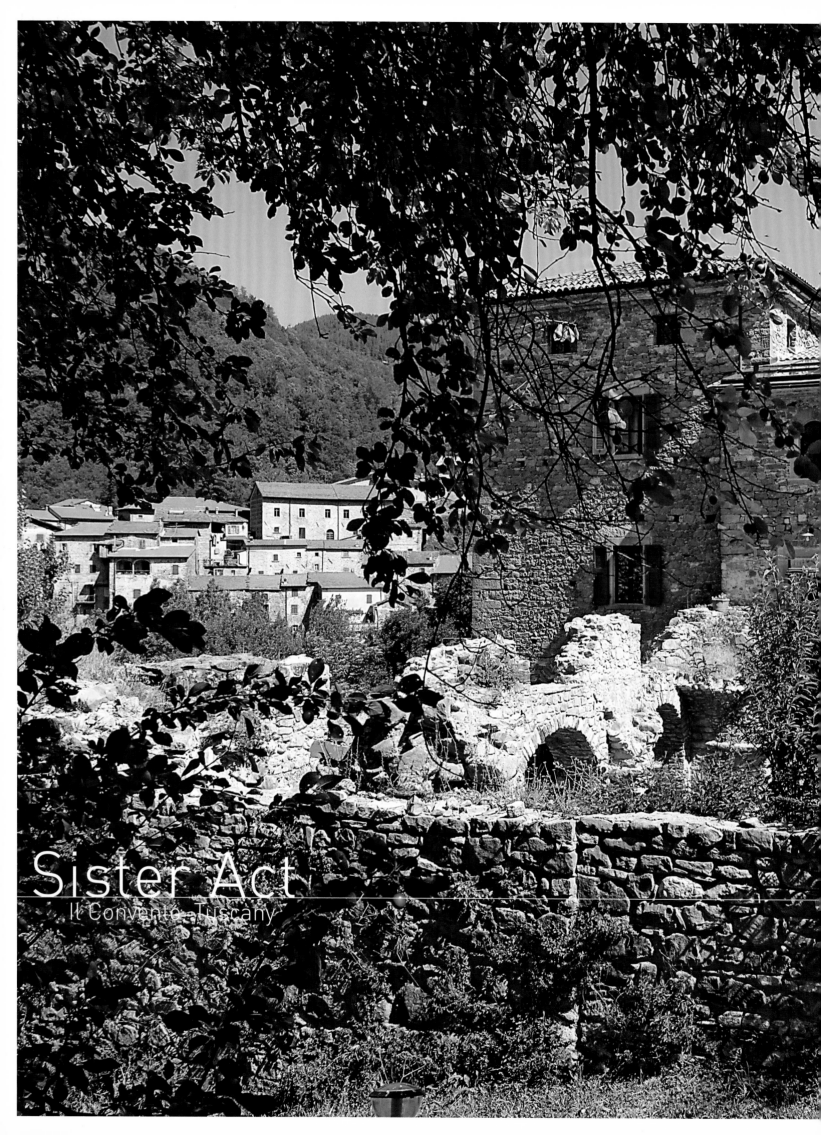

Sister Act
Il Convento, Tuscany

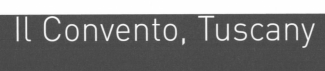

Il Convento, Tuscany

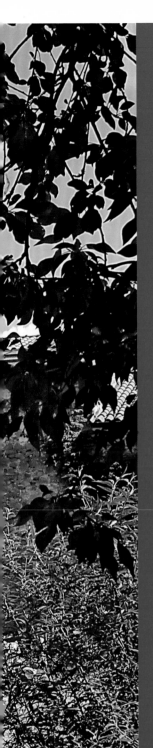

Sister Act

When a dancer and a meditating Marxist look for a place to stay together, a former convent is really the only thing that fits the bill. Il Convento, built in 1549, accommodated the nuns of Santa Marta for over three centuries. St Martha is the patron saint of housekeeping and often depicted with cooking utensils and a bunch of keys, but she is also responsible for painters and sculptors. Lunigiana, an area of countryside between Parma and Florence as yet little developed for tourism, captivates through its green hills, vineyards, endless chestnut forests, olive groves and river sources, the mountain pasture of the Apennines and the peaks of the Apuan Alps on the horizon. Time and time again, friends and relations lent money to the couple, who brought up their children here, until from the half-dilapidated masonry a charming place of retreat emerged. In the vault of the former wine cellar, Yoga is now practised; guests sleep in simple whitewashed rooms and read by the fireplace. The overall impression is still somewhat monastic, but in compensation the view into the valley is anything but restrained, and the cuisine is sensually Italian. You can, by the way, also find accommodation as a working guest and participate intellectually and materially, directly or indirectly in this small family's big project to create a place of peace and contemplation. But don't worry: the sisters of Santa Marta are sure to have giggled on occasion, too.

Books to pack: "The Name of the Rose" by Umberto Eco and "The Palace" by Lisa St. Aubin de Terán.

Il Convento	
Casola in Lunigiana, 54014	
Italy	
Tel. +39 585 900 75	
Fax +39 585 900 75	
convento.seminar@tin.it	
www.il-convento.net	

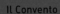

DIRECTIONS	Il Convento in Casola lies 2 hrs north of Florence Airport.
YOGA	Workshops only.
TEACHERS	QBI, Mahashakti Veronika, Planetyoga.
ROOMS	15 rooms for max. 35 guests.
FOOD	Vegetarian Lunigianan and Tuscan cuisine with artichokes, green asparagus, peppers, stuffed zucchini, porcini, chestnuts with sage, rosemary and bay leaf.
RECREATION	Meditation, hiking.

Sister Act

Wenn eine Tänzerin und ein meditierender Marxist zusammen eine Bleibe suchen, kann eigentlich nichts anderes herauskommen als ein ehemaliges Kloster. Il Convento, 1549 gebaut, beherbergte über drei Jahrhunderte den Frauenorden Santa Marta, der heiligen Martha, die als Patronin der Häuslichkeit gerne mit Kochgerät und Schlüsselbund dargestellt wird, aber auch für Maler und Bildhauer zuständig ist. Die Lunigiana, eine touristisch noch wenig erschlossene Landschaft zwischen Parma und Florenz, besticht durch ihre grünen Hügel, Weinberge, endlosen Kastanienwälder, Olivenhaine und Quellflüsse – am Horizont die Bergwiesen des Appenins und die Gipfel der Apuanischen Alpen. Freunde und Verwandte haben dem Paar, das hier seine Kinder aufzog, immer wieder Geld geliehen, bis aus dem halb verfallenen Gemäuer ein bezaubernder Ort des Rückzugs wurde. Im Gewölbe des ehemaligen Weinkellers wird jetzt Yoga geübt, in weiß gekalkten, schlichten Zimmern wird geschlafen, am Kaminfeuer gelesen. Die gesamte Anmutung ist noch immer etwas klösterlich, dafür ist der Blick ins Tal alles andere als zurückhaltend und die Küche sinnlich italienisch. Man kann übrigens auch als Working Guest unterkommen und sich gedanklich und materiell, direkt oder indirekt beteiligen am großen Lebensprojekt der kleinen Familie, einen Ort der Ruhe und Selbstbesinnung zu schaffen. Aber keine Angst: Die Schwestern von Santa Marta haben sicher auch gelegentlich gekichert.

Buchtipps: »Der Name der Rose« von Umberto Eco und »Der Palast« von Lisa St. Aubin de Terán.

Sister Act

Quand une danseuse et un marxiste épris de méditation cherchent ensemble un logis, il ne peut s'agir que d'un ancien cloître. Il Convento, construit en 1549, hébergea pendant plus de trois siècles l'ordre religieux féminin Santa Marta, de sainte Marthe patronne des foyers, souvent représentée munie d'ustensiles de cuisine et d'un trousseau de clés, mais protégeant aussi les peintres et les sculpteurs. La Lunigiana, région encore peu ouverte aux touristes entre Parme et Florence, séduit par ses vertes collines, ses vignobles, ses infinies forêts de châtaigniers, ses bosquets d'oliviers, ses sources jaillissantes, et, à l'horizon, les prairies de l'Appenin et les sommets des Alpes apuanes. Des amis et parents ont régulièrement prêté de l'argent au couple, qui a élevé ses enfants ici, jusqu'à ce que ces murs en ruine se transforment en un lieu de retraite envoûtant. Sous la voûte de l'ancien cellier ont lieu désormais des séances de yoga, les austères chambres blanchies à la chaux invitent au sommeil, les feux de cheminée à la lecture. Si l'atmosphère générale est restée quelque peu monastique, le panorama de la vallée est des plus vastes et la cuisine italienne succulente à souhait. De plus, il est possible d'y séjourner en tant que working guest, en participant sur le plan spirituel et matériel, directement ou indirectement, au grand projet d'ensemble de la petite famille : créer un lieu de paix et de recueillement. Mais n'ayez crainte : il est sûrement arrivé aussi aux religieuses de sainte Marthe de rire en douce.

Livres à emporter : « Le Nom de la rose » d'Umberto Eco et « The Palace » de Lisa St. Aubin de Terán.

ANREISE	Il Convento in Casola liegt 2 Std. nördlich des Flughafens Florenz.
YOGA	Nur Workshops.
GASTLEHRER	QBI, Mahashakti Veronika, Planetyoga.
ZIMMER	15 Zimmer für max. 35 Gäste.
KÜCHE	Vegetarische lunigianische und toskanische Küche mit Artischocken, grünem Spargel, Paprika, gefüllten Zucchini, Steinpilzen, Kastanien mit Salbei, Rosmarin und Lorbeer.
FREIZEIT	Meditation, Wandern.

ACCÈS	Il Convento in Casola est à 2 h au nord de l'aéroport de Florence.
YOGA	Stages uniquement.
PROFESSEURS	QBI, Mahashakti Veronika, Planetyoga.
CHAMBRES	15 chambres pour 35 hôtes max.
RESTAURATION	Cuisine végétarienne, lunigianaise et toscane. Artichauts, asperges vertes, poivrons, courgettes farcies, cèpes, marrons à la sauge, au romarin et au laurier.
ACTIVITÉS	Méditation, randonnées.

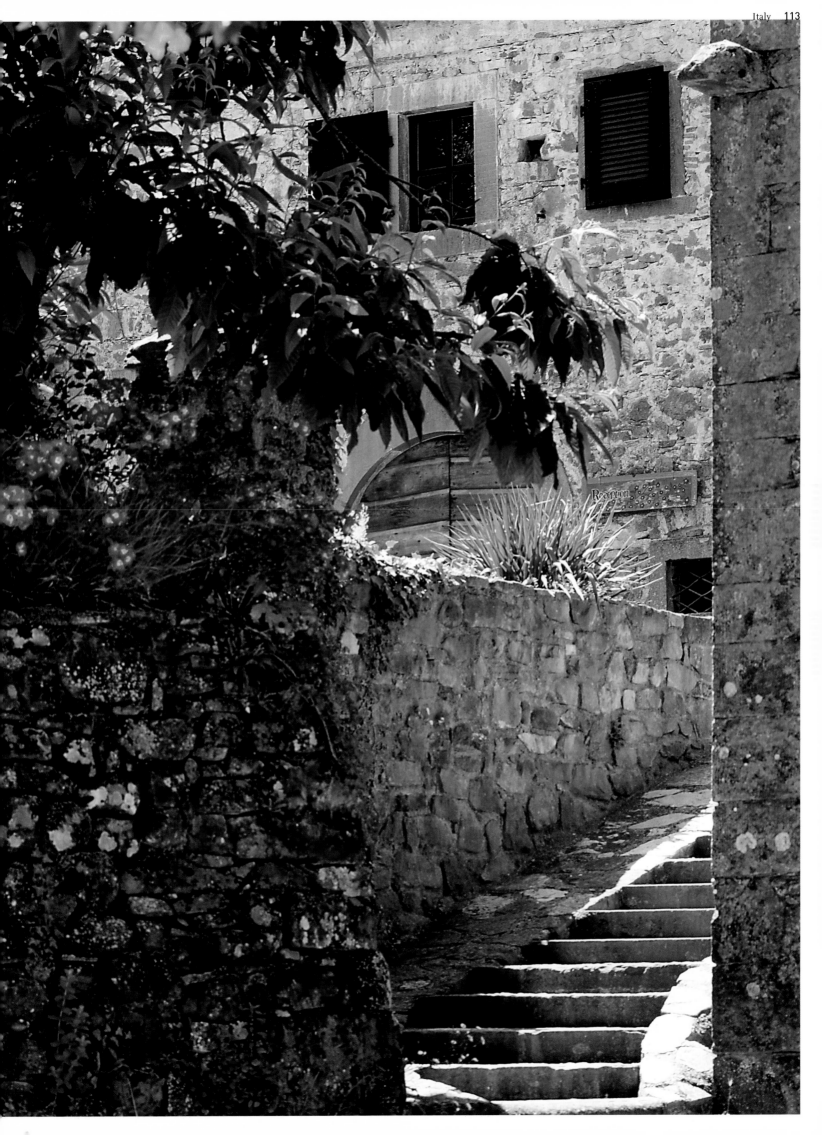

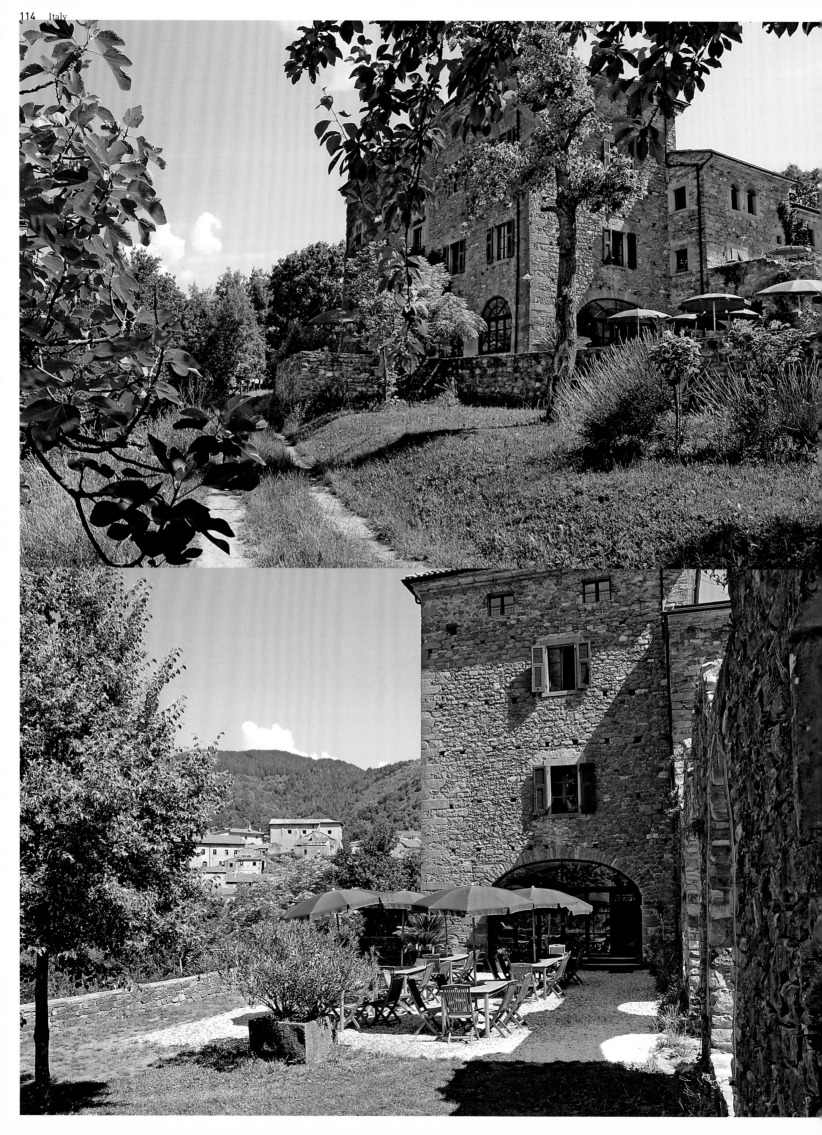

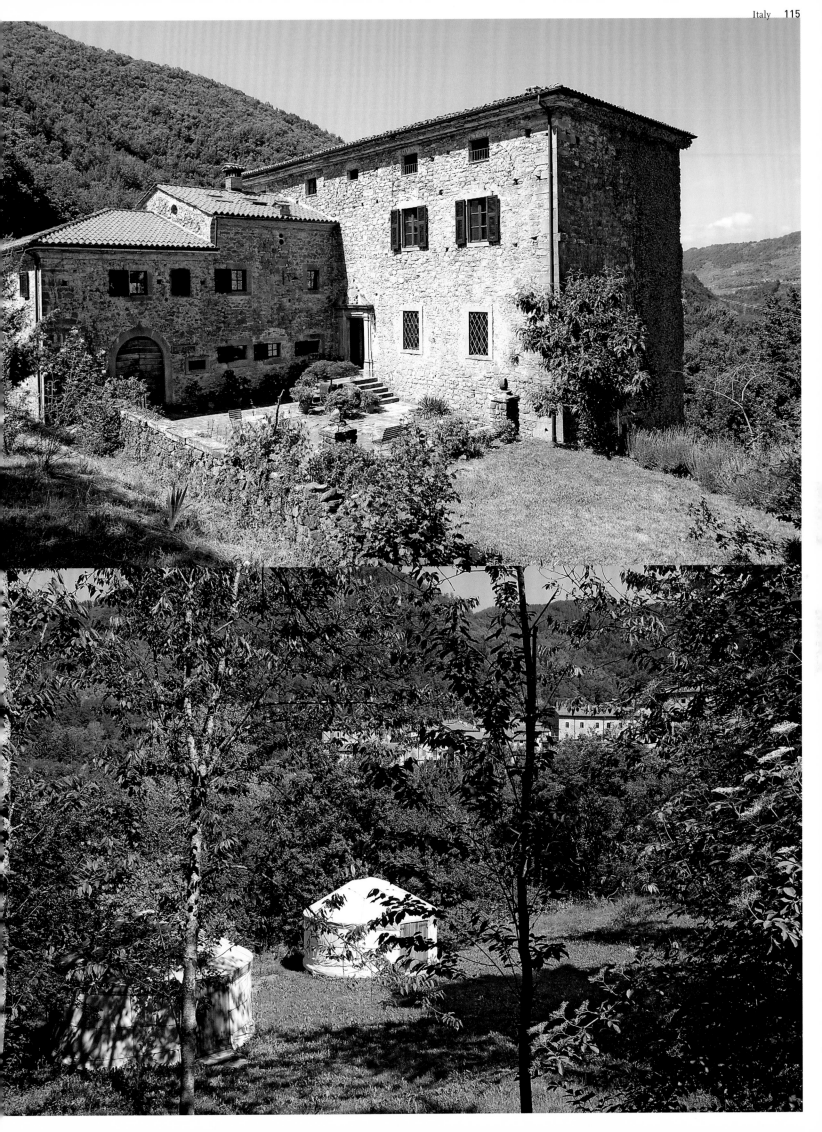

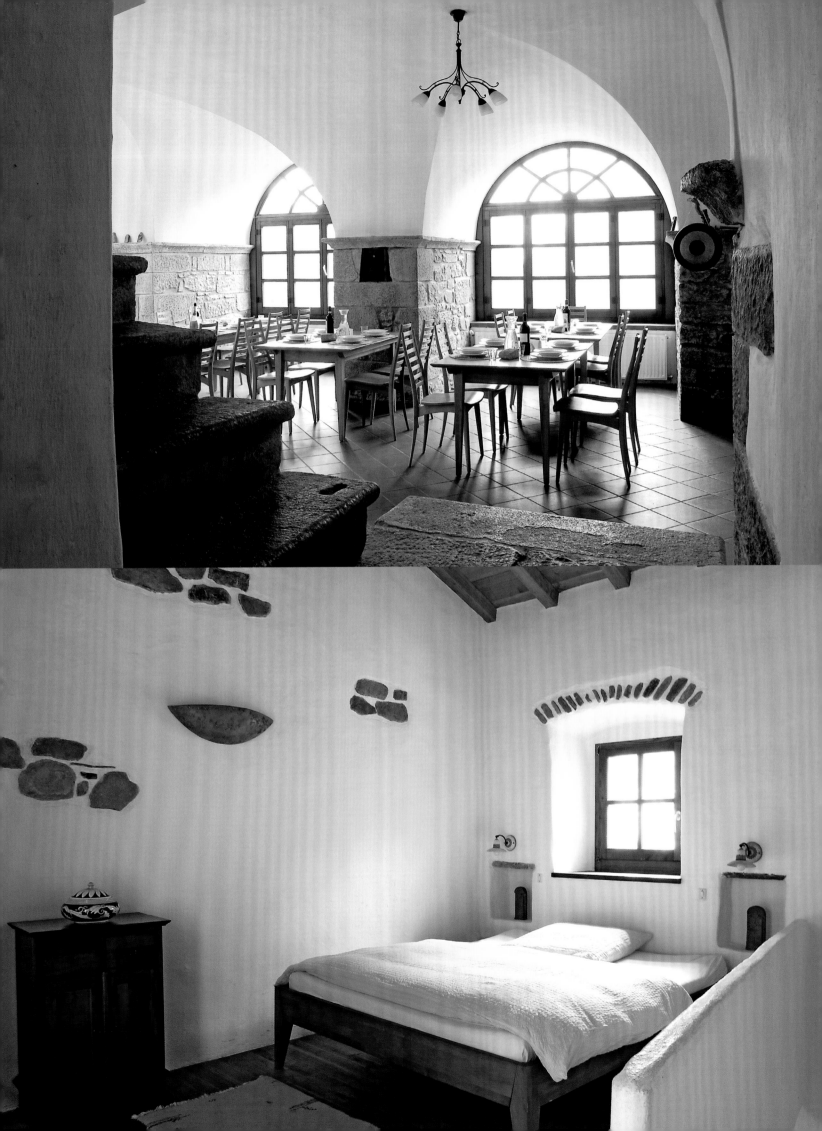

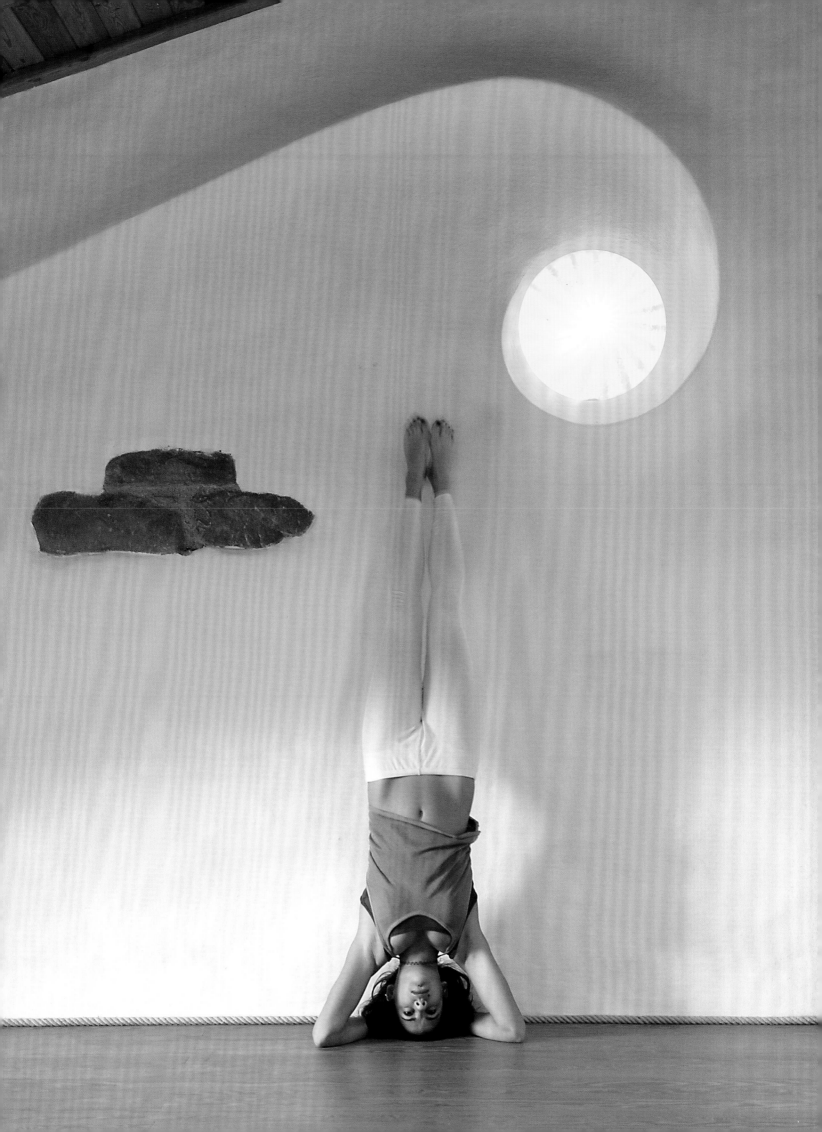

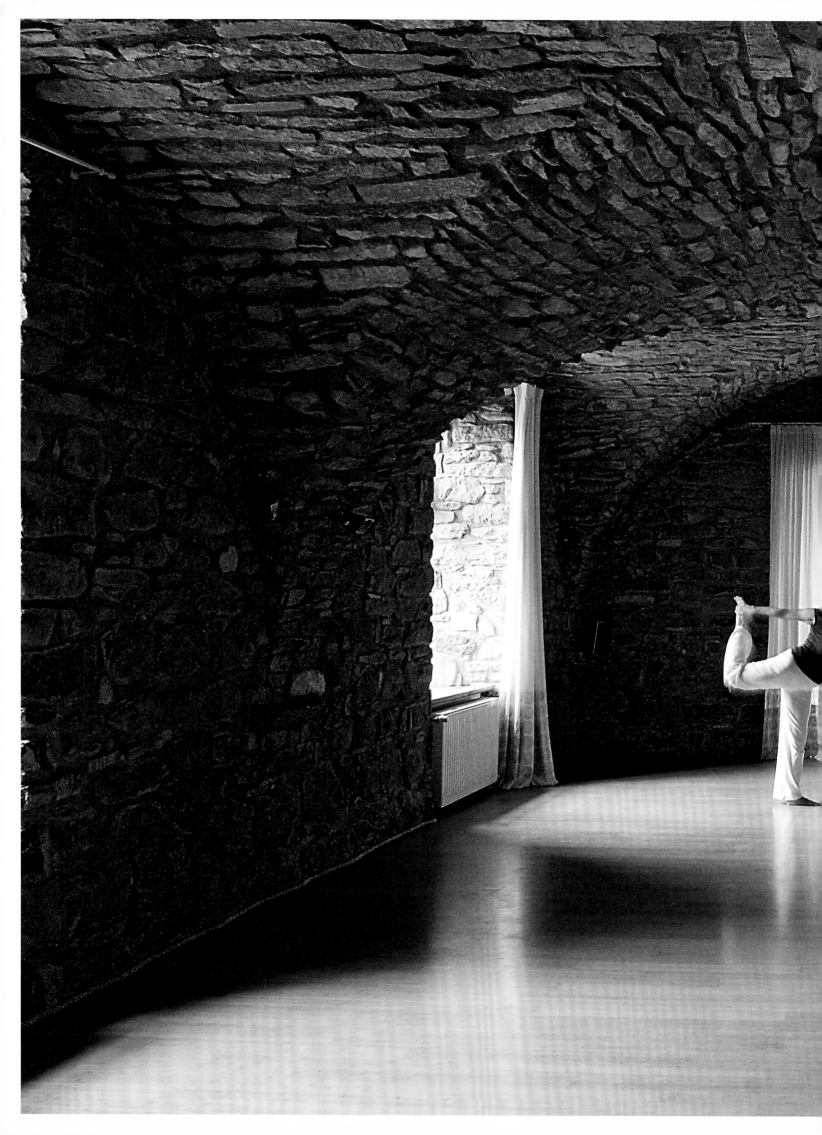

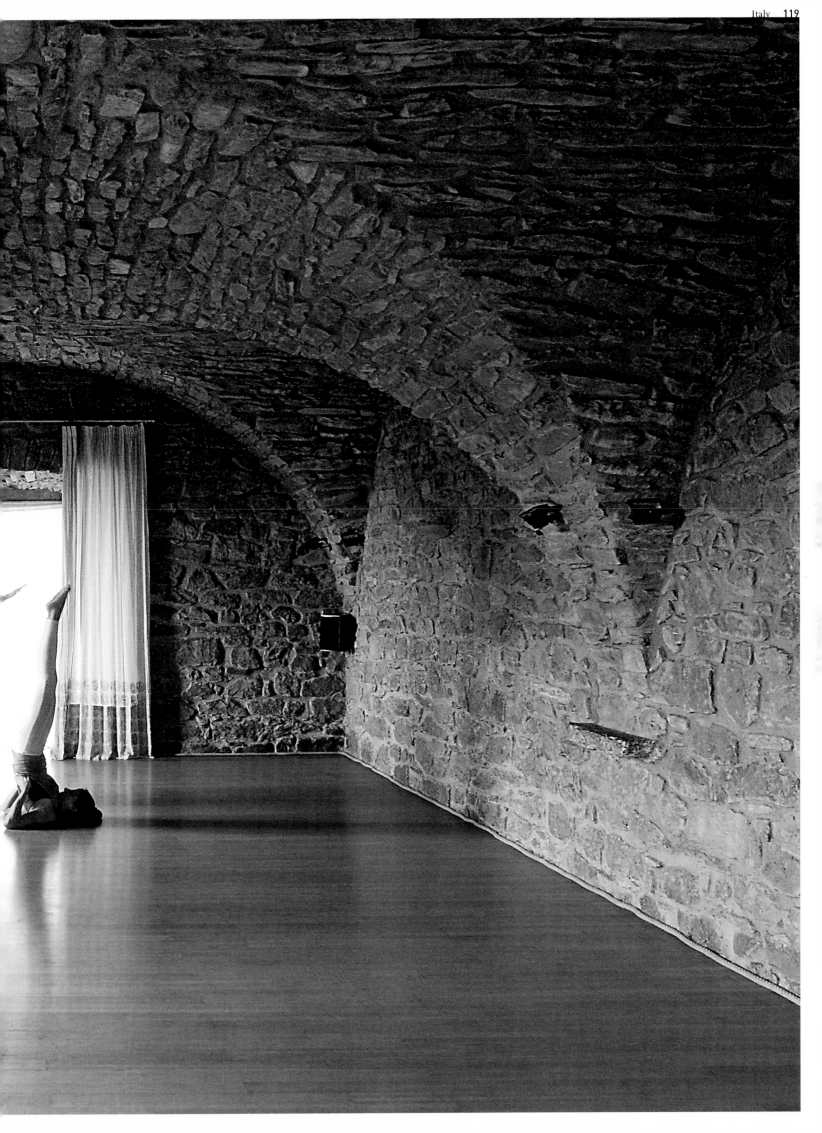

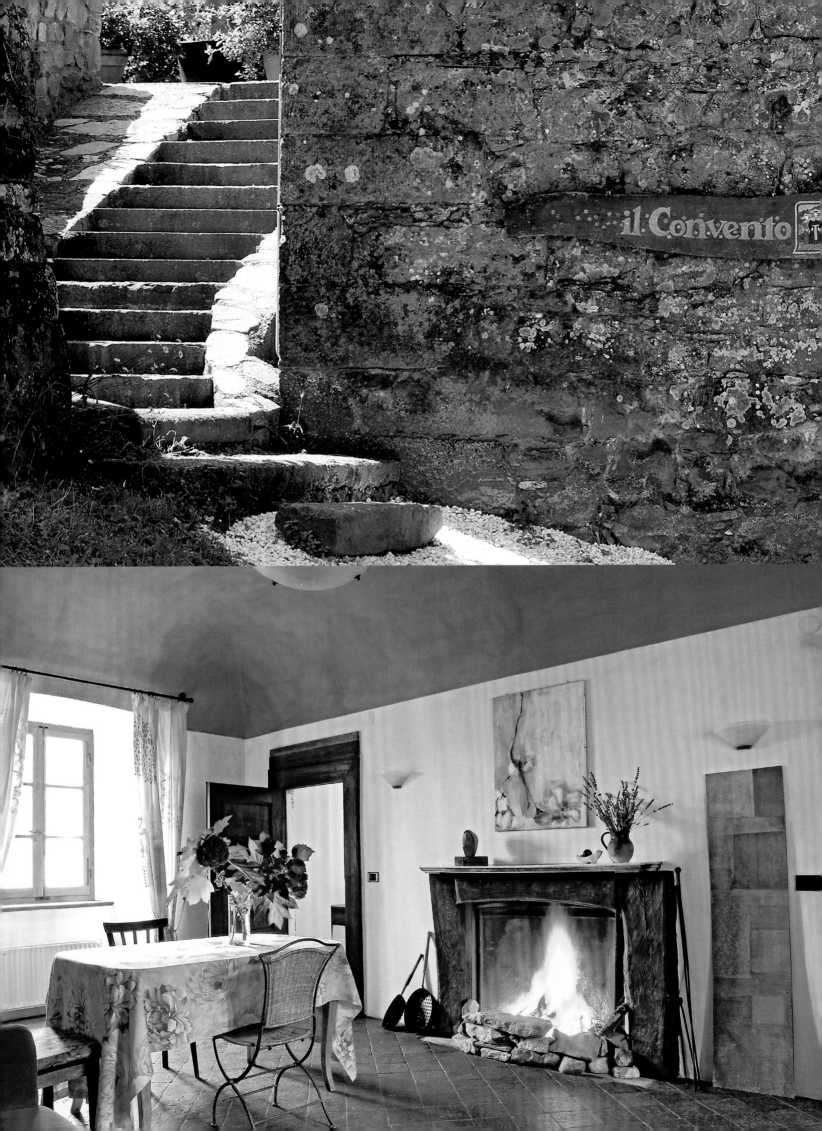

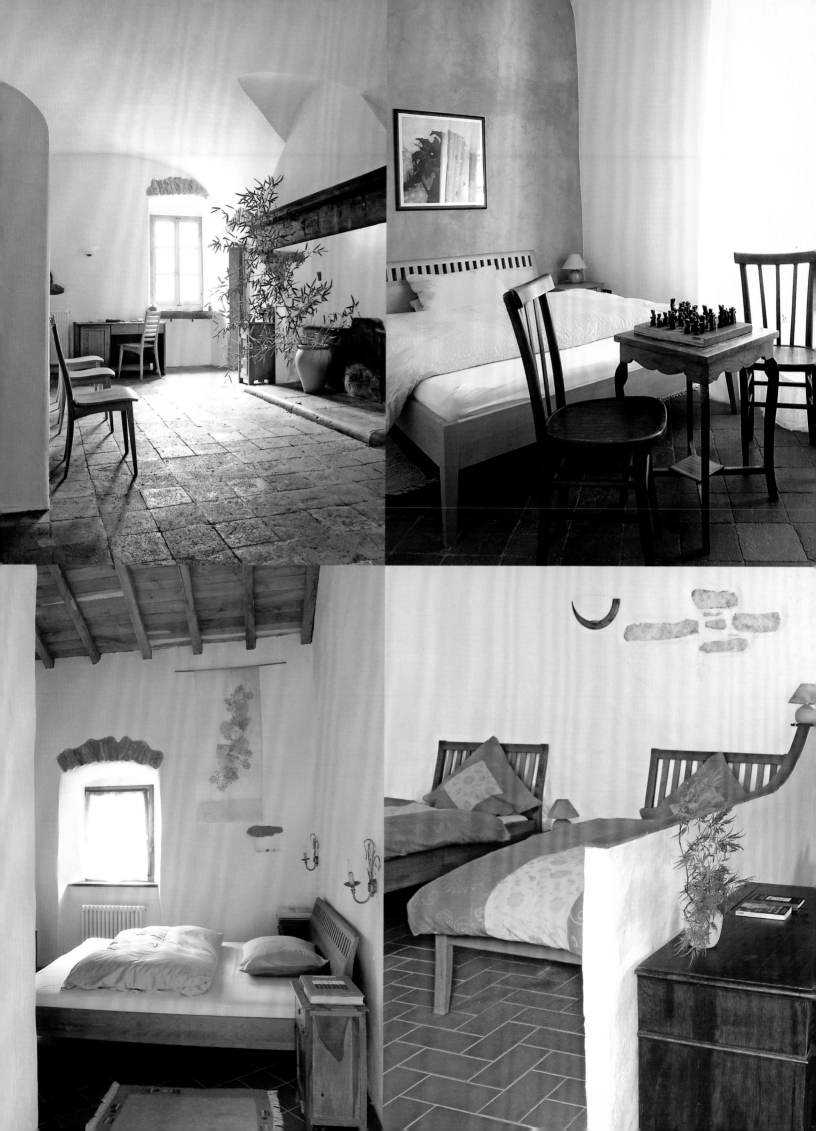

In the Here and Now for Ete

In Sabina, Latium

In Sabina, Latium

In the Here and Now for Eternity

If Rome is the Eternal City, then In Sabina, less than an hour away, has even more of a claim to eternity. Because that's how long you would like to stay within these old 17th-century walls. Located not far from the medieval village of Torri in Sabina between olive groves and fruit trees, from each of the three terraces there is an amazing view of the sunset that stirs even the most unshakable of yogis. Simply and lovingly furnished inside, hammocks and loungers at the pool, a richly laid table in the garden and even a cinema screen in the open air for occasional evening entertainment turn this place into a second home that makes you forget the passing time. The Yoga deck, in the midst of the greenery, is protected from the sun by a light, white canvas. Yoga arises from the observation of nature, as Patañjali said more than two millennia ago. Another reason to transform yourself into Vrksasana, the tree, and hope that you can stay an eternity.
Books to pack: "One Last Ride on the Merry-Go-Round" by Tiziano Terzani and "Invisible Cities" by Italo Calvino.

In Sabina	
Via Pizzuti 53	
Torri in Sabina Rieti, 02049	
Italy	
Tel. +39 340 387 6028	
www.insabina.com	

DIRECTIONS	47 miles north of Rome, 1 1/2 hrs away from Rome Airport.
YOGA	Ashtanga, Sivananda, Iyengar, Scaravelli, Jivamukti, Anusara.
TEACHERS	Glenn Ceresoli, John Stirk, Gingi Lee, Heather Elton.
ROOMS	1–3-bed rooms for max. 22 people.
FOOD	Organic cuisine with self-grown produce.
TREATMENTS	Massages in specially built tree-house hut.
RECREATION	Day trips to Orvieto, Assisi, Spoleto and Rome, and to the hot springs of Viterbo. Hiking and horseback riding.

Im Hier und Jetzt für eine Ewigkeit

Wenn Rom die ewige Stadt ist, dann hat In Sabina, weniger als eine Stunde entfernt, erst Recht Anspruch auf Ewigkeit. So lange möchte man nämlich bleiben in diesen alten Gemäuern aus dem 17. Jahrhundert. Nicht weit von dem mittelalterlichen Dorf Torri in Sabina, zwischen Olivenhainen und Obstbäumen gelegen, hat man von jeder der drei Terrassen einen umwerfenden Blick auf Sonnenuntergänge, die selbst den unerschütterlichsten Yogi rühren. Schlichte, liebevolle Ausstattung im Inneren, Hängematten und Liegestühle am Pool, eine reich gedeckte Tafel im Garten und sogar eine Kinoleinwand im Freien für gelegentliche Abendunterhaltungen machen diesen Platz zu einem Zuhause, das einen die Zeit vergessen lässt. Das mitten ins Grüne gebaute Yoga-Deck wird von einem luftigen weißen Segel gegen die Sonne geschützt. Yoga entsteht aus der Beobachtung der Natur, sagte Patañjali vor über 2000 Jahren. Ein Grund mehr, sich in Vrksasana, den Baum, zu verwandeln und zu hoffen, dass man bleiben darf.

Buchtipps: »Noch eine Runde auf dem Karussell: Vom Leben und Sterben« von Tiziano Terzani und »Die unsichtbaren Städte« von Italo Calvino.

Ici et maintenant pour l'éternité

Si Rome est la Ville éternelle, In Sabina, située à moins d'une heure, peut légitimement prétendre à l'éternité. Car on aimerait rester pour toujours entre ces vieux murs du 17e siècle. A proximité du village médiéval de Torri in Sabina entre les bosquets d'oliviers et les arbres fruitiers, on a, de chacune des trois terrasses, une vue époustouflante sur des couchers de soleil qui émeuvent même le yogi le plus inébranlable. Un intérieur simple, aménagé avec amour, des hamacs et des chaises longues au bord de la piscine, une table copieusement garnie dans le jardin et même un écran de cinéma pour les soirées en plein air donnent à celui qui séjourne ici et oublie le temps, l'impression d'être chez soi. La plate-forme de yoga bâtie dans la verdure est protégée du soleil par une voile blanche aérienne. Le yoga naît de l'observation de la nature, a dit Patañjali il y a plus de 2000 ans. Raison de plus pour se métamorphoser en arbre, en Vrksasana, et espérer qu'on pourra rester.

Livres à emporter : « Un autre tour de manège » de Tiziano Terzani et « Les Villes invisibles » d'Italo Calvino.

ANREISE	75 km nördlich von Rom, 1,5 Std. vom Flughafen Rom entfernt.
YOGA	Astanga, Sivananda, Iyengar, Scaravelli, Jivamukti, Anusara.
GASTLEHRER	Glenn Ceresoli, John Stirk, Gingi Lee, Heather Elton.
ZIMMER	1–3 Bett-Zimmer für max. 22 Personen.
KÜCHE	Biologische Küche mit Produkten aus eigenem Anbau.
ANWENDUNGEN	Massagen im eigens gebauten Baumhaus.
FREIZEIT	Ausflüge nach Orvieto, Assisi, Spoleto und Rom, zu den heißen Quellen von Viterbo. Wandern und Reiten.

ACCÈS	Situé à 75 km au nord de Rome, à 1h30 de l'aéroport de Rome.
YOGA	Ashtânga, Shivananda, Iyengar, Scaravelli, Jivamukti, Anusara.
PROFESSEURS	Glenn Ceresoli, John Stirk, Gingi Lee, Heather Elton.
CHAMBRES	Chambres de 1 à 3 lits pour 22 personnes max.
RESTAURATION	Cuisine bio à base de produits cultivés sur place.
TRAITEMENTS	Massages dans la maison-arbre spécialement conçue.
ACTIVITÉS	Excursions à Orvieto, Assise, Spolète et Rome, aux sources chaudes de Viterbe. Randonnées et équitation.

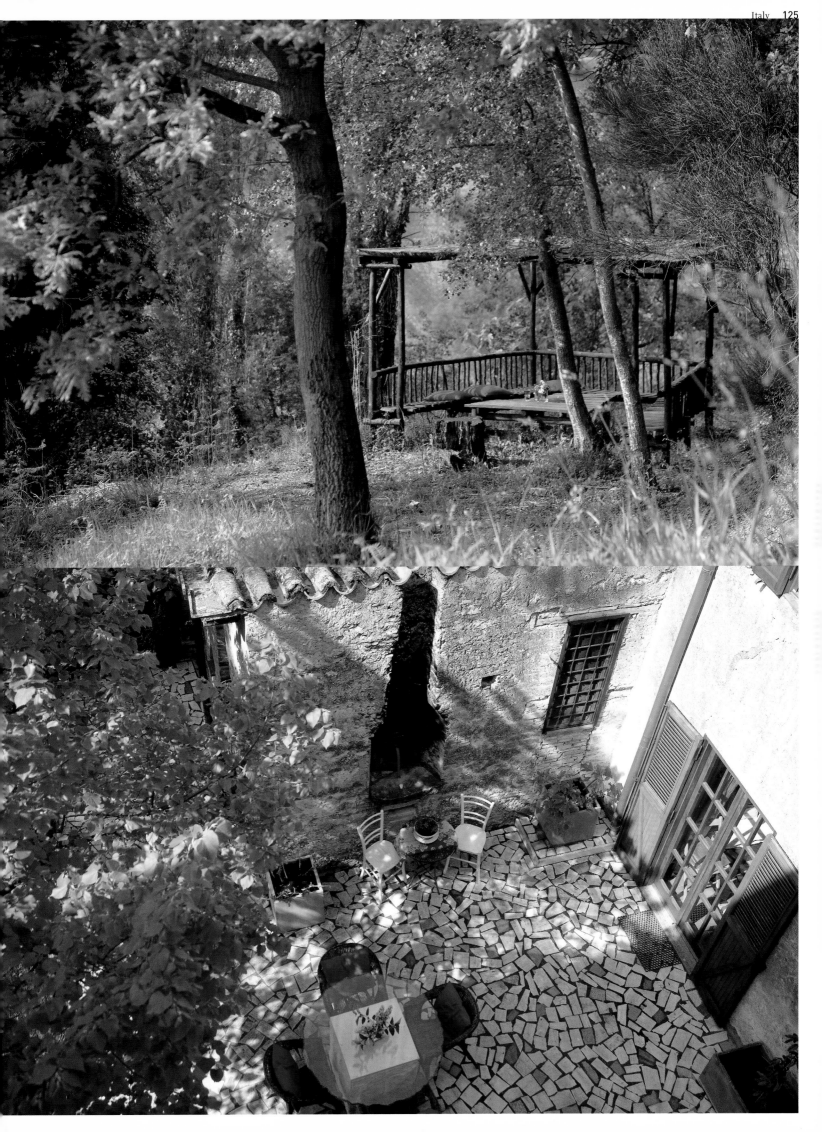

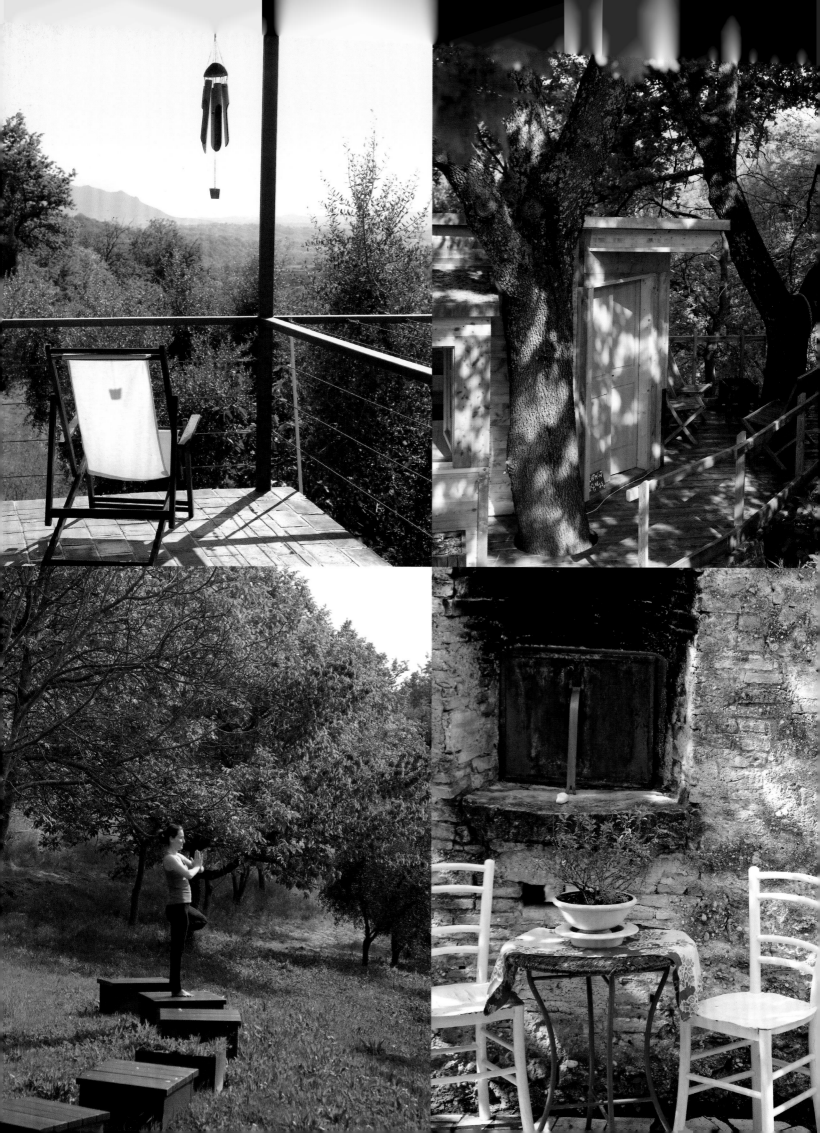

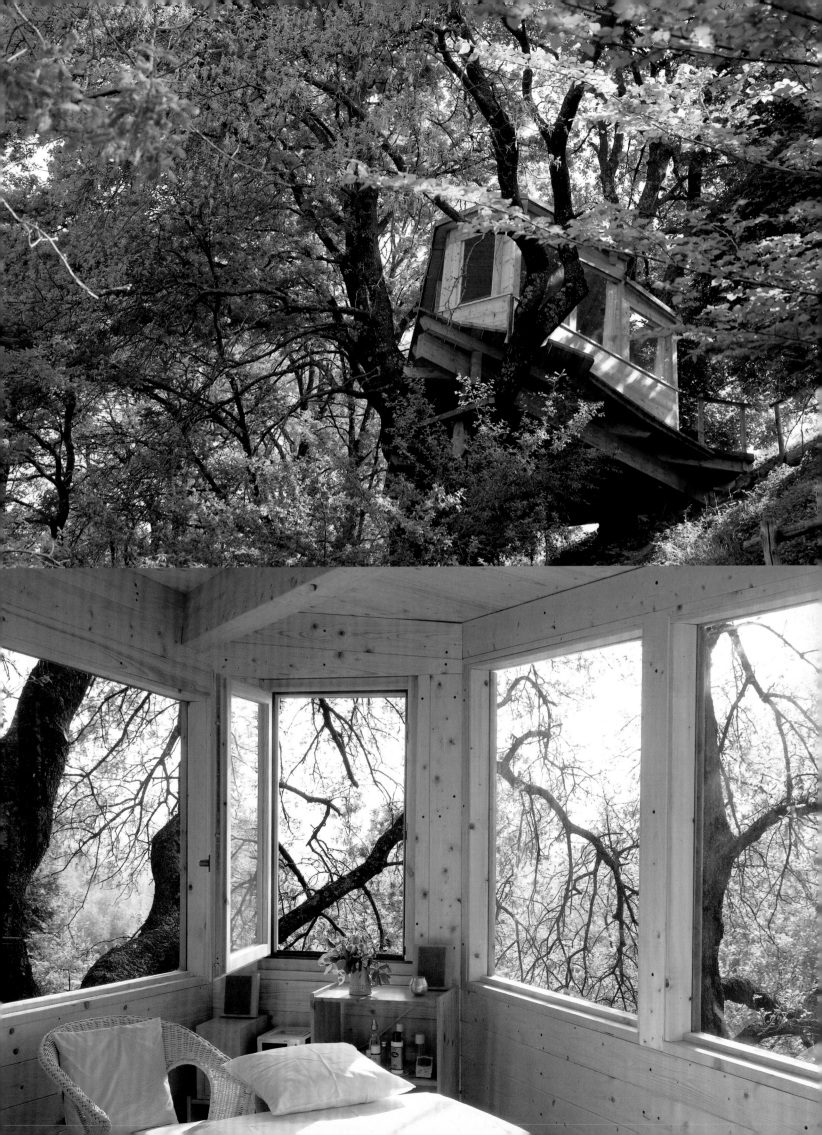

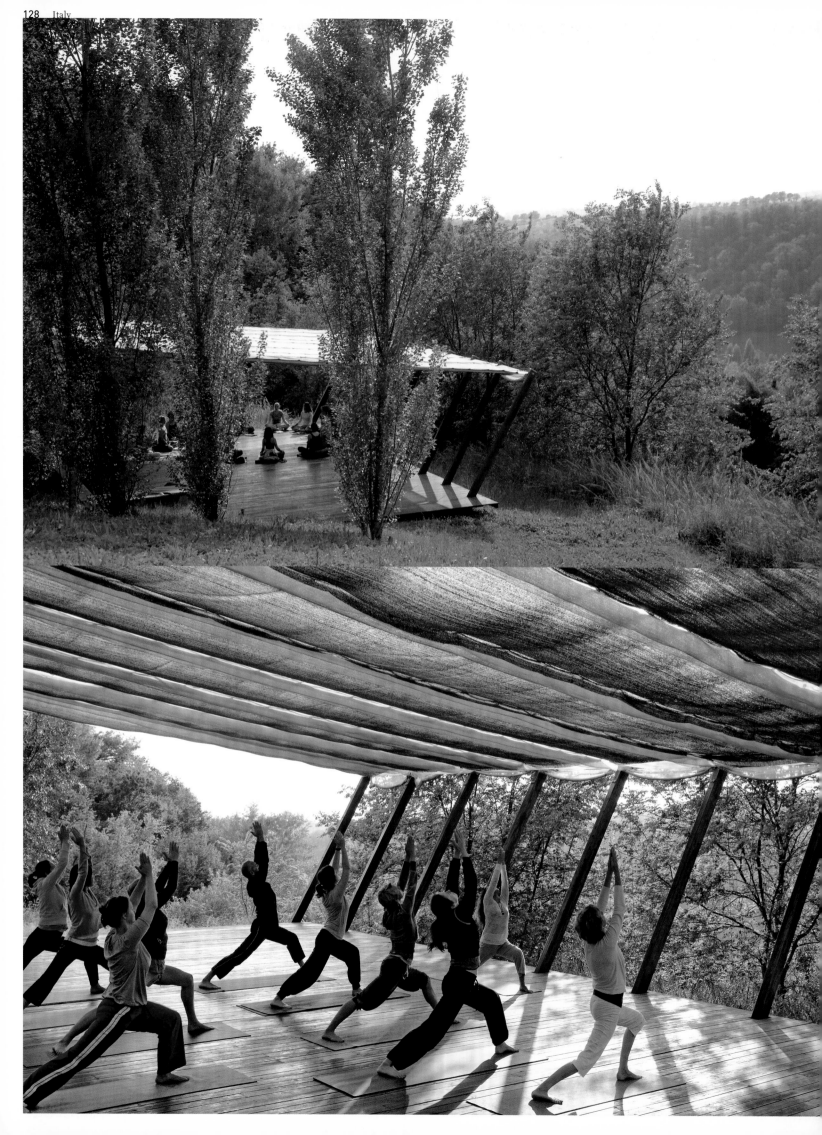

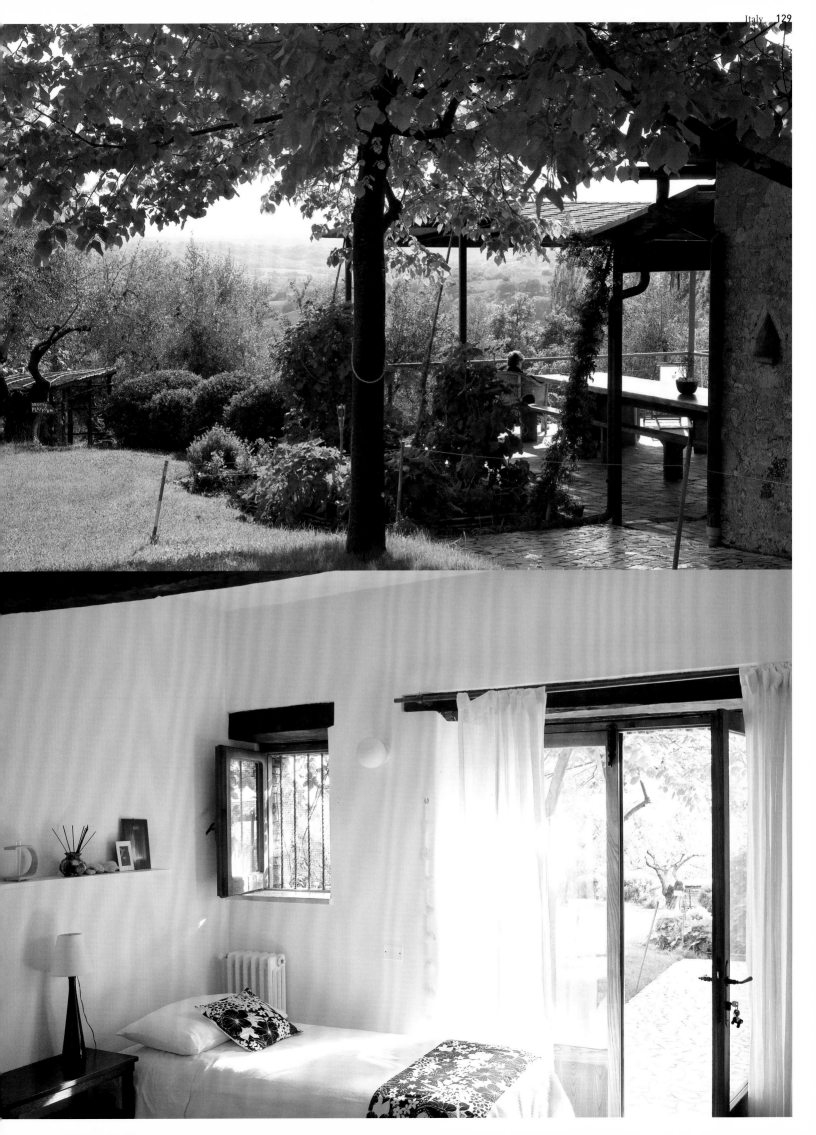

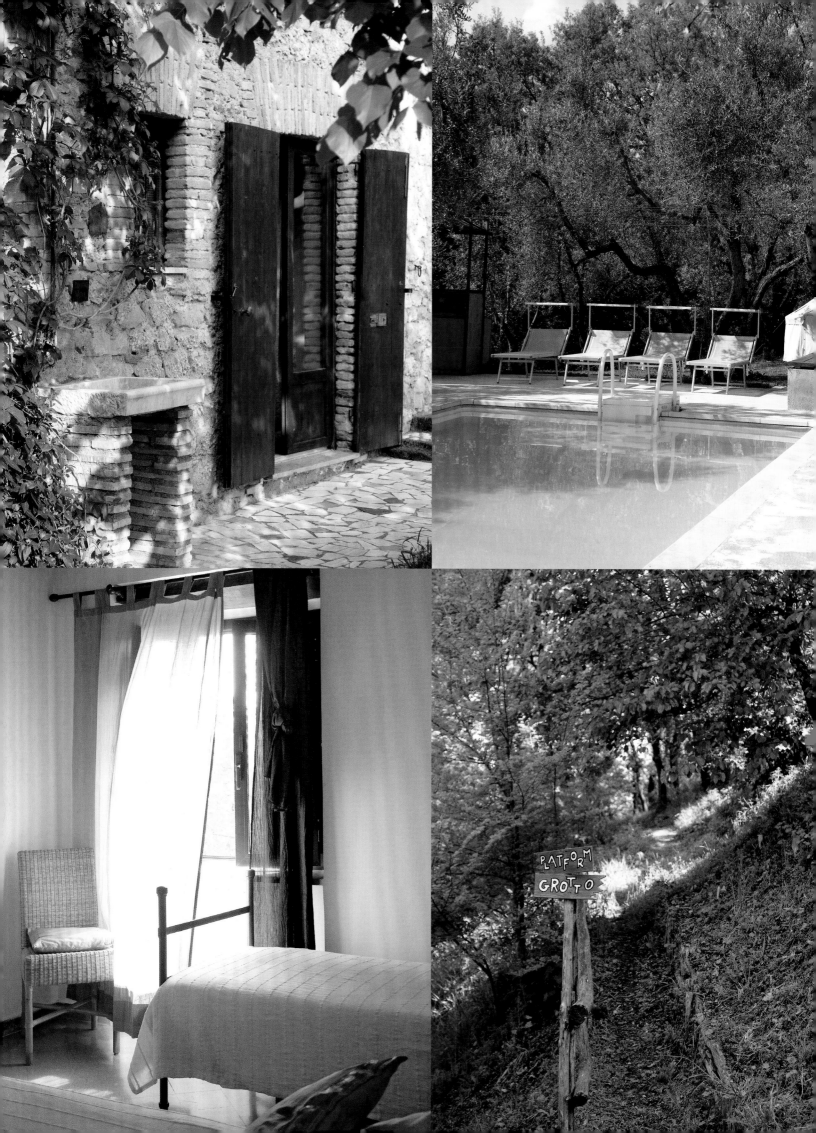

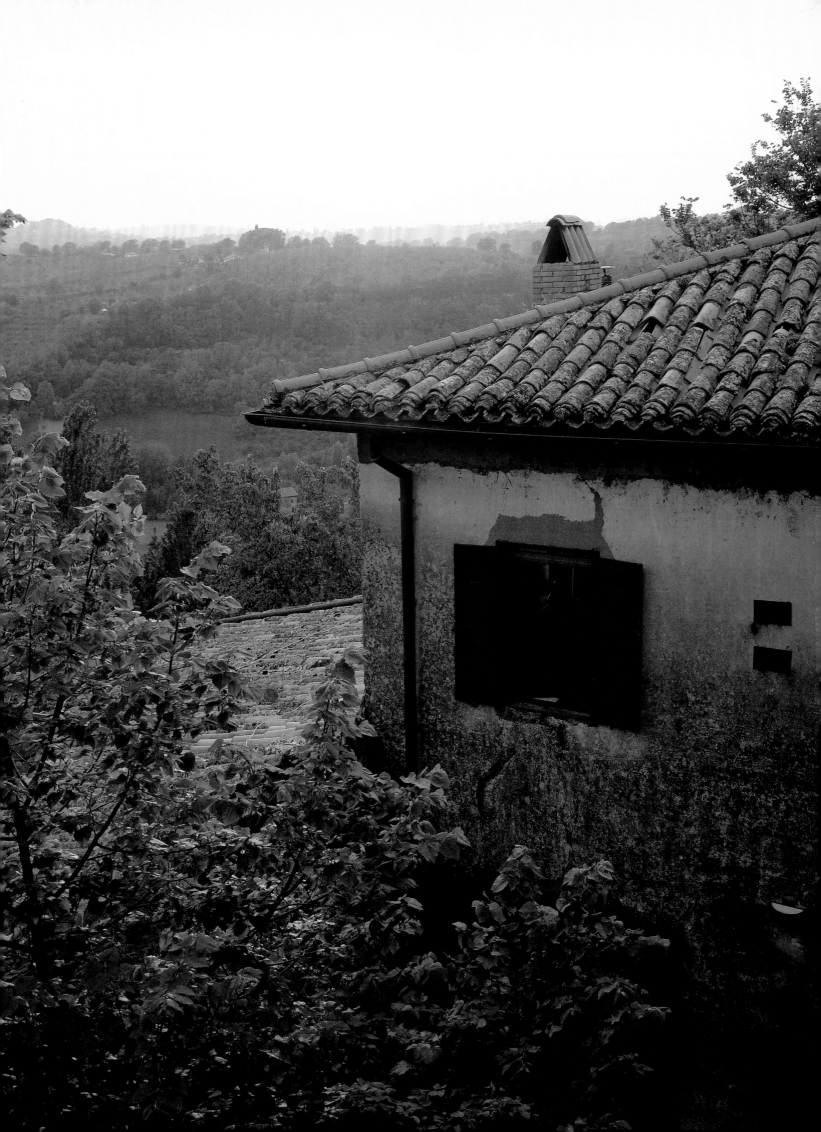

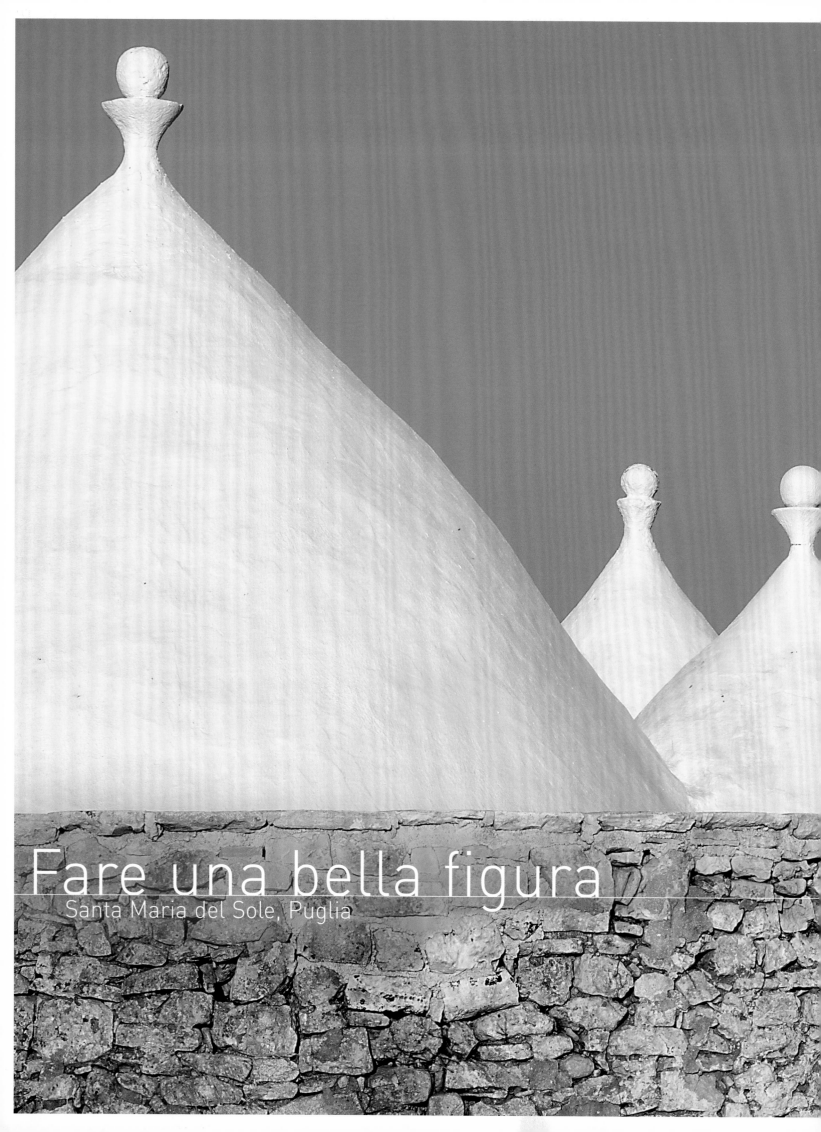

Fare una bella figura
Santa Maria del Sole, Puglia

Santa Maria del Sole, Puglia

Fare una bella figura
Gleaming white like forgotten pieces of laundry, the little houses of the masseria lie on the plain and defy the Apulian sun. Like a fortress of happiness, the small, whitewashed dwellings of the estate, with their conical roofs, pit themselves against the endlessly blue sky. Between the 17th and 19th centuries, farmers lived in these so-called trulli. The walls, up to three feet thick, served as protection from cold and heat and are freshly whitewashed every year as a means of disinfection. Olive trees, grapevines, orange, lemon and almond trees thrive, and dusty blackberry bushes entwine themselves between the low stone walls. The food comes direct from the garden onto the plate and is generously sprinkled with olive oil. Yoga is taught on the hard parquet floor in a fantastically appointed vault, which can also be heated if necessary. Those who are admitted through the stone gate of Santa Maria del Sole today are part of the large hippy community, which – as befits Italy – is splendidly good-looking. Women of all ages with open locks and intelligent smiles offer proof that the earth is female – wouldn't you agree?
Books to pack: "Peace Is Every Step" by Thich Nhat Hanh and "A Walk in the Dark" by Gianrico Carofiglio.

Santa Maria del Sole
Via Monti del Duca 302
Martina Franca, 74014
Italy
Tel. +39 080 449 0224
info@santamariadelsole.it
www.santamariadelsole.it

DIRECTIONS	40 min from Brindisi Airport, 1 hr from Bari Airport; the next railway station is Ostuni.
YOGA	Hatha, Ashtanga, Iyengar, Kirtan.
TEACHERS	Anna Pilotti, Faustomaria Dorelli, Elizabeth Bunker.
ROOMS	2- and 3-bed rooms for max. 25 guests.
FOOD	Macrobiotic, homemade organic pasta, pizza, cheese from the surrounding region.
RECREATION	Swimming, hiking, horseback riding, day trips to the sea.

Fare una bella figura

Gleißend weiß wie vergessene Wäschestücke liegen die Häuschen der Masseria in der Ebene und trotzen der apulischen Sonne. Wie ein Fort der Fröhlichkeit stemmen sich die kleinen, gekalkten Zipfelmützenhäuser des Landguts dem endlos blauen Himmel entgegen. In diesen sogenannten Trulli wohnten zwischen dem 17. und 19. Jahrhundert Bauern. Die bis zu einem Meter dicken Mauern dienten zum Schutz vor Kälte und Hitze und werden jedes Jahr frisch gekalkt als Mittel der Desinfektion. Olivenbäume, Weinreben, Orangen-, Zitronen- und Mandelbäume blühen, staubige Brombeerbüsche ranken zwischen den steinernen Mäuerchen hervor. Das Essen kommt direkt aus dem Garten auf den Teller und wird großzügig mit Olivenöl besprenkelt. Yoga wird auf hartem Parkett in einem fantastisch hergerichteten Gewölbe unterrichtet, das bei Bedarf sogar geheizt werden kann. Wer heute durch das steinerne Tor von Santa Maria del Sole eingelassen wird, ist Teil der großen Hippiegemeinde, die, wie sollte es in Italien anders sein, blendend aussieht. Frauen jeden Alters mit offenem langem Haar und klugem Lächeln beweisen, die Erde ist weiblich – oder etwa nicht?

Buchtipps: »Ich pflanze ein Lächeln« von Thich Nhat Hanh und »In freiem Fall« von Gianrico Carofiglio.

Fare bella figura

D'une blancheur éblouissante, comme des pièces de linge qu'on aurait oubliées, les maisonnettes en pierre à chaux de la Masseria ornent la plaine, bravant le soleil des Pouilles. Telle une citadelle du bonheur, les petites maisons en forme de bonnet de lutin se dressent vers l'azur infini. Entre le 17e et le 19e siècle, des paysans logèrent dans ces « trulli ». Les murs, dont l'épaisseur va jusqu'à un mètre, protégeaient du froid et de la chaleur et sont, chaque année, assainis à la chaux. Oliviers, vignes, orangers, citronniers et amandiers fleurissent, des buissons de mûres grimpent le long des murets en pierre. Les aliments, généreusement aspergés d'huile d'olive, passent directement du jardin à la table. Les cours de yoga ont lieu sur parquet dur dans une salle voûtée magnifiquement restaurée qui peut, au besoin, être chauffée. Quiconque, aujourd'hui, est admis à franchir la porte en pierre de Santa Maria del Sole devient membre de la grande communauté hippie qui, mais comment pourrait-il en être autrement en Italie, est d'une beauté rayonnante. Les femmes, tous âges confondus, aux longs cheveux défaits et au sourire subtil sont bien la preuve vivante que la Terre est une femme, non ?

Livres à emporter : « La paix en marche. La paix en soi » de Thich Nhat Hanh et « Les yeux fermés » de Gianrico Carofiglio.

ANREISE	40 min Fahrt vom Flughafen Brindisi entfernt, 1 Std. vom Flughafen Bari, nächster Bahnhof Ostuni.
YOGA	Hatha, Astanga, Iyengar, Kirtan.
GASTLEHRER	Anna Pilotti, Faustomaria Dorelli, Elizabeth Bunker.
ZIMMER	2–3-Bettzimmer für max. 25 Gäste.
KÜCHE	Makrobiotisch, hausgemachte biologische Pasta, Pizza, Käse aus der Umgebung.
FREIZEIT	Schwimmen, Wandern, Reiten, Ausflüge ans Meer.

ACCÈS	Situé à 40 min de l'aéroport de Brindisi, à 1 h de l'aéroport de Bari, gare la plus proche : Ostuni.
YOGA	Hatha, Ashtânga, Iyengar, Kirtan.
PROFESSEURS	Anna Pilotti, Faustomaria Dorelli, Elizabeth Bunker.
CHAMBRES	Chambres à deux et trois lits pour 25 personnes max.
RESTAURATION	Cuisine macrobiotique, pâtes bio maison, pizza, fromages de la région.
ACTIVITÉS	Natation, randonnées, équitation, promenades en mer.

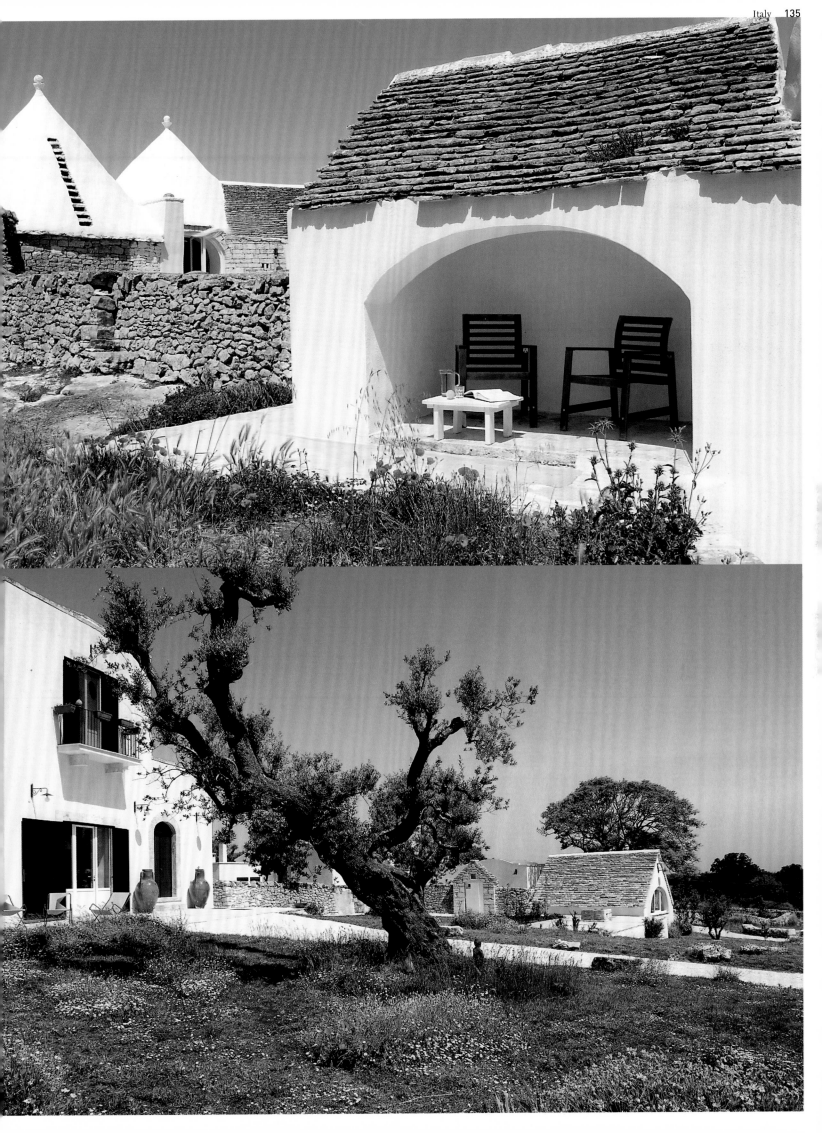

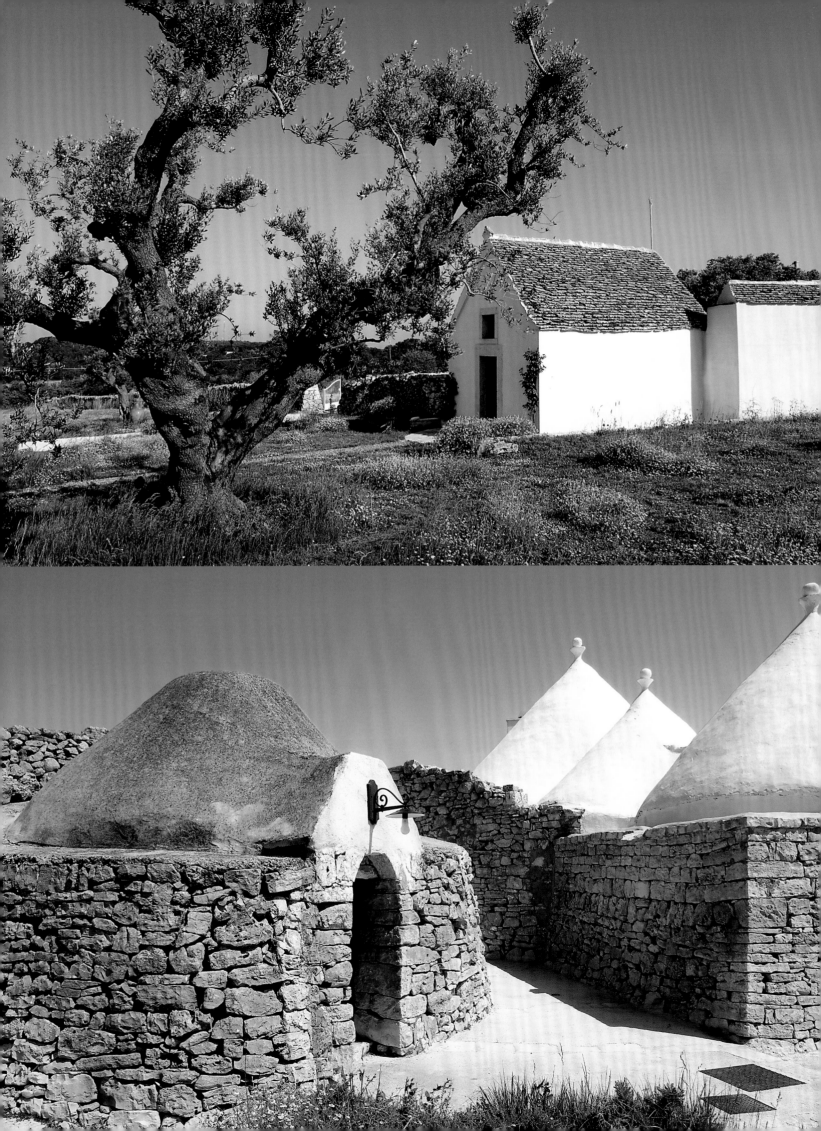

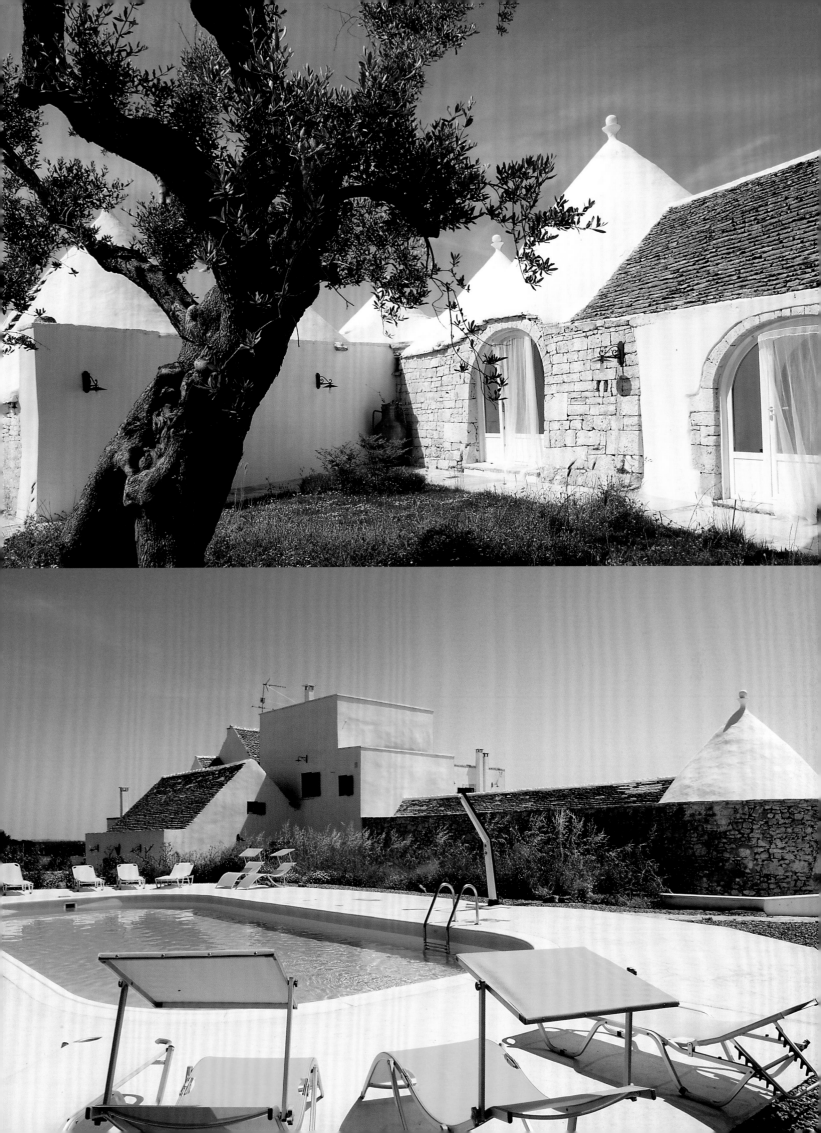

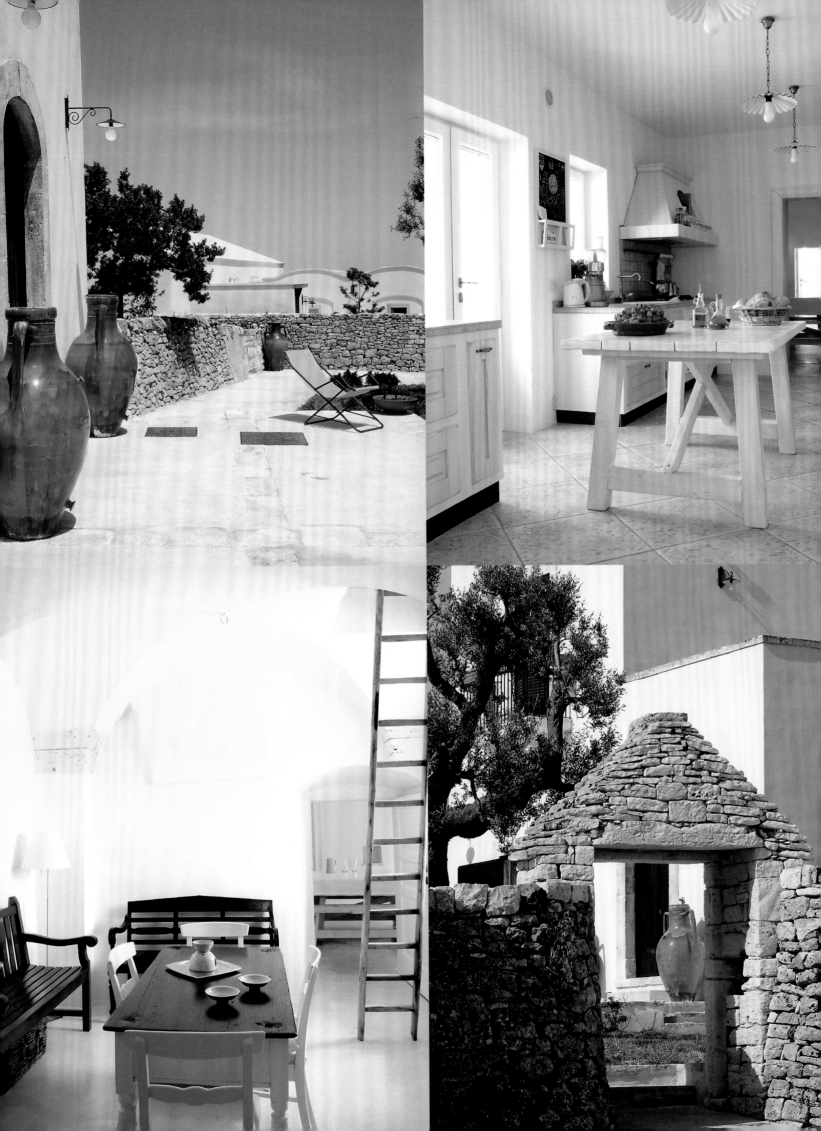

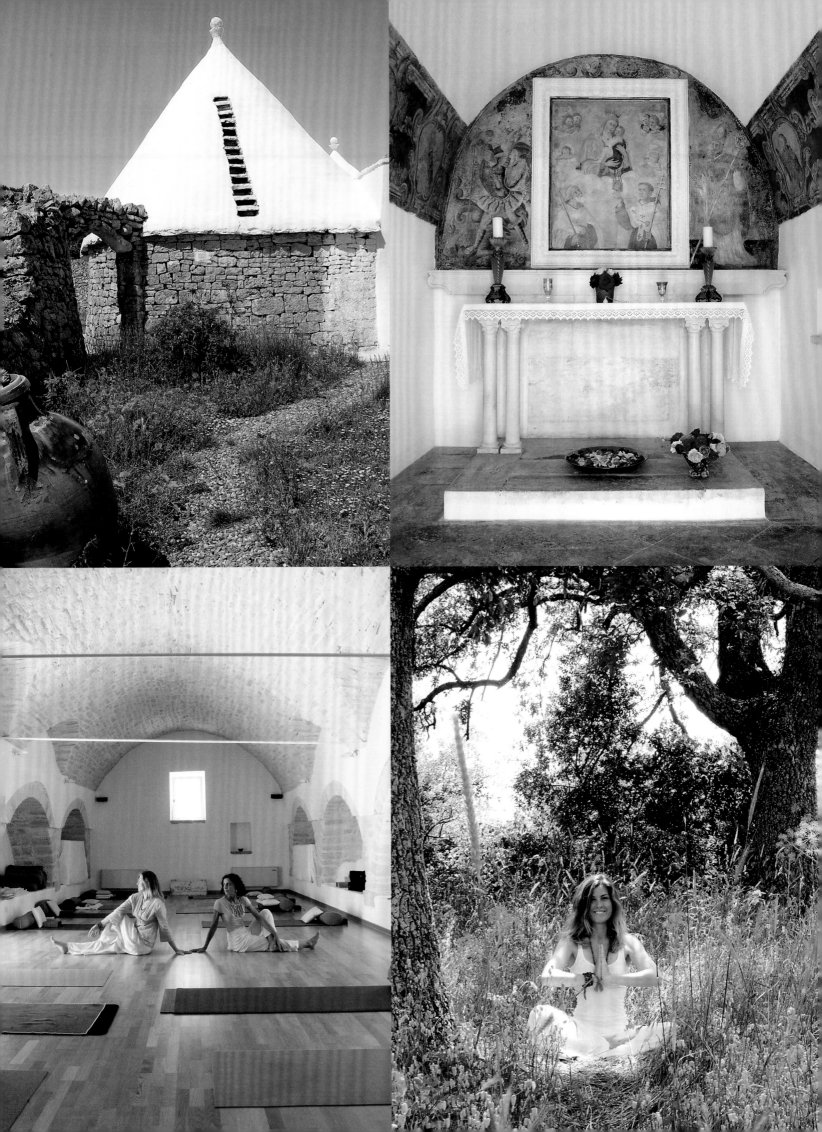

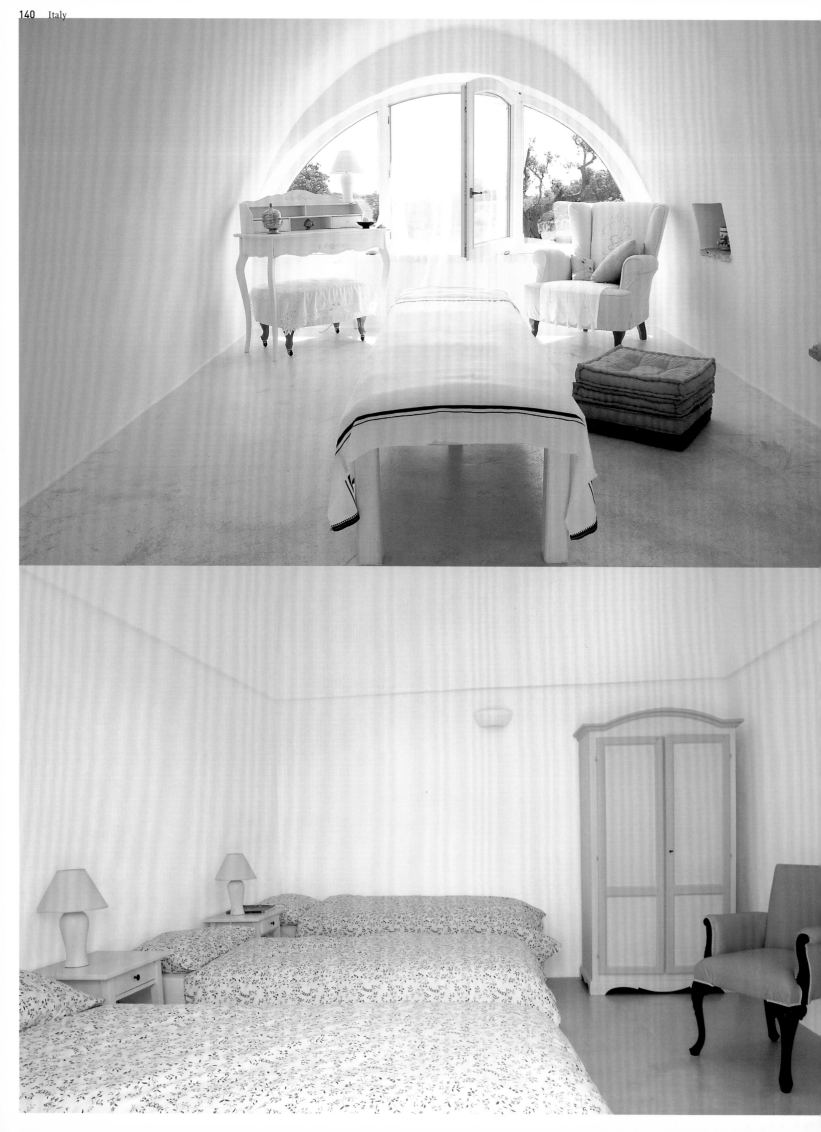

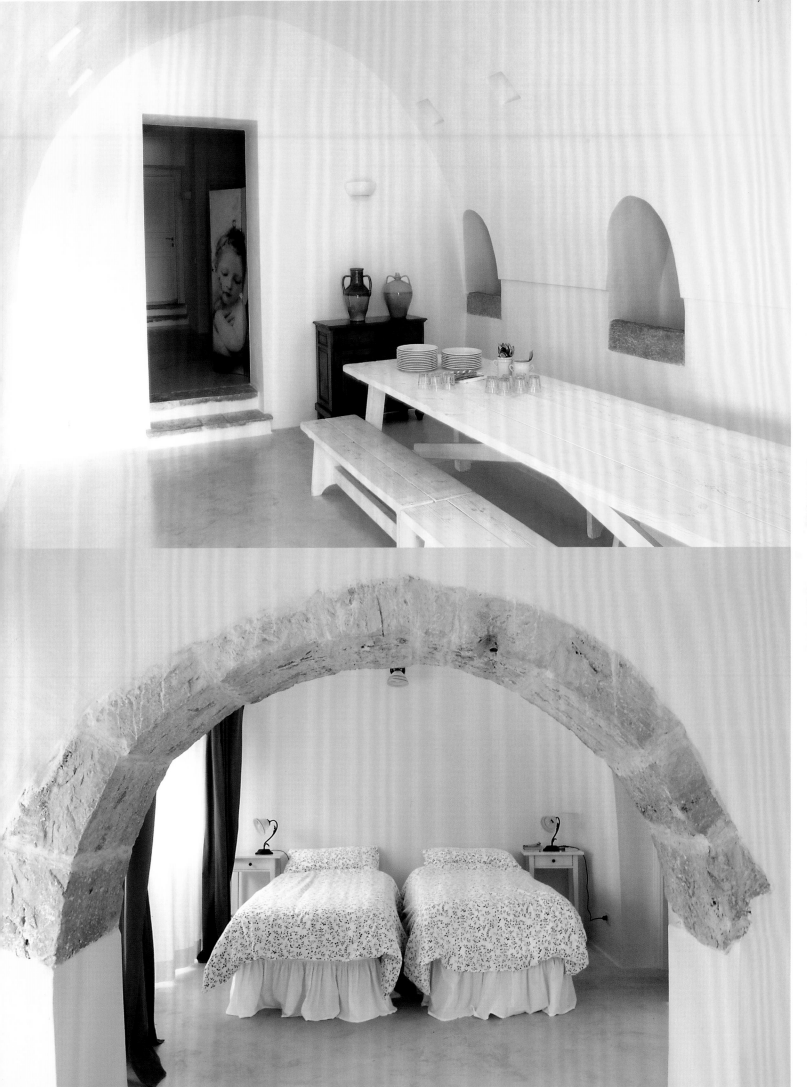

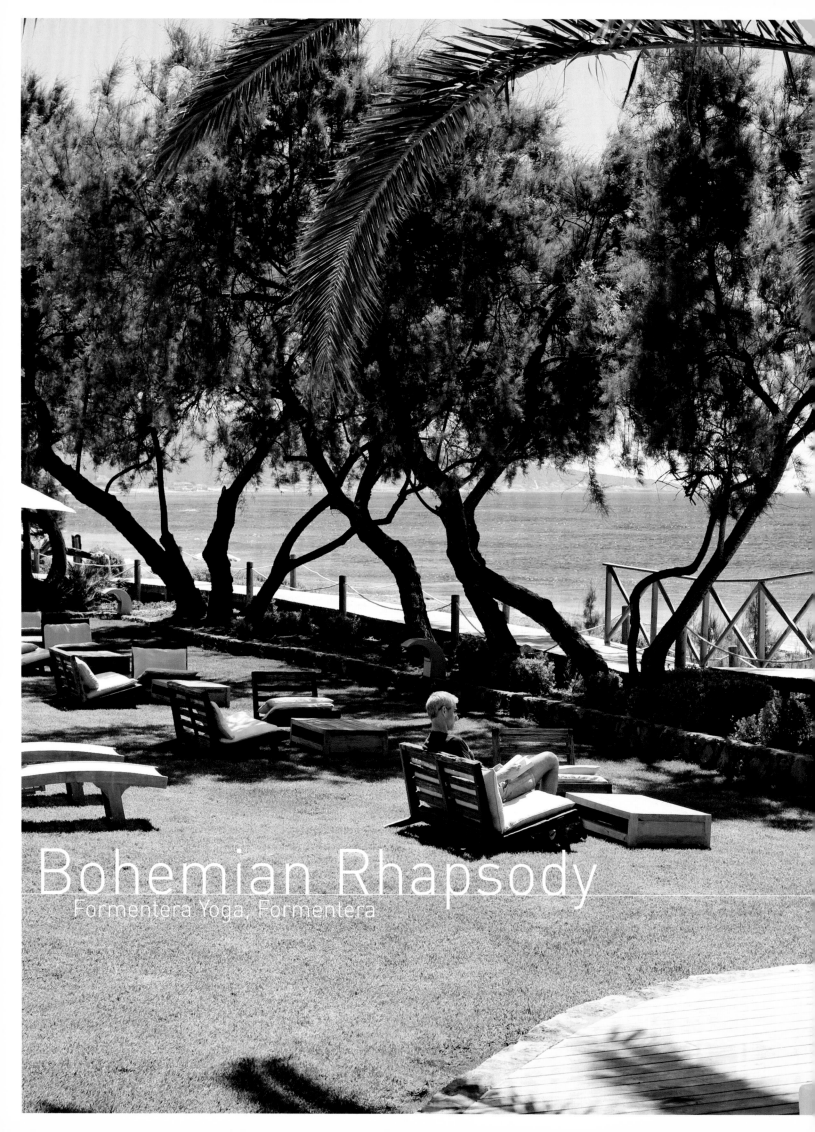

Bohemian Rhapsody
Formentera Yoga, Formentera

Formentera Yoga, Formentera

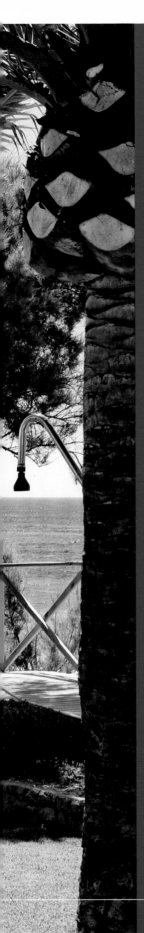

Bohemian Rhapsody

For all our appreciation of elaborate design sometimes we simply want to walk along an unmade track to the beach, stay in an inconspicuous deluxe barrack and practise Yoga to loud disco music – put on by Sundara from New York, one of the self-styled Yoga teachers, to hot things up for her students, who have travelled from London. Ibiza is within spitting distance and yet far enough away not to interfere with its little sister Formentera. Tiny, enchanted fishing coves, unspoilt hinterland, transparent, turquoise water and endless beaches onto which at most an old shoe is washed up from the mainland: even if word has long got around that Kate and Co. secretly relax here after the hustle and bustle of the party, the Balearic island, which is on UNESCO's World Cultural Heritage list, is still a little Mediterranean treasure. The Romans knew that, and so did Bob Dylan; the Bohemians know it, too, when after two hours of hefty Asana practice they wander over to the Blue Bar at the Playa Migjorn, where every evening cool DJs from Scotland spin discs as the sun goes down.

Books to pack: "It's Here Now (Are You?)" by Bhagavan Das and "Speaking with the Angel" by Nick Hornby (ed.).

Formentera Yoga	
Platja de Migjorn	
Formentera, The Balearics	
Spain	
Tel. +34 606 117 373 and +44 7956 854 922	
info@formenterayoga.com	
www.formenterayoga.com	

DIRECTIONS	Located 11 miles south of the island of Ibiza. Go by boat from Ibiza Old Town Port to La Savina Port Formentera; continue from there by taxi.
YOGA	Restorative, Vinyasa, Yin Yoga, Ashtanga, Jivamukti.
TEACHERS	Jax Lysycia, Bryan Kest, Liz Lark, Jean Hall, Sundara.
ROOMS	10 double rooms, 5 3-bed rooms, 7 twin rooms for max. 40 people.
FOOD	Vegetarian, Ayurvedic cuisine possible.
TREATMENTS	Facials, pedicure, massage.
RECREATION	Sailing, water-skiing, cookery courses, volleyball, cycling, swimming.

Bohemian Rhapsody

Bei aller Liebe zu ausgetüfteltem Design, manchmal ist einem einfach danach, auf einem ungeteerten Feldweg zum Strand zu laufen, in einer unaufdringlichen Luxusbaracke unterzukommen und bei lauter Discomusik Yoga zu üben. Die legt Sundara aus New York auf, eine der selbsternannten Yogalehrerinnen, die ihren aus London angereisten Schülern einheizt. Ibiza ist in Spuckweite und doch weit genug entfernt, um der kleinen Schwester Formentera nicht dazwischenzureden. Verträumte, winzige Fischerbuchten, unberührtes Hinterland, durchsichtiges, türkisfarbenes Wasser, endlose Strände, an die höchstens mal ein alter Schuh vom Festland angeschwemmt wird: Auch wenn sich längst herumgesprochen hat, dass Kate und Co. hier heimlich vom Partyrummel entspannen, ist die balearische Insel, von der UNESCO zum Weltkulturerbe erklärt, noch immer ein kleiner Schatz im Mittelmeer. Das wussten die Römer, das wusste Bob Dylan, das weiß die Bohème, wenn sie nach zwei Stunden saftiger Asana-Übung zur Blue Bar an der Playa Migjorn schlendert, wo jeden Abend coole DJs aus Schottland zum Sonnenuntergang auflegen.
Buchtipps: »It's Here Now (Are You?)« von Bhagavan Das und »Speaking with the Angel« von Nick Hornby (Hrsg.)

Rhapsodie bohémienne

Sans renier le goût du design raffiné, la simple envie vous prend parfois de marcher sur un chemin de campagne non goudronné menant à la plage, de loger dans une baraque luxueuse et de faire du yoga dans le tapage d'une musique disco. C'est cette musique que choisit Sundara de New York, l'une des professeurs de yoga autoproclamées, pour stimuler ses élèves venus tout droit de Londres. Ibiza est à deux pas et pourtant assez éloignée pour ne pas couvrir la voix de Formentera, la petite sœur. De minuscules criques de pêche romantiques, un arrière-pays encore intact, une eau transparente couleur turquoise, des plages à perte de vue où vient seulement, de temps à autre, échouer du continent une vieille chaussure : même si, depuis longtemps, ce n'est plus un secret que Kate et compagnie viennent ici incognito se reposer du tourbillon des fêtes, cette île des Baléares, inscrite au patrimoine mondial de l'UNESCO, demeure un petit joyau de la Méditerranée. Les Romains le savaient, de même que Bob Dylan, de même que les bohèmes de passage qui, après deux heures d'Âsana, flânent en direction du Blue Bar de la Playa Migjorn où, chaque soir, des DJ écossais branchés passent leurs disques face au coucher du soleil.
Livres à emporter : « It's Here Now (Are You?) » de Bhagavan Das et « Conversation avec l'ange » de Nick Hornby (éditeur).

ANREISE	18 km südlich von der Insel Ibiza gelegen. Mit dem Boot von Ibiza Old Town Port zum La Savina Port von Formentera und von dort aus weiter mit dem Taxi.
YOGA	Restorative, Vinyasa, Yin Yoga, Astanga, Jivamukti.
GASTLEHRER	Jax Lysycia, Bryan Kest, Liz Lark, Jean Hall, Sundara.
ZIMMER	10 Doppelzimmer, 5 Dreibettzimmer, 7 Twins für max. 40 Personen.
KÜCHE	Vegetarisch, ayurvedische Küche möglich.
ANWENDUNGEN	Facials, Pediküre, Massage.
FREIZEIT	Segeln, Wasserski, Kochkurse, Volleyball, Radfahren, Schwimmen.

ACCÈS	Situé à 18 km de l'île d'Ibiza. Accessible en bateau d'Ibiza Old Town Port à La Savina Port Formentera et, de là, transfert par taxi.
YOGA	Restoratif, Vinyasa, Yin Yoga, Ashtânga, Jivamukti.
PROFESSEURS	Jax Lysycia, Bryan Kest, Liz Lark, Jean Hall, Sundara.
CHAMBRES	10 chambres doubles, 5 chambres à 3 lits, 7 Twins pour 40 personnes max.
RESTAURATION	Cuisine végétarienne ayurvédique possible.
TRAITEMENTS	Soins du visage, pédicurie, massages.
ACTIVITÉS	Voile, ski nautique, volley-ball, cyclisme, natation.

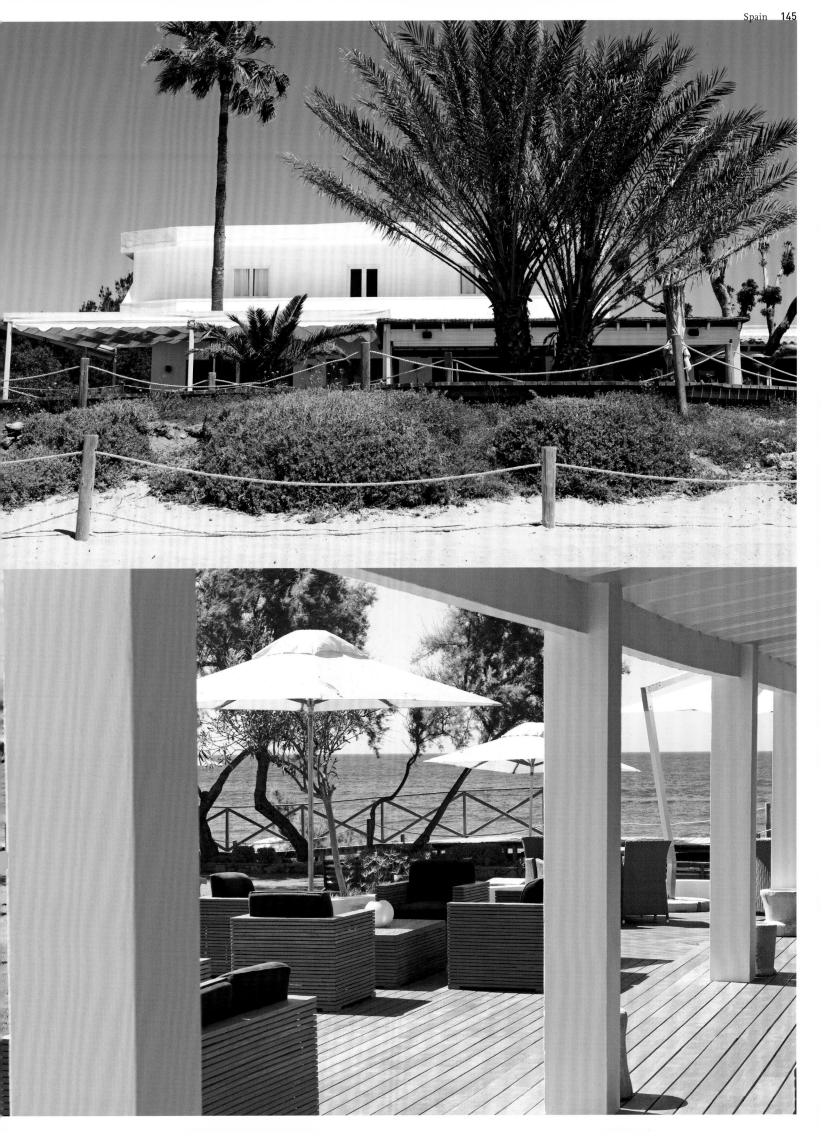

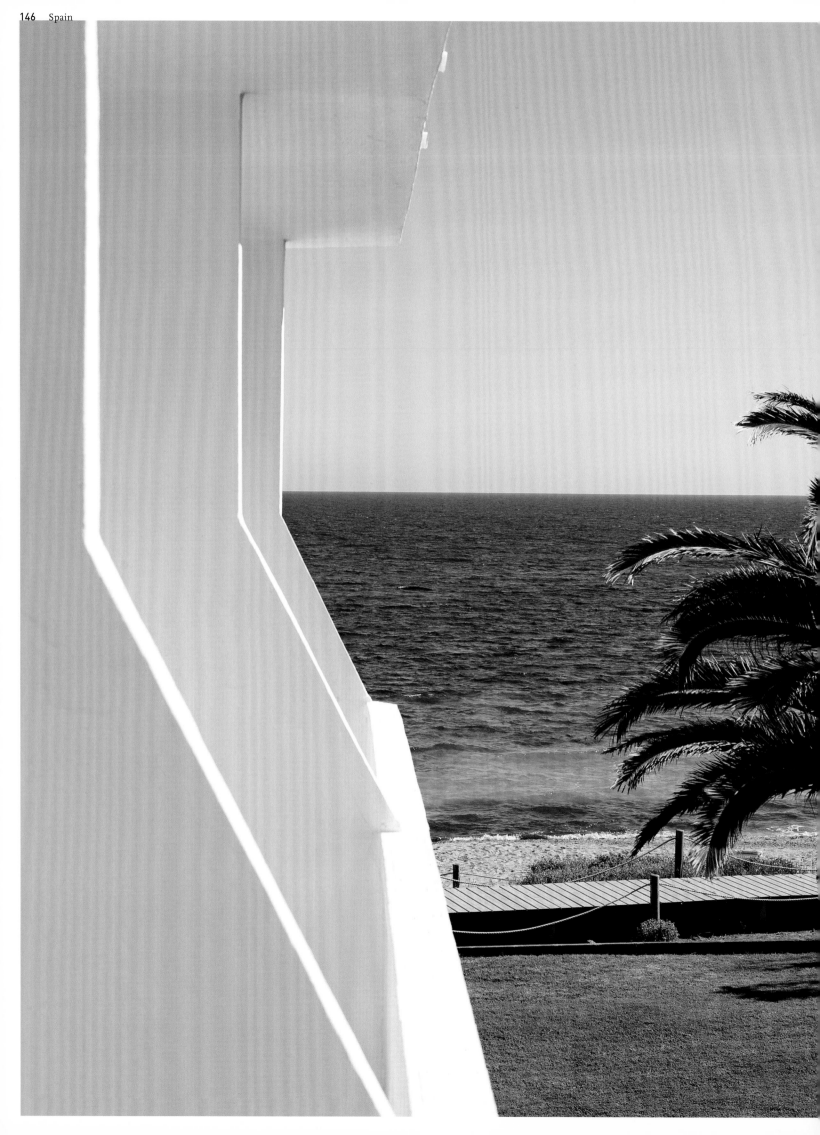

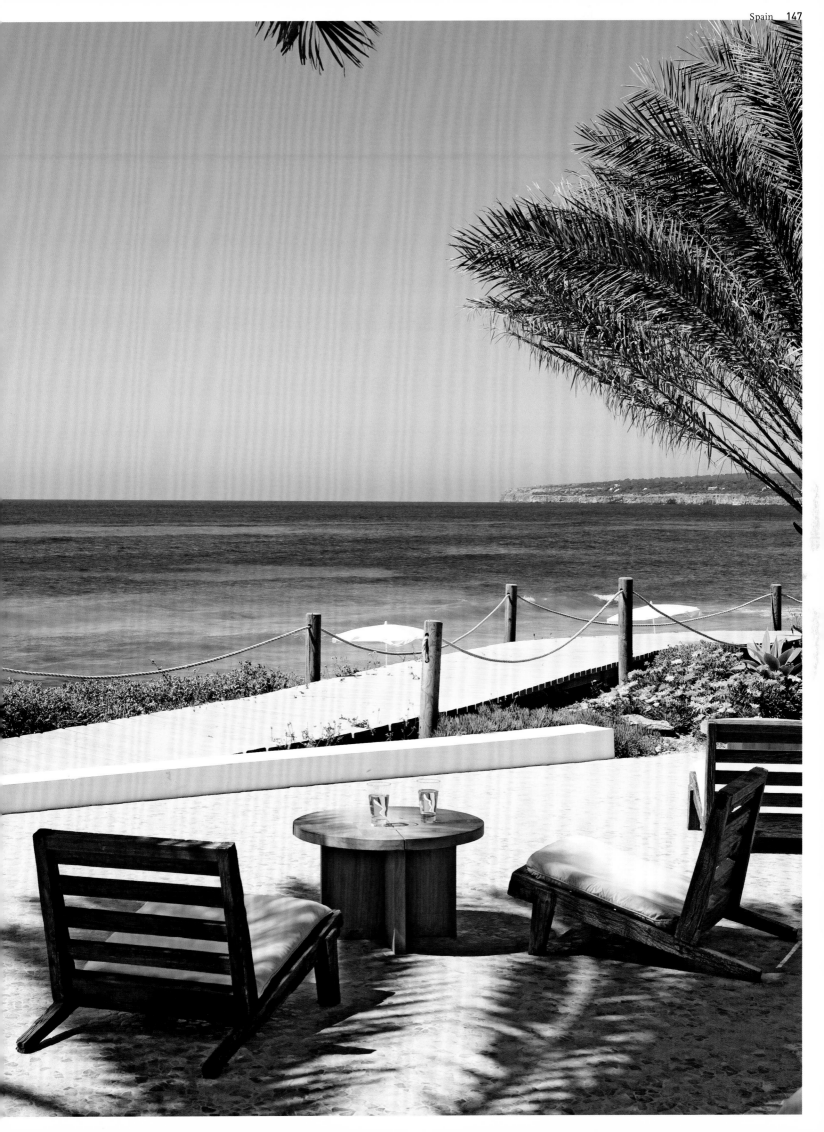

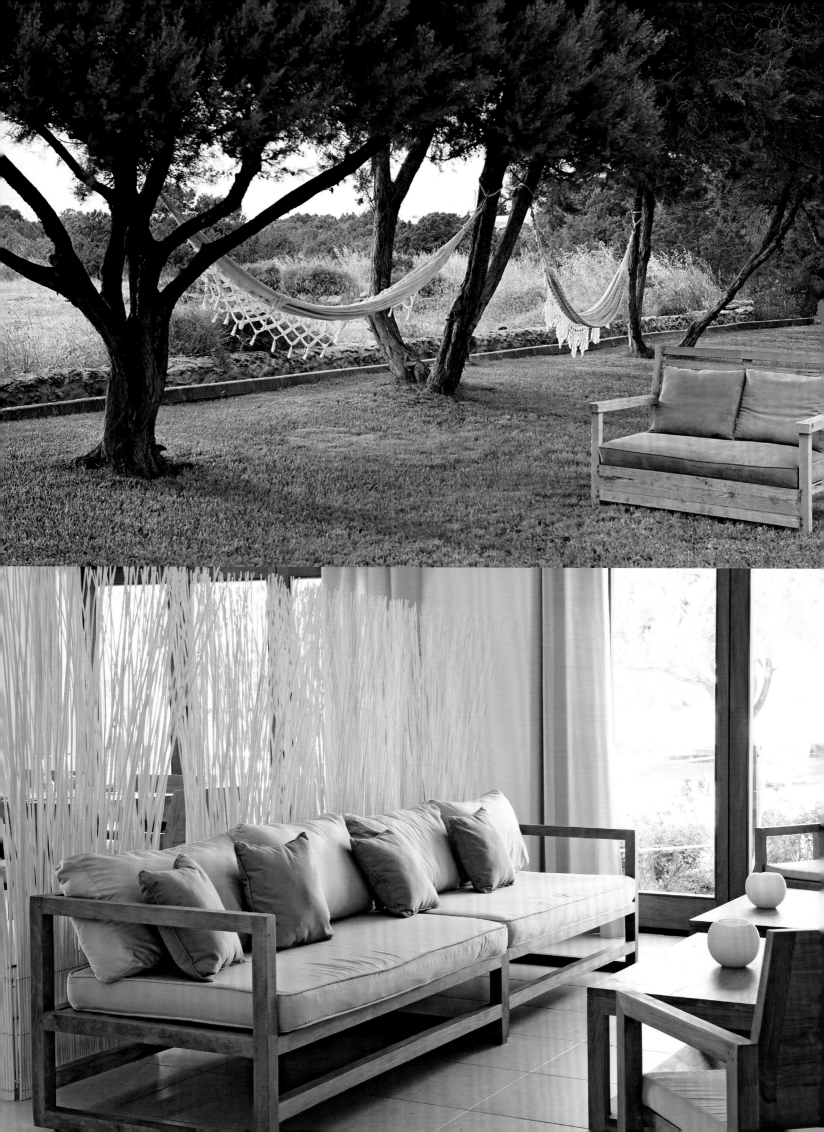

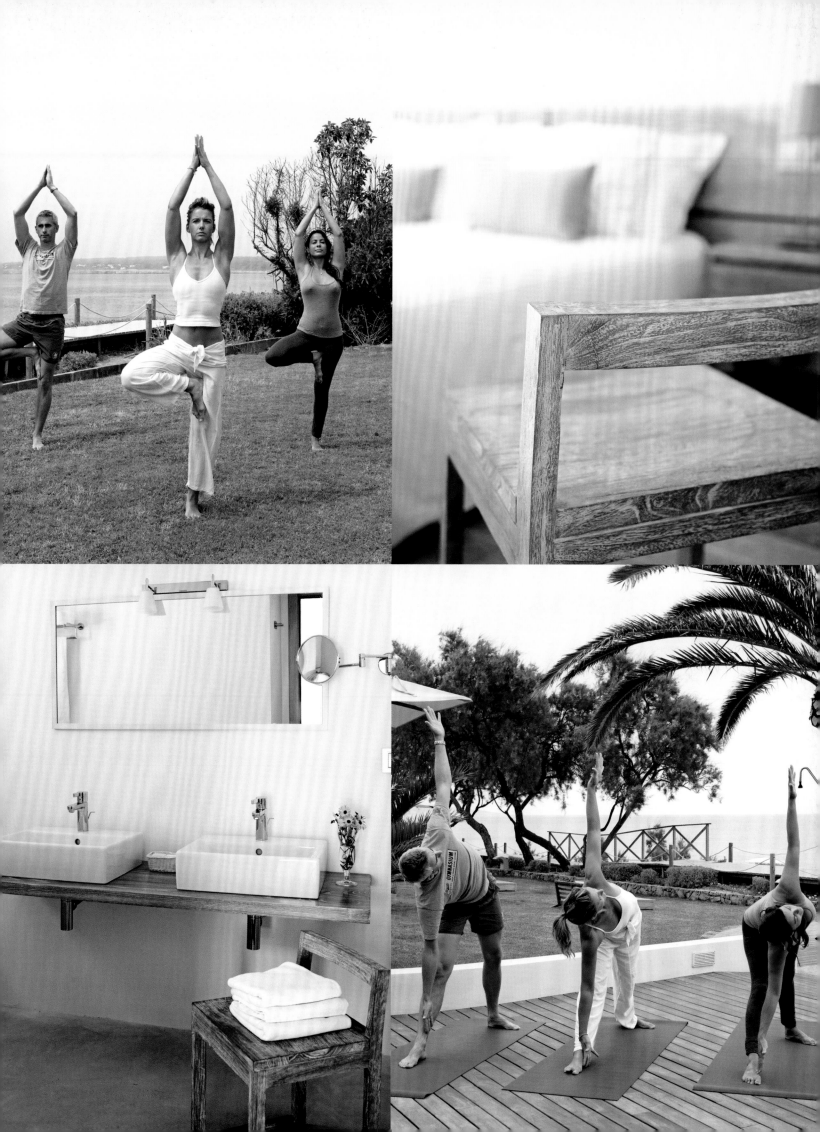

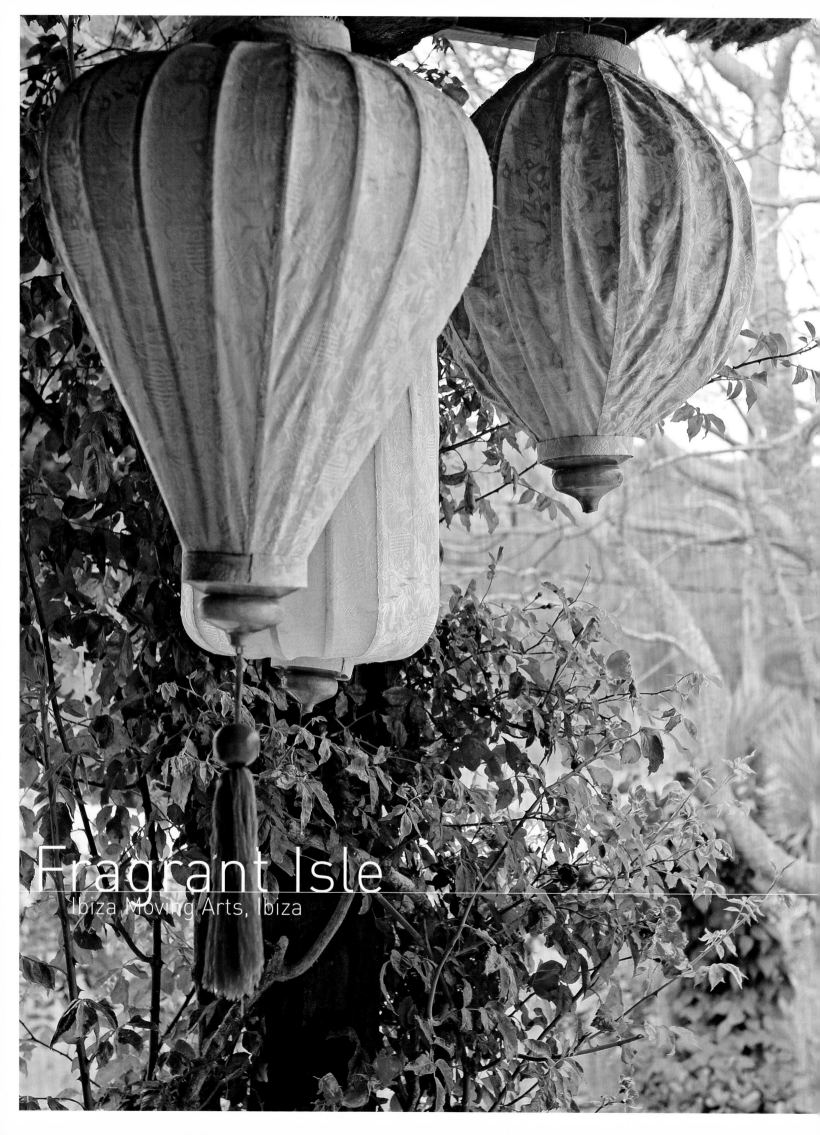

Fragrant Isle
Ibiza Moving Arts, Ibiza

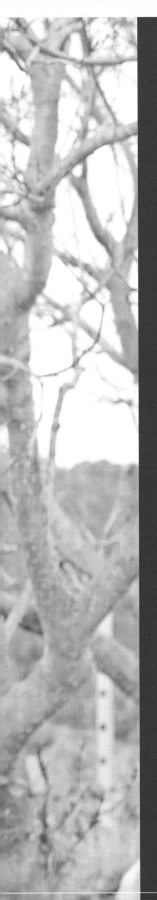

Ibiza Moving Arts, Ibiza

Fragrant Isle

In the quiet north of the island, far from the English tourists who come to dance, stands a 400-year-old Ibizan finca, bedded in between orange and apricot groves. Nothing here is reminiscent of the hyped-up nervousness that Ibiza owes to its unique reputation as a party island. Ancient olive trees, brought here by the Phoenicians, entwine the white walls, along with mint and jasmine. The name Ibiza comes from the Phoenician god Bes, responsible for fertility, dance and music. Another derivation translates the original meaning as "island of perfumes". An intensive Hatha Yoga session, some craniosacral therapy and a long stroll across the neighbouring fields while the almond trees are in bloom lifts the spirits so far that the evening's programme of dance and music reveals its own unstoppable charm, and may even persuade you to set foot on the dance floor in one of the legendary clubs at the end of the holiday after all. A leap into the delightful pool the next morning, and your spiritual peace is restored.

Books to pack: "The Yoga-Sûtra of Patañjali" by Georg Feuerstein and "On Love and Death" by Patrick Süskind.

Ibiza Moving Arts	
P.O. Box 144	
07815 San Miguel, San Juan, Ibiza	
Spain	
Tel. +34 971 324 275 and +34 637 269 884	
info@ibizamovingarts.com	
www.ibizamovingarts.com	

DIRECTIONS	15 1/2 miles from Ibiza Airport in the north of the island.
YOGA	Hatha, Vinyasa Flow, meditation.
TEACHERS	Sarah Cullen, Mark Ansari, Marte Kamzelas, Lara Baumann.
ROOMS	7 rooms for up to 15 people.
FOOD	Mediterranean organic vegetarian cuisine.
TREATMENTS	Massage, craniosacral therapy, foot reflexology massage, rebalancing massage, somato emotional release.
RECREATION	Swimming, hiking, sailing, diving, horseback riding, cycling, free climbing.

Insel des Wohlgeruchs

Im ruhigen Norden der Insel, weit weg von den englischen Touristen, die zum Tanzen kommen, liegt eingewachsen zwischen Orangen- und Aprikosenhainen eine 400 Jahre alte ibizenkische Finca. Nichts erinnert hier an die überdrehte Nervosität, der Ibiza seinen einzigartigen Ruf als Partyinsel verdankt. Uralte Olivenbäume, von den Phöniziern hergebracht, Minze und Jasmin umranken das weiße Gemäuer. Der Name Ibiza verdankt sich dem phönizischen Gott Bes, verantwortlich für Fruchtbarkeit, Tanz und Musik. Eine andere Ableitung übersetzt die ursprüngliche Bedeutung als »Insel des Wohlgeruchs«. Während der Mandelblüte eine intensive Hatha-Yogastunde, eine Cranio-Sacral-Therapie und einen langen Spaziergang über die angrenzenden Felder zu machen, hebt die Stimmung so weit, dass die abendlichen Tanz- und Musikprogramme ihren eigenen ungebremsten Charme entfalten können und einen vielleicht sogar so weit bringen, am Ende der Ferien doch noch die Tanzfläche einer der legendären Clubs zu betreten. Ein Sprung in den entzückenden Pool am nächsten Morgen – und die Stille im Geist ist wiederhergestellt.

Buchtipps: »Patañjali: Das Yogasutra« von R. Sriram und »Über Liebe und Tod« von Patrick Süskind.

L'île aux fragrances

Au nord de l'île, au calme, bien loin des touristes anglais qui viennent pour danser, entre les bosquets d'orangers et d'abricotiers se trouve enracinée depuis 400 ans une finca ibizienne. Ici, rien ne rappelle l'extrême fébrilité à laquelle Ibiza doit sa réputation exclusive d'île fêtarde. Les oliviers ancestraux, importés autrefois par les Phéniciens la menthe et le jasmin recouvrent les murailles blanches. Le nom Ibiza remonte au dieu phénicien Bès, divinité de la fécondité, de la danse et de la musique. Une autre dérivation traduit le sens originel comme « île aux fragrances ». Au moment de la floraison de l'amandier, une heure intensive de Hatha-yoga, une thérapie cranio-sacrale et une longue promenade à travers les champs avoisinants vous mettent de si bonne humeur que les programmes de danse et de musique du soir peuvent déployer leur charme sans retenue et vous amener peut-être même, à la fin des vacances, à risquer quelques pas sur la piste de danse d'un des clubs légendaires. Le lendemain, un plongeon dans la merveilleuse piscine et la paix de l'esprit est revenue.

Livres à emporter : « Yoga-Sutras de Patanjali » de Françoise Mazet et « Sur l'amour et la mort » de Patrick Süskind.

ANREISE	25 km vom Ibiza-Flughafen entfernt, im Norden der Insel gelegen.
YOGA	Hatha, Vinyasa Flow, Meditation.
GASTLEHRER	Sarah Cullen, Mark Ansari, Marte Kamzelas, Lara Baumann.
ZIMMER	7 Zimmer für bis zu 15 Personen.
KÜCHE	Mediterrane biologisch-vegetarische Küche.
ANWENDUNGEN	Massage, Cranio-Sacral-Therapie, Fussreflexzonen-Massage Rebalancing-Massage, Somato Emotional Release.
FREIZEIT	Schwimmen, Wandern, Segeln, Tauchen, Reiten, Radfahren, Freeclimbing.

ACCÈS	Situé au nord de l'île, à 25 km de l'aéroport d'Ibiza.
YOGA	Hatha, Vinyasa Flow, méditation.
PROFESSEURS	Sarah Cullen, Mark Ansari, Marte Kamzelas, Lara Baumann.
CHAMBRES	7 chambres pouvant accueillir jusqu'à 15 personnes.
RESTAURATION	Cuisine méditerranéenne, bio-végétarienne.
TRAITEMENTS	Massage, thérapie cranio-sacrale, massage réflexe du pied, massage rééquilibrant, Somato Emotional Release.
ACTIVITÉS	Natation, randonnées, voile, plongée, équitation, bicyclette, escalade.

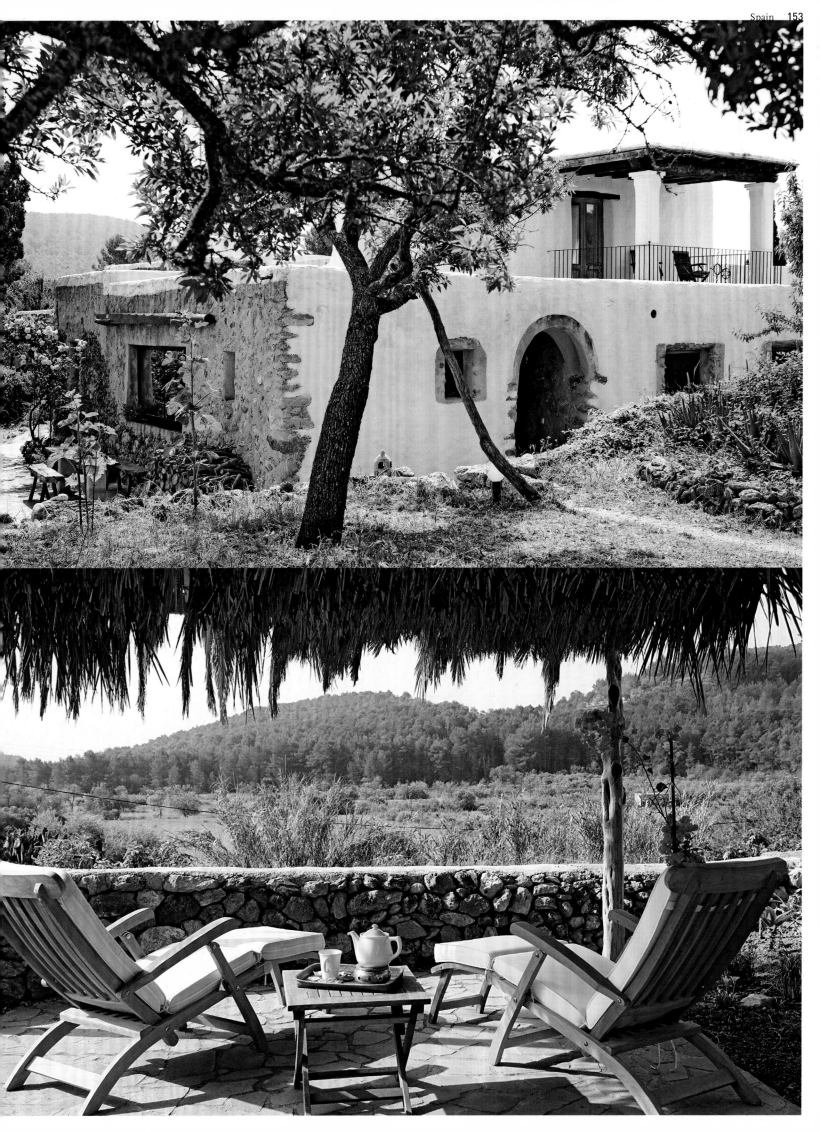

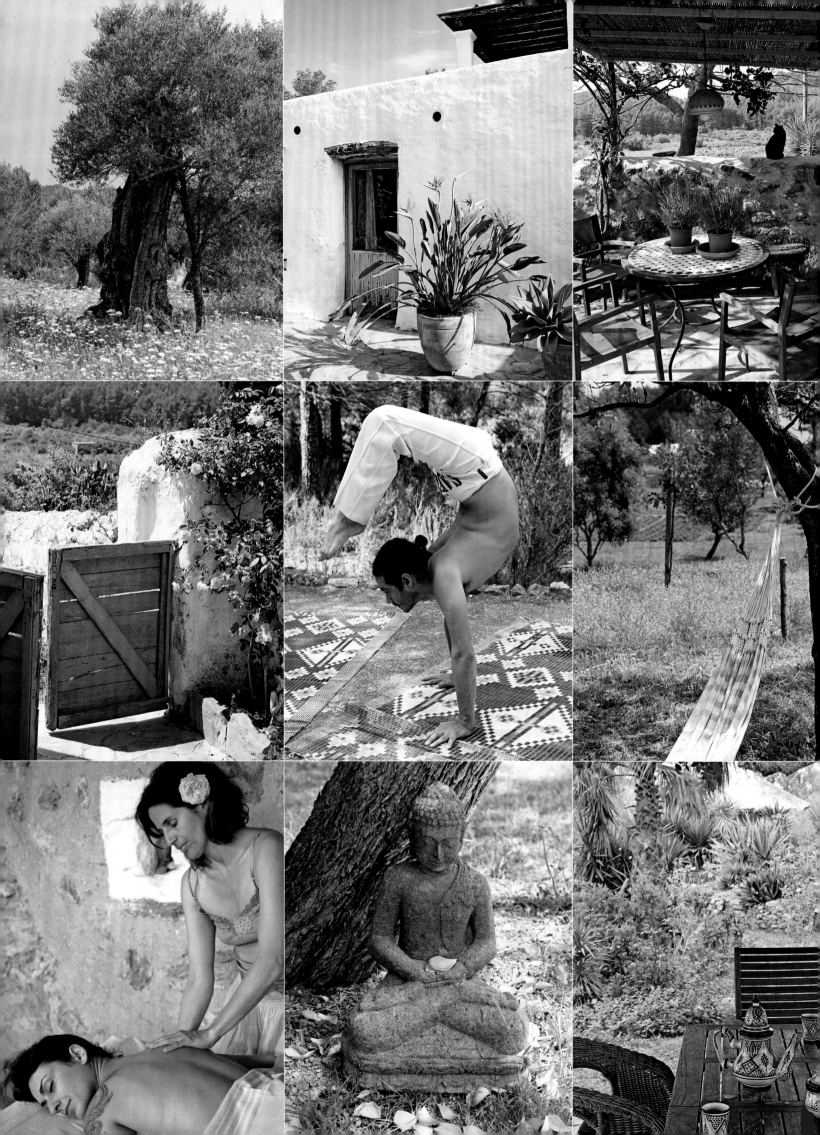

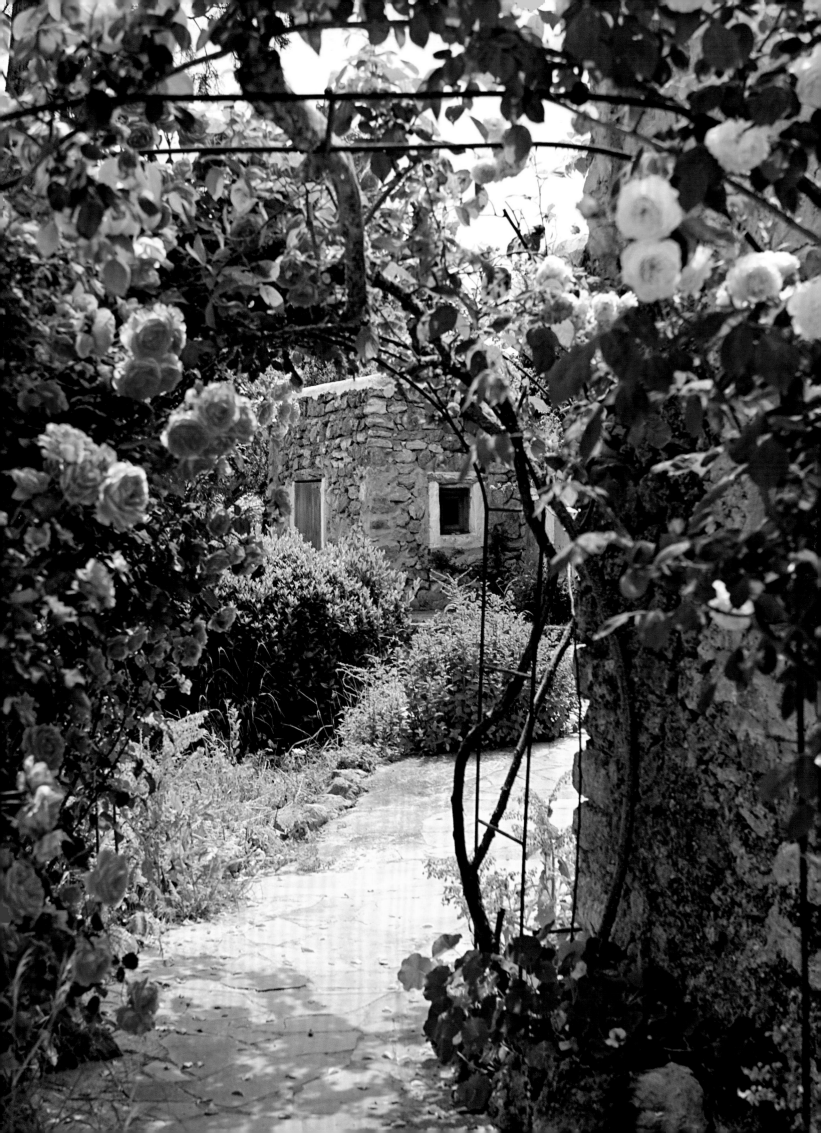

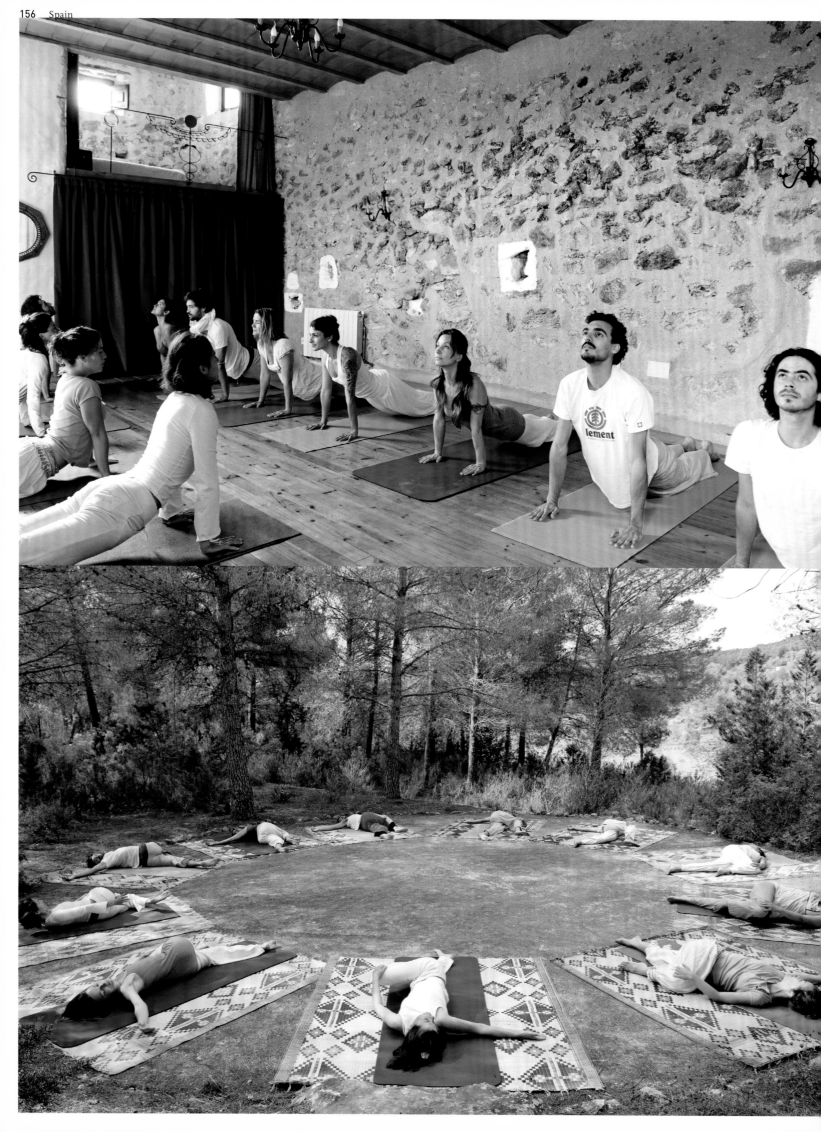

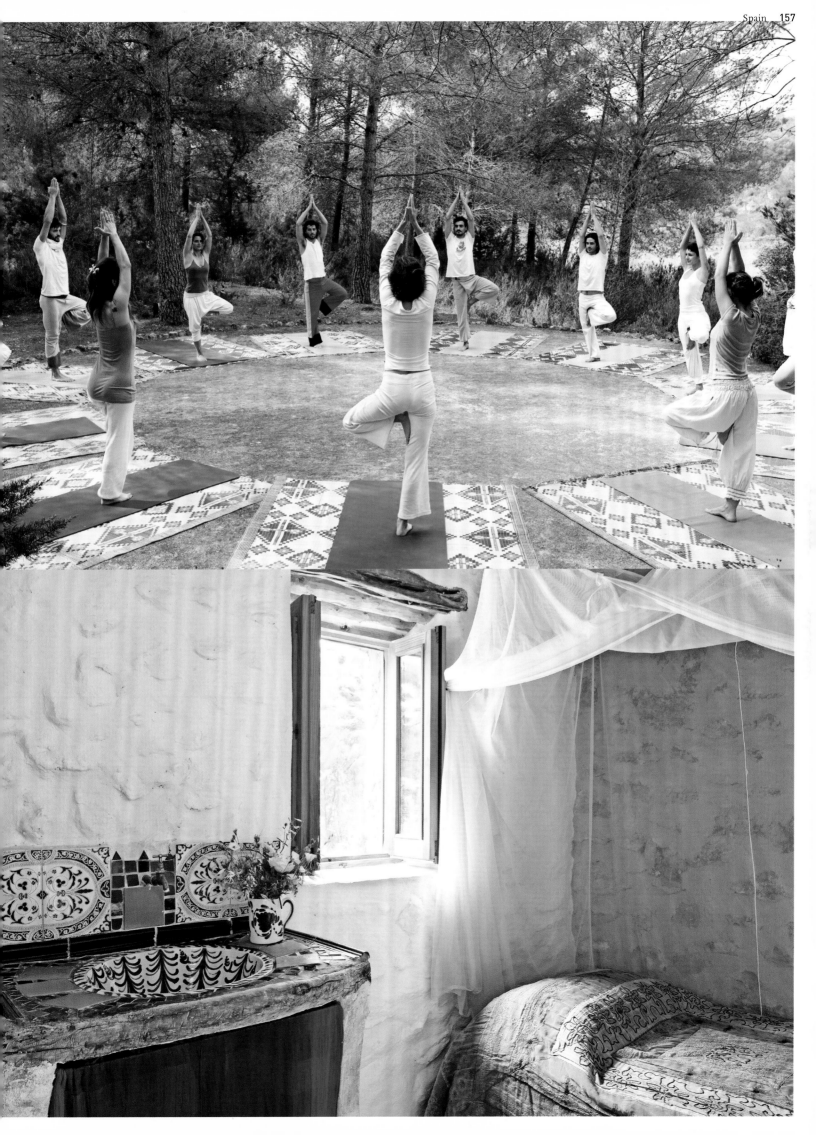

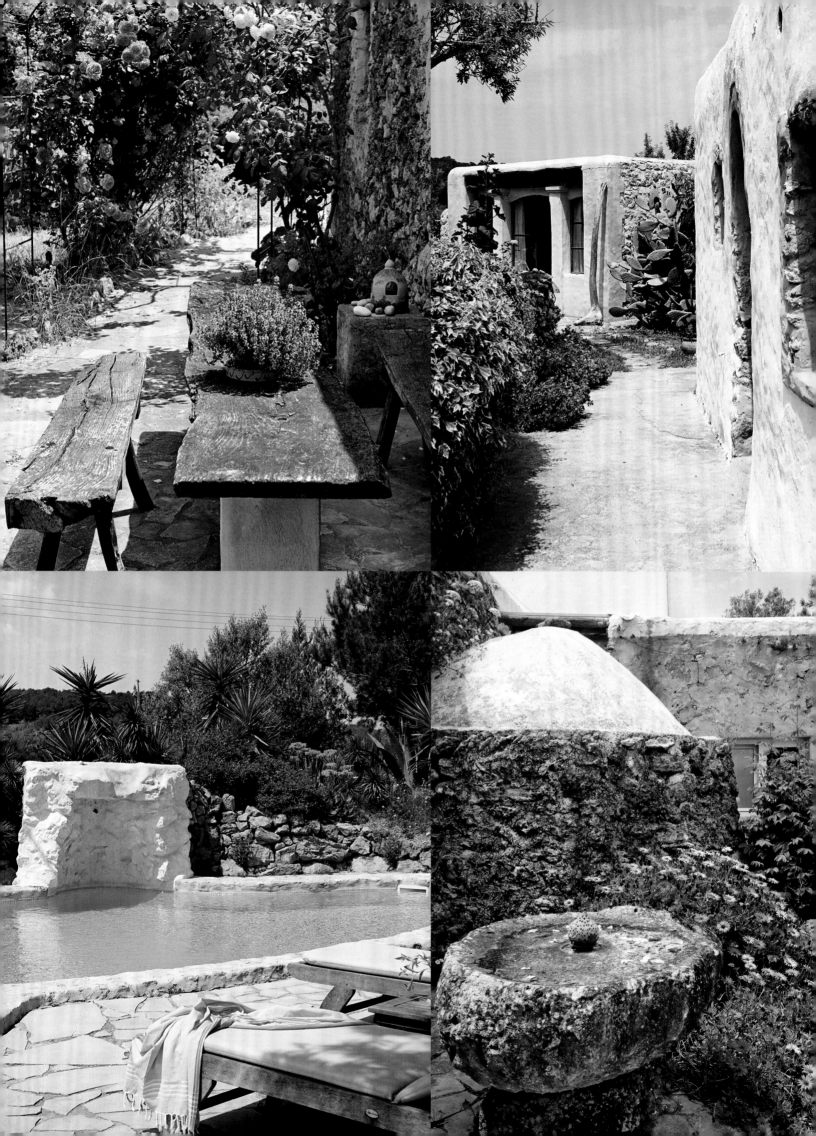

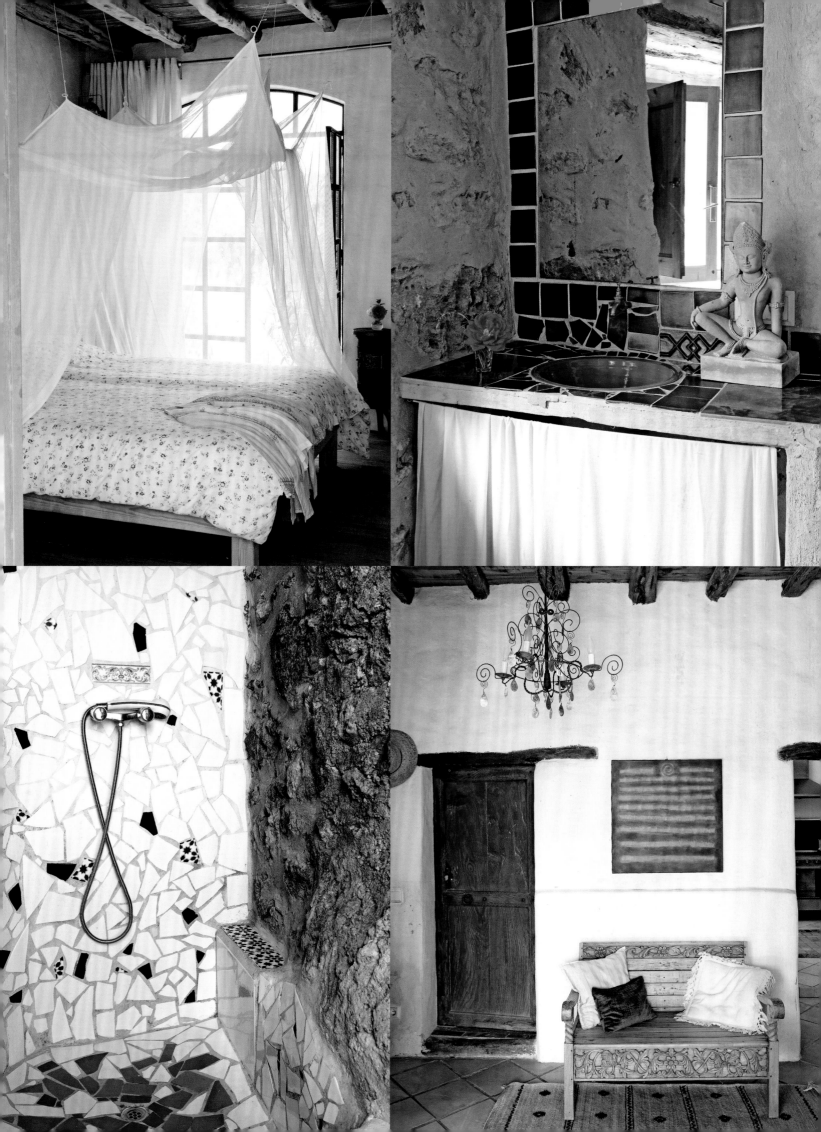

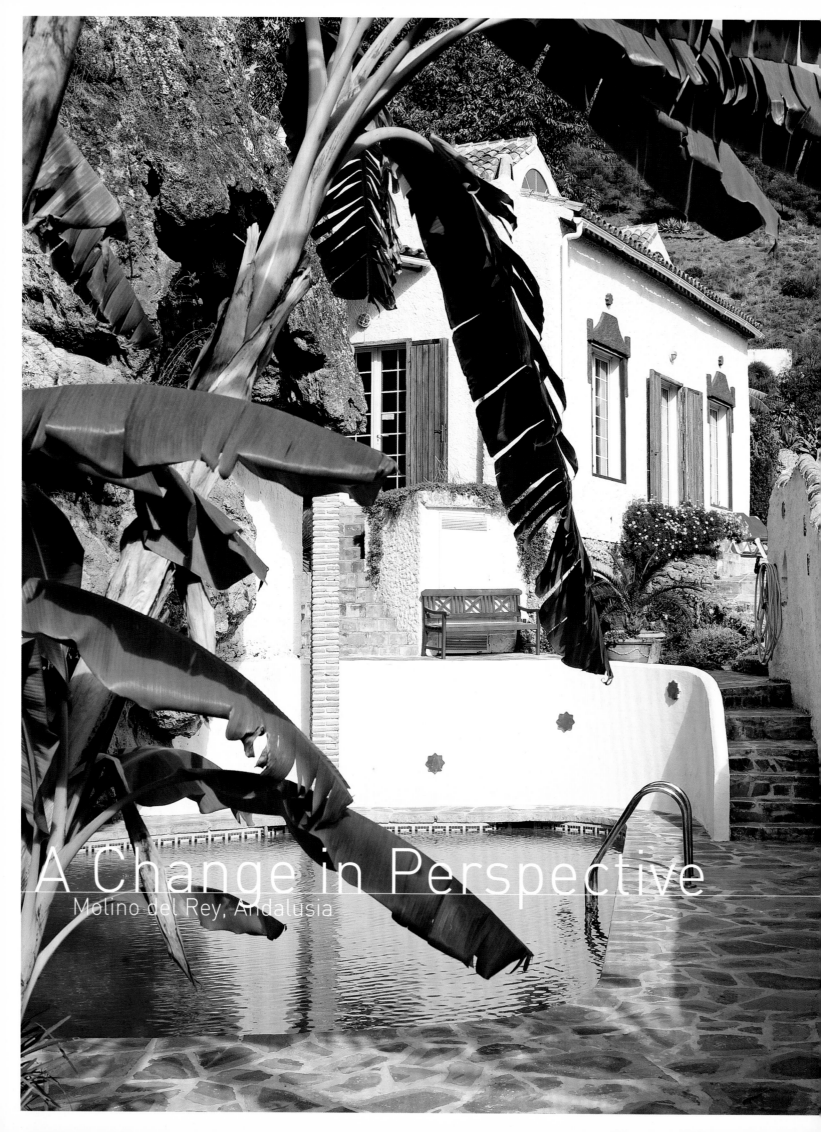

A Change in Perspective
Molino del Rey, Andalusia

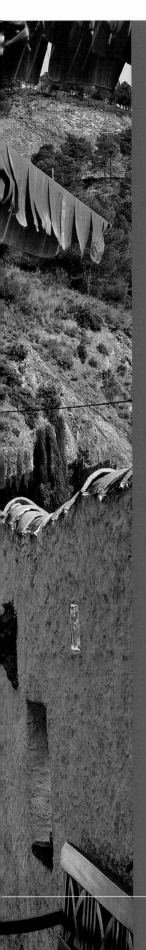

Molino del Rey, Andalusia

A Change in Perspective

Whichever king it was that these two former mills belonged to, you can't feel sorry enough for him. Of course he would have felt pride and love for his land as he looked towards the horizon across the deep green Andalusian hills and the orange and avocado groves. But however rich he might have been, his was the fate of those born too soon. He was never to enjoy being taught by famous English gurus in the Yoga Shala carved into the mountain; he would never meditate in the cave in the rock, never swim by candlelight in the seawater pool. With the conversion work undertaken by the owners themselves, these mills, which lie at the source of one of the tributaries of the Rio Grande, attract an enthusiastic clientele from all over the world. The guests here are spoilt for choice: a trip between Yoga lessons to Granada, Seville, Córdoba or Ronda, a trek through the breathtaking conservation area next door or simply a hot stone massage in the shade. The place itself is a source for new ideas and a change in perspective.

Books to pack: "Health, Healing & Beyond: Yoga and the Living Tradition of Krishnamacharya" by T. K. V. Desikachar and "Raquel, the Jewess of Toledo" by Lion Feuchtwanger.

Molino del Rey	
Valle de Jorox	
Alozaina-Málaga 29567	
Spain	
Tel. +34 952 480 009	
molinodelrey@hotmail.com	
www.molinodelrey.com	

DIRECTIONS	60 min west of Malaga Airport.
YOGA	Ashtanga, Kundalini, Vinyasa Flow, Iyengar.
TEACHERS	Simon Low, Clive Sherida, Yogateam Berlin.
ROOMS	Total of 20 beds, 1 single room, 6 double rooms and one room with 3 beds, 2 two-bed houses some distance away.
FOOD	Vegetarian; specialities: chocolate muffins, Spanish tortilla, paella.
TREATMENTS	Traditional Thai massage, royal oil massage, aromatherapy, Japanese facial massage, Thai foot massage, hot stone massage, Chavutti Thirumal massage, Swedish massage.
RECREATION	Hiking, meditation cave, pool.

Perspektivenwechsel

Welchem König diese beiden ehemaligen Mühlen auch immer gehört haben mögen, man kann ihn gar nicht genug bedauern. Sicherlich blickte er mit Stolz über die tiefgrünen Hügel Andalusiens, die Orangen- und Avocadohaine zum Horizont und liebte sein Land, doch so reich er auch gewesen sein mochte, ihn ereilte das Schicksal des zu früh Geborenen. Nie kam er in den Genuss, in der in den Berg hineinge-hauenen Yoga-Shala von berühmten englischen Gurus unterrichtet zu werden, in der Höhle im Fels zu meditieren oder im Seewasserpool bei Kerzenlicht zu schwimmen. Diese von den Besitzern eigenhändig umgebauten Mühlen, die an der Quelle eines der Seitenflüsse des Rio Grande liegen, ziehen ein begeistertes Publikum aus der ganzen Welt an, das die Qual der Wahl hat: ein Ausflug zwischen den Yogastunden nach Granada, Sevilla, Córdoba oder Ronda oder doch lieber eine Wanderung durch das angren-zende atemberaubende Naturschutzgebiet oder einfach eine Heiße-Stein-Massage im Schatten. Der Platz selbst wird zur Quelle für neue Ideen und einen Wechsel der Perspektive.
Buchtipps: »Yoga. Gesundheit von Körper und Geist: Leben und Lehren Krishnamacharyas« von T. K. V. Desikachar und »Die Jüdin von Toledo« von Lion Feuchtwanger.

Changement de perspective

Quel que soit le roi à qui ces deux anciens moulins aient pu appartenir, on ne pourra jamais le plaindre assez. Certes, son regard glissait fièrement sur les collines d'un vert pro-fond de l'Andalousie, les orangers et avocatiers se profilant à l'horizon et il aimait son pays, pourtant aussi riche qu'il ait pu être, le fait d'être né trop tôt lui fut fatal. Jamais il ne put se délecter de l'enseignement d'un célèbre guru anglais dans la yoga-shala implantée sur la montagne, d'une méditation au cœur d'une caverne ou d'un bain d'eau de mer en piscine, à la lueur de bougies. Ces moulins, situés à la source d'un affluent du Rio Grande et transformés grâce au travail per-sonnel de leurs propriétaires, attirent du monde entier un public enthousiaste qui n'a que l'embarras du choix : entre les séances de yoga faire une excursion à Grenade, Séville, Cordoue ou Ronda ou plutôt une randonnée à travers la réserve naturelle avoisinante, d'une beauté époustouflante, ou simplement profiter d'un massage aux pierres chaudes à l'ombre. L'endroit lui-même, induisant un changement de perspective, devient source d'idées nouvelles.
Livres à emporter : « Le yoga du yogi : L'héritage de T. Krishnamacharya » de Kausthub Desikachar et « La Juive de Tolède » de Lion Feuchtwanger.

ANREISE	60 min westlich vom Flughafen Malaga entfernt.
YOGA	Astanga, Kundalini, Vinyasa Flow, Iyengar.
GASTLEHRER	Simon Low, Clive Sherida, Yogateam Berlin.
ZIMMER	Insgesamt 20 Betten, 1 Einzelzimmer, 6 Doppel- und 1 Dreibettzimmer, 2 abgelegene Zweibetthäuschen.
KÜCHE	Vegetarisch, Spezialitäten: Schokoladenmuffins, spa-nische Tortilla, Paella.
ANWENDUNGEN	Traditionelle Thai-Massage, Royal-Oil-Massage, Aromatherapie, Japanische Gesichtsmassage, Thai-Fußmassage, Heiße-Steine-Massage, Chavutti-Thirummai-Massage, Schwedische Massage.
FREIZEIT	Wandern, Meditationshöhle, Pool.

ACCÈS	À 60 min à l'ouest de l'aéroport de Malaga.
YOGA	Ashtânga, Kundalini, Vinyasa Flow, Iyengar.
PROFESSEURS	Simon Low, Clive Sherida, Yogateam Berlin.
CHAMBRES	En tout 20 lits, 1 chambre individuelle, 6 chambres doubles et à trois lits, 2 bungalows en retrait avec 2 lits.
RESTAURATION	Végétarienne, spécialités : muffins au chocolat, tortillas espagnoles, paëlla.
TRAITEMENTS	Massage thaïlandais traditionnel, massage à l'huile royale, aromathérapie, massage facial japonais, mas-sage de pieds thaïlandais, massage aux pierres chaudes, massage chavutti thirumal, massage suédois.
ACTIVITÉS	Randonnées, caverne de méditation, piscine.

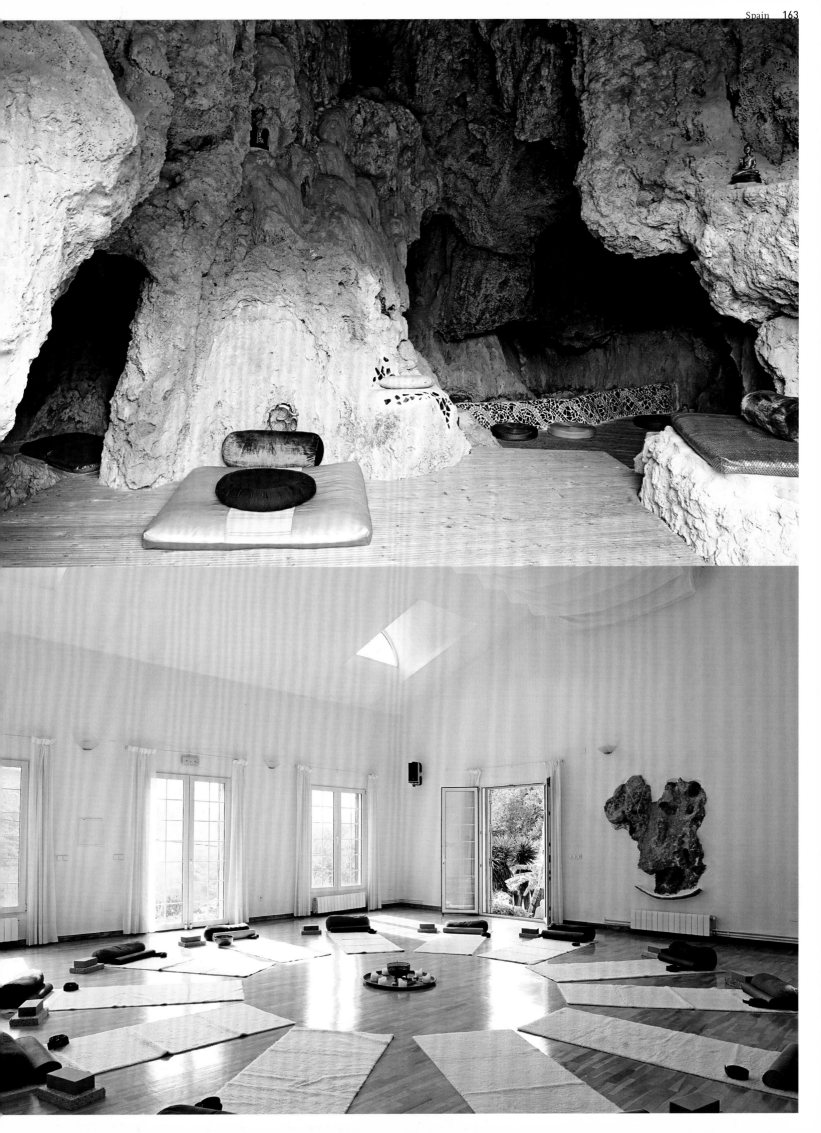

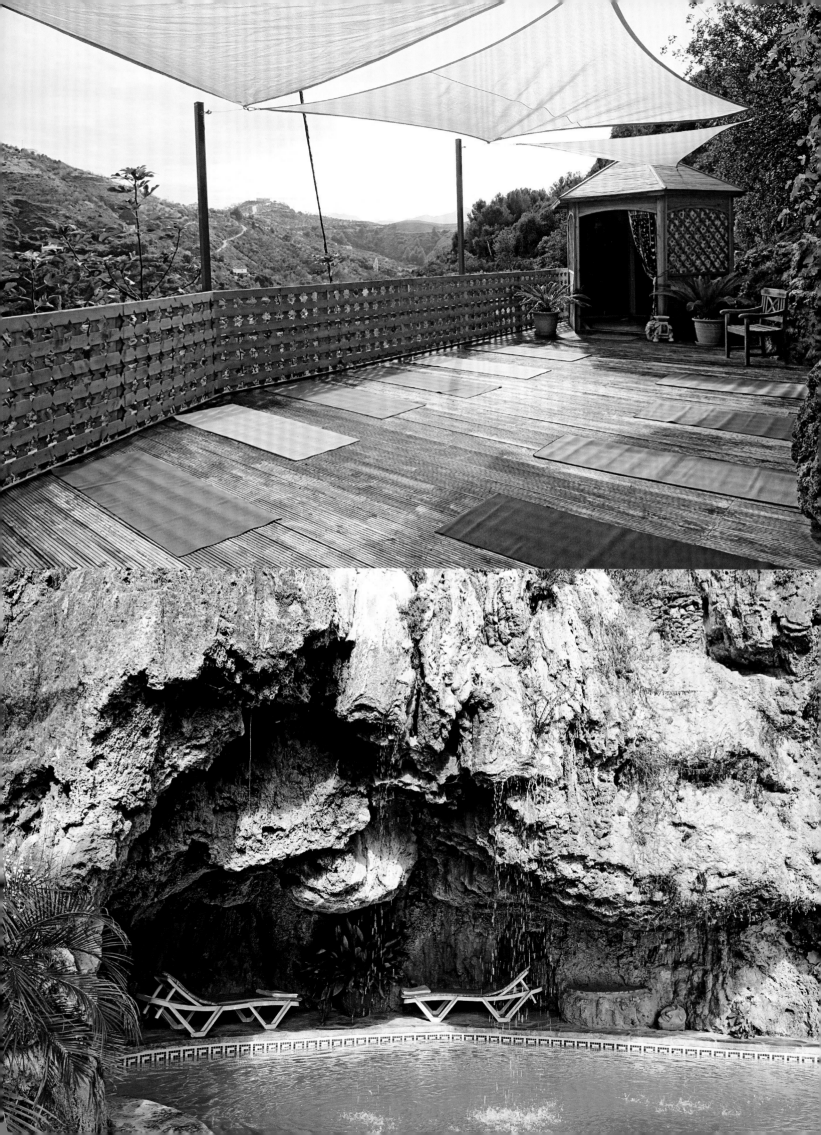

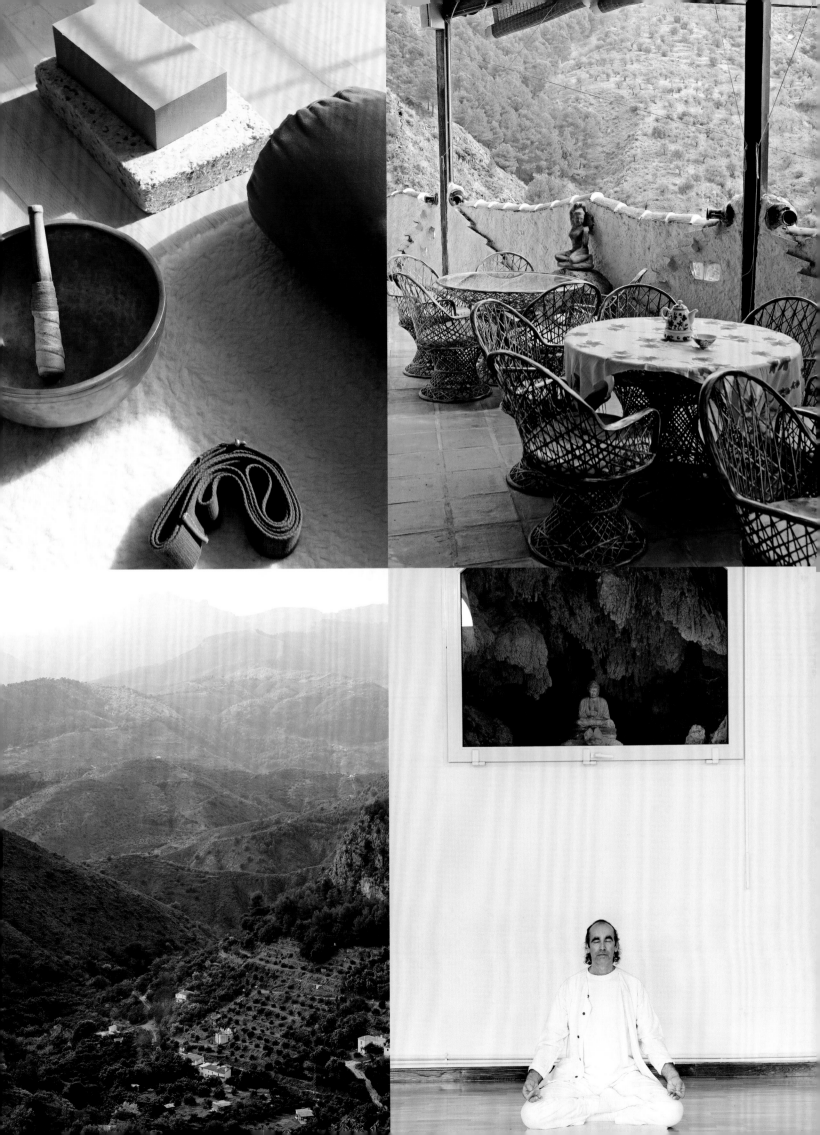

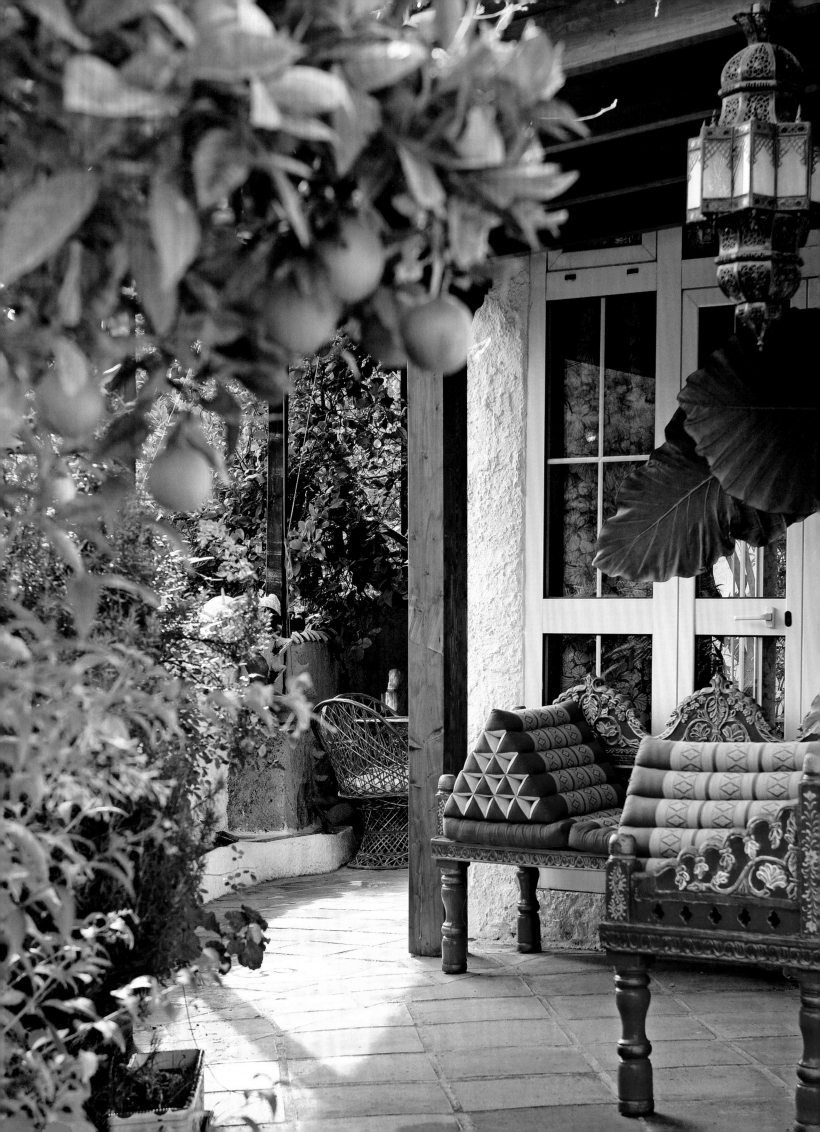

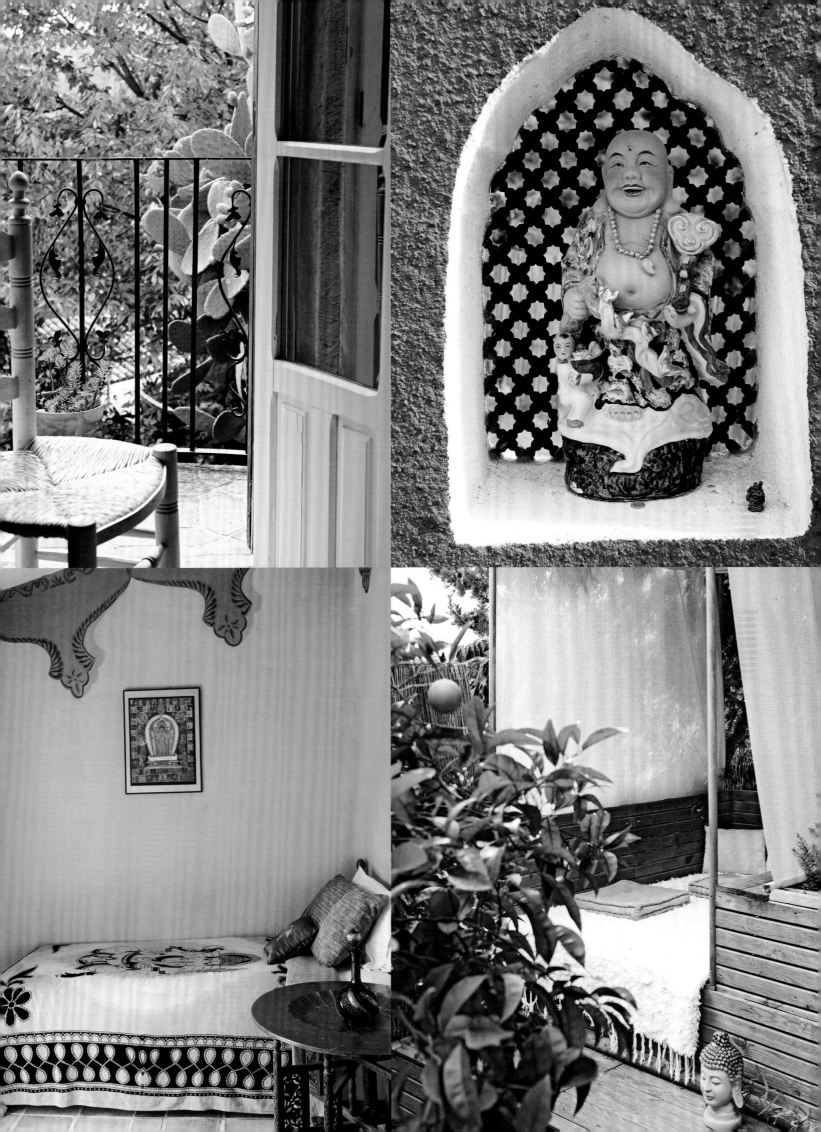

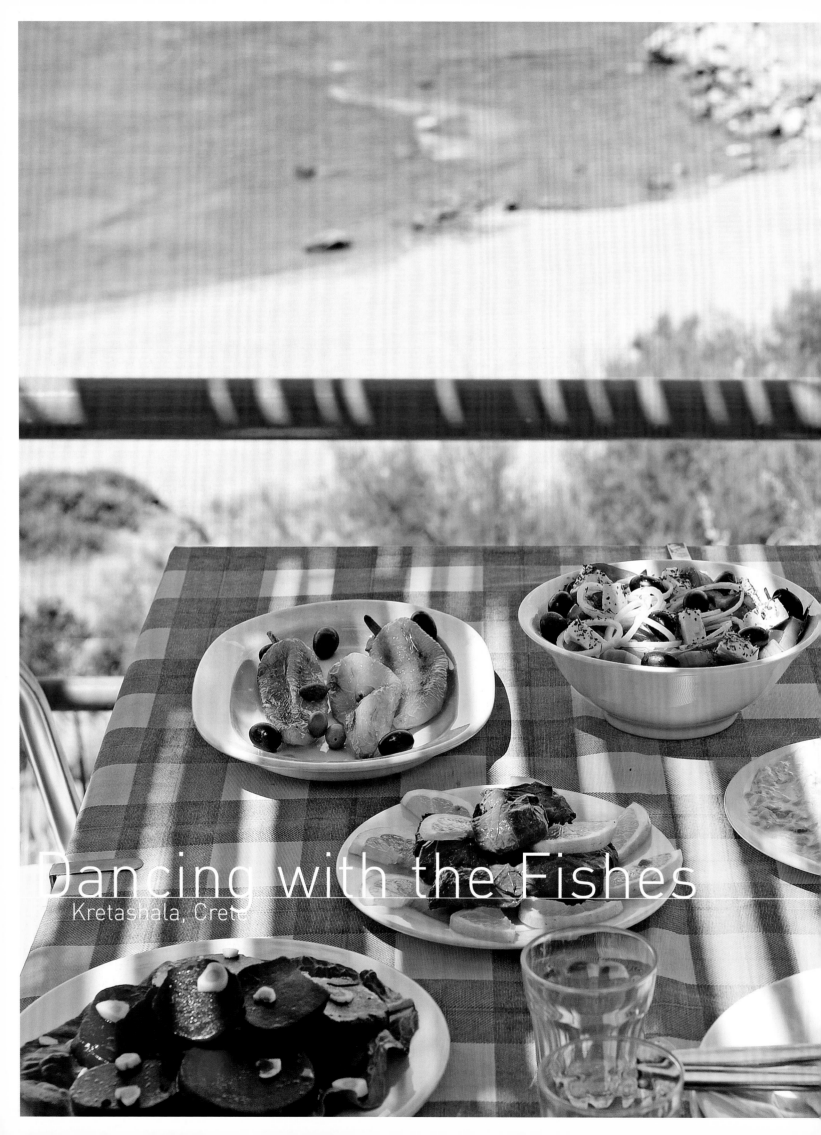

Dancing with the Fishes
Kretashala, Crete

Kretashala, Crete

Dancing with the Fishes

High on a cliff behind a high mountain chain, on which goats live an arduous life between dusty foliage and bristly bushes, stands Pavlos's guest house, a little oasis of humanity. "Handstand," orders the Greek Yoga teacher Petros in a light Bavarian accent and all at once, to the sound of Moby, the world stands on its head: the endless expanse of the Libyan Sea and the three rocks that give the region its name. No wonder that one of the most popular places for Vinyasa Yoga in Europe has developed here. The tiny tavern with checked table cloths, the terrace grown over with oleander bushes, deep-red geraniums and palm trees, the bright Yoga room and the small, comfortable rooms with their light-blue varnished doors is run by Pavlos and his family. If Prometheus had not set light to the common giant fennel that also grows here and thus, against the will of Zeus, given the people fire, it would surely have been Pavlos. You couldn't wish for a more attentive host. After working up a sweat during a Yoga session, an extended stroll along the long, solitary bay and an evening meditation session, there is baked fennel, stuffed vine leaves, sweet pita with pears, pomegranate and figs. It can even happen that Petros reaches for the guitar afterwards, and everybody starts to dance.

Books to pack: "The Odyssey" by Homer and "Gods and Heroes: Myths and Epics of Ancient Greece" by Gustav Schwab.

Kretashala	
Pavlos Kakogiannakis, Triopetra	
74100 Rethymnon, Crete	
Greece	
Tel. +49 89 333 295	
info@kretashala.de	
www.kretashala.de	

DIRECTIONS	Located in the west of the south coast of Crete. About 2 hrs from Heraklion Airport.
YOGA	Jivamukti, Anusara, Ashtanga, Kirtan, Nada Yoga.
TEACHERS	Patrick Broome, Petros Haffenrichter, Gabriela Bozic, Antje Schäfer, Mark Whitwell, Bryan Kest, Dave Stringer.
ROOMS	21 rooms for max. 45 guests.
FOOD	Vegetarian, authentic Cretan cuisine.
TREATMENTS	Massages, Thai massage, Shiatsu.
RECREATION	Hiking, swimming, walks along the beach.

Mit den Fischen tanzen

Hinter einer hohen Bergkette, auf der Ziegen ein mühseliges Leben zwischen staubigen Kräutern und borstigen Sträuchern führen, liegt hoch oben auf einem Kliff Pavlos' Pension, eine kleine Oase der Menschlichkeit. »Handstand« befiehlt Petros, der griechische Yogalehrer, in leichtem Bayerisch, und auf einmal steht die Welt zum Sound von Moby auf dem Kopf: die unendliche Weite der Libyschen See und die drei Felsen, die der Gegend den Namen gaben. Kein Wunder, dass sich dies zu einer der beliebtesten Adressen für Vinyasa Yoga in Europa entwickelt hat. Die winzige Taverne mit ihren karierten Tischdecken, der von Oleanderbüschen, tiefroten Geranien und Palmen bewachsenen Terrasse, dem lichten Yogaraum und den gemütlichen, kleinen Zimmern mit ihren hellblau lackierten Türen wird von Pavlos und seiner Familie geführt. Hätte nicht Prometheus das hier ebenfalls wachsende gemeine Steckenkraut entflammt und so den Menschen gegen den Willen von Zeus Feuer geschenkt, wäre es wohl Pavlos gewesen. Fürsorglicher kann man sich einen Wirt nicht wünschen. Nach schweißtreibenden Yogastunden, ausgedehnten Spaziergängen durch die lang gestreckte, einsame Bucht und Abendmeditation gibt es gebackenen Fenchel, gefüllte Weinblätter, süße Pita mit Birnen, Granatäpfeln und Feigen. Es kann einem sogar passieren, dass Petros danach zur Gitarre greift und alle anfangen zu tanzen.

Buchtipps: »Die Odyssee« von Homer und »Sagen des klassischen Altertums« von Gustav Schwab.

Danse avec les poissons

Derrrière une haute chaîne de montagnes, là où les chèvres mènent une vie rude entre herbes poussiéreuses et buissons épineux, tout en haut d'une falaise, est perchée la pension Pavlos, un petit havre d'humanité. « Faites le poirier », ordonne Petros, le professeur de yoga grec, avec un léger accent bavarois et, tout à coup, sur la musique de Moby, le monde est à l'envers : l'espace infini de la mer Lybienne et les trois rochers qui ont donné leur nom à la région. Rien d'étonnant que l'une des adresses les plus prisées du yoga Vinyasa en Europe ait pris ici son essor. La minuscule taverne avec ses nappes à carreaux, sa terrasse envahie de buissons de laurier rose, de géraniums rouge foncé et de palmiers, sa salle de yoga baignée de lumière et ses petites chambres confortables aux portes laquées en bleu clair est dirigée par Pavlos et sa famille. Si Prométhée n'avait pas allumé la férule commune, qui pousse ici aussi, et ainsi, contre la volonté de Zeus, apporté le feu aux hommes, c'est bien Pavlos qui s'en serait chargé. Impossible de trouver un hôtelier plus attentionné. Après les séances de yoga sudorifiques, les longues promenades sur l'immense crique solitaire et la méditation, place aux fenouils au four, aux feuilles de vigne farcies, à la pita sucrée aux poires, aux pommes et aux figues. Il peut même arriver que Pavlos prenne ensuite sa guitare et que tous se mettent à danser.

Livres à emporter : « L'Odyssée » d'Homère et « Légendes de l'Antiquité classique » de Gustav Schwab.

ANREISE	Im Westen der Südküste von Kreta gelegen. Etwa 2 Std. vom Flughafen Heraklion entfernt.
YOGA	Jivamukti, Anusara, Astanga, Kirtan und Nada Yoga.
GASTLEHRER	Patrick Broome, Petros Haffenrichter, Gabriela Bozic, Antje Schäfer, Mark Whitwell, Bryan Kest, Dave Stringer.
ZIMMER	21 Zimmer für max. 45 Gäste.
KÜCHE	Vegetarisch, authentische kretische Küche.
ANWENDUNGEN	Massage, Thai-Massage, Shiatsu.
FREIZEIT	Wandern, Schwimmen, Strandspaziergänge.

ACCÈS	Situé à l'ouest de la côte sud de la Crète. A environ 2 h de l'aéroport d'Héraklion.
YOGA	Jivamukti, Anusara, Ashtânga, Kirtan et Nada Yoga.
PROFESSEURS	Patrick Broome, Petros Haffenrichter, Gabriela Bozic, Antje Schäfer, Mark Whitwell, Bryan Kest, Dave Stringer.
CHAMBRES	21 chambres pour 45 personnes max.
RESTAURATION	Cuisine végétarienne, cuisine crétoise régionale authentique.
TRAITEMENTS	Massage, massage thaïlandais, shiatsu.
ACTIVITÉS	Randonnées, natation, promenades sur la plage.

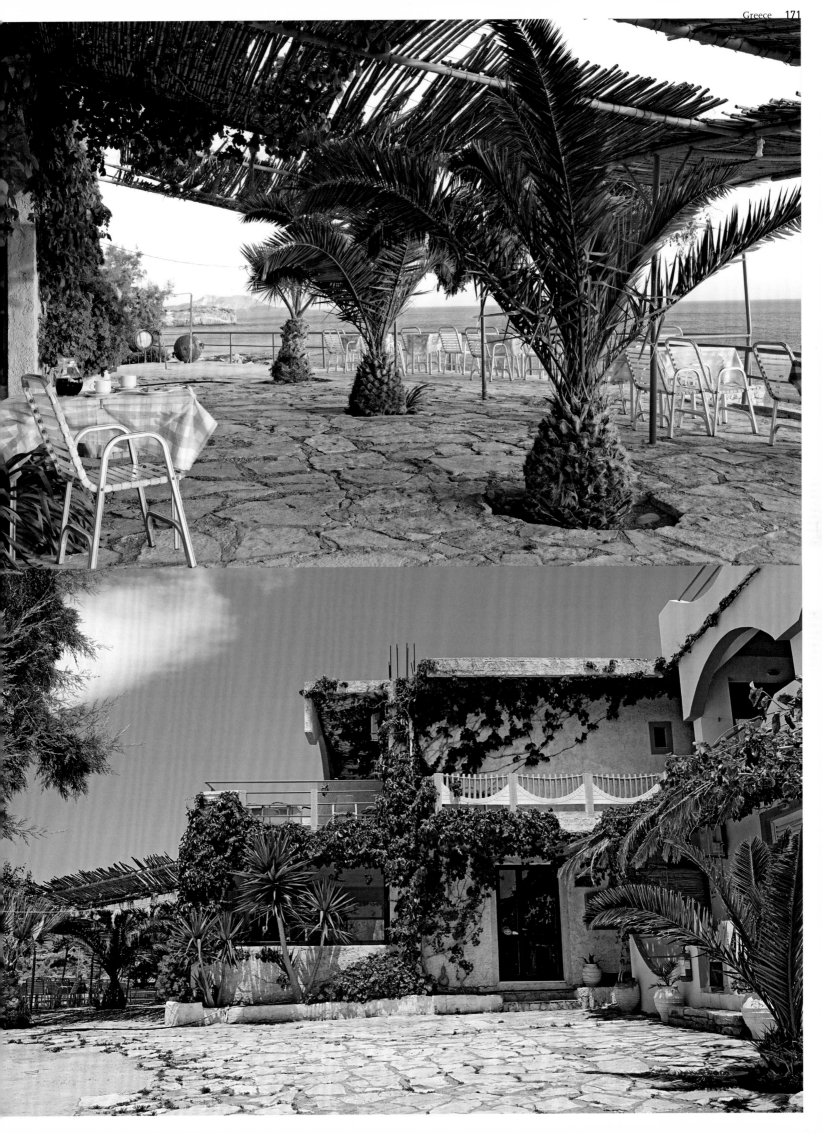

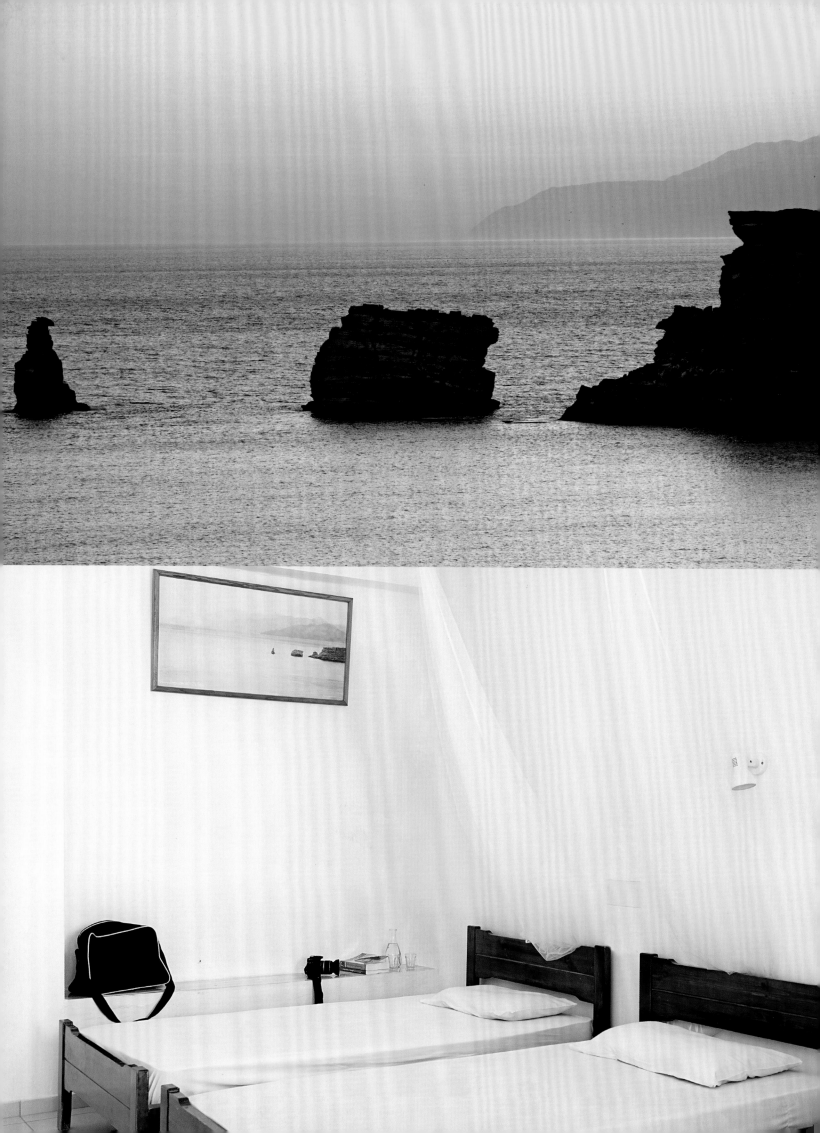

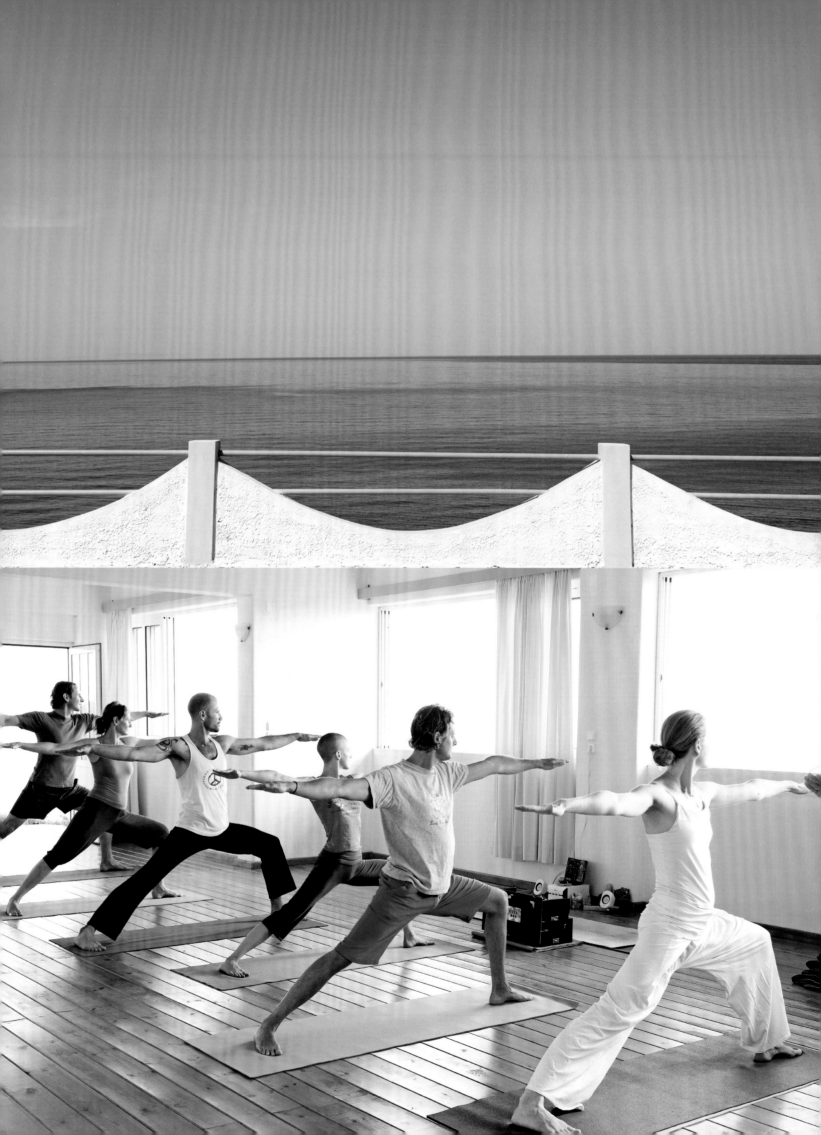

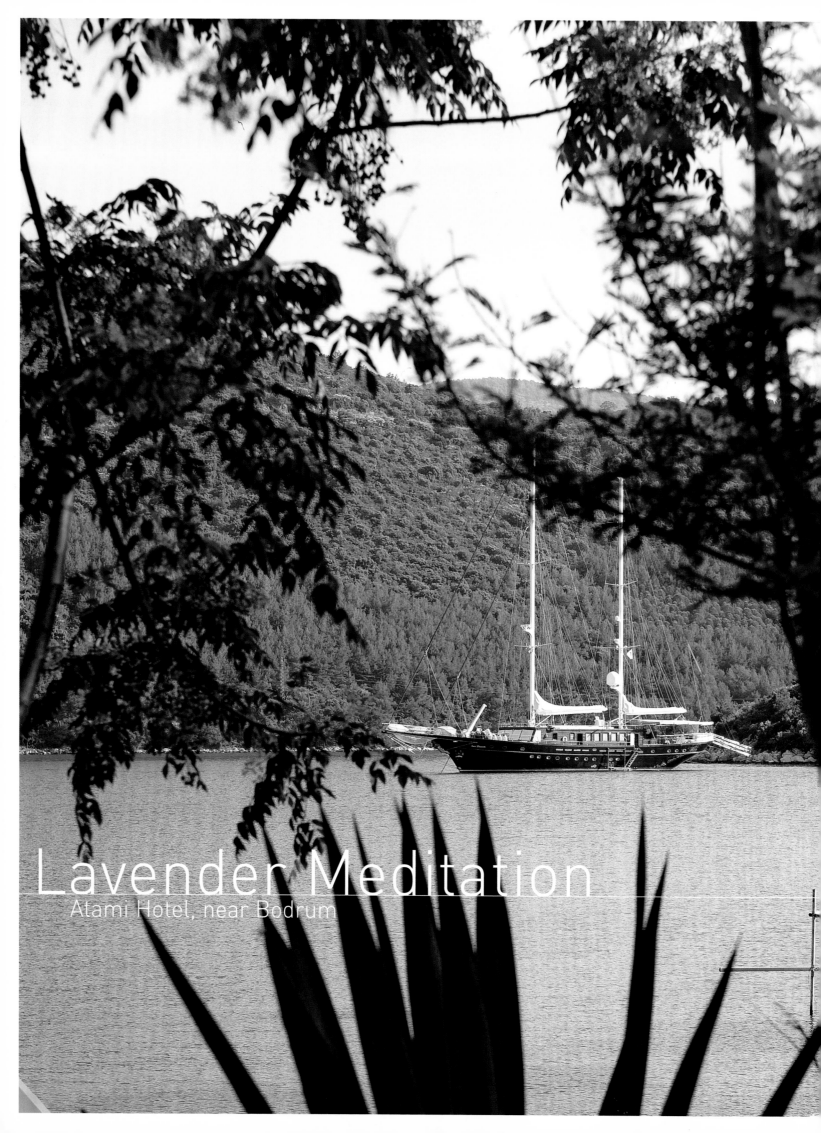

Lavender Meditation
Atami Hotel, near Bodrum

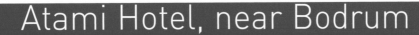

Atami Hotel, near Bodrum

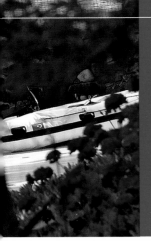

Lavender Meditation

When a beach bears the name paradise, caution is most often advised. But the bay on which the small luxury hotel Atami lies has surely earned the name: crystal-clear water, a sea like an aquarium in which the widest variety of fish can be marvelled at, even without a snorkel, a lovely little beach and a view onto the surrounding hilly coastal landscape prove that you have come to the right place. Run by Japanese-Turkish owners, the Atami Hotel is a likeable establishment whose mix of minimalist style and classic massive furnishings is perhaps not to everyone's taste. All the better in contrast is the cuisine, which along with Turkish specialities also includes excellent vegetarian and Japanese dishes, served outside on the terrace under a starry sky. Behind all this stands the grande dame of the hotel, a former Lufthansa stewardess, who has also planted the artful garden with over 50 different varieties of plant. The early-morning stroll along the lavender bushes, a challenging Yoga session next to the pool and the awareness that the owners give their very generous support to a Turkish animal protection organisation make holidays here on the Turkish Riviera not only relaxing, but also mutually beneficial.

Books to pack: "The Museum of Innocence" by Orhan Pamuk and "Salman the Solitary" by Yaşar Kemal.

Atami Hotel
Cennet Koyu n. 48
Gölköy
48400 Bodrum Muğla
Turkey
Tel. +90 252 357 7416 and +90 252 357 7417
Fax +90 252 357 7421
yoga@atamihotel.com or info@atamihotel.com
www.atamihotel.com

DIRECTIONS	Located in the north of the Bodrum peninsula. 28 miles from Bodrum Airport.
YOGA	Hatha, Jivamukti, Sivananda, Iyengar, Anusara, Energy.
TEACHERS	Durga Devi, Emma Henry, Lizzy Giles, Carin Zahn, Susan Desmarais.
ROOMS	29 rooms for max. 58 guests.
FOOD	Mediterranean cuisine. Japanese salads, lunch, snacks. Vegetarian/vegan options.
TREATMENTS	Massage.
RECREATION	Swimming, hiking and day trips to bazaars, hammams and to sample the night life of the Turkish St. Tropez, Türkbükü.

Lavendel-Meditation

Wenn ein Strand Paradies heißt, ist meistens Vorsicht geboten.
Doch die Bucht, an der das kleine Luxushotel Atami liegt,
hat den Namen durchaus verdient: kristallklares Wasser, ein
Meer wie ein Aquarium, in dem die verschiedensten Fische
auch ohne Schnorchel zu bestaunen sind, ein lieblicher kleiner Strand und ein Blick auf die hügelige Küstenlandschaft
ringsum, der beweist, dass man am richtigen Ort ist. In
japanisch-türkischer Hand ist das Atami Hotel eine sympa-
thische Adresse, deren Stilmischung aus minimalistischer
und klassisch wuchtiger Einrichtung vielleicht nicht jeder-
manns Geschmack ist. Umso gelungener dagegen präsentiert
sich die Küche, die außer türkischen Spezialitäten ausge-
zeichnete vegetarische und japanische Gerichte anbietet, die
draußen auf der Terrasse unterm Sternenhimmel serviert
werden. Dahinter steckt die Grande Dame des Hauses, eine
ehemalige Lufthansa-Stewardess, die auch den kunstvollen
Garten mit über 50 verschiedenen Pflanzensorten angelegt
hat. Der frühmorgendliche Spaziergang entlang der Lavendel-
büsche, eine herausfordernde Yogastunde neben dem Pool
und das Bewusstsein, dass die Eigentümer sehr großzügig
eine türkische Tierschutzorganisation unterstützen, machen
Ferien an der türkischen Riviera nicht nur erholsam, sondern
in jeder Hinsicht wohltuend.

Buchtipps: »Über Freiheit und Meditation. Das Yoga Sûtra
des Patañjali« von T. K. V. Desikachar, »Das Museum der
Unschuld« von Orhan Pamuk und »Der Sturm der Gazellen«
von Yaşar Kemal.

Méditation au parfum de lavande

Quand une plage est appelée paradis, le plus souvent la pru-
dence est de mise. Et pourtant, la baie où se trouve le petit
hôtel de luxe Atami mérite amplement son nom : une eau
cristalline, une mer où, comme dans un aquarium, on peut
contempler même sans tuba les poissons les plus variés, une
délicieuse petite plage et une vue sur les côtes vallonnées
alentour, autant de preuves que nous sommes au bon endroit.
L'hôtel Atami, sous direction turco-japonaise, est une sympa-
thique adresse dont l'aménagement, à la fois minimaliste et
classique, n'est peut-être pas du goût de tous. En revanche,
la cuisine n'en est que plus appréciable, qui, en plus de
spécialités turques, propose de succulents plats végétariens
et japonais, servis dehors sur la terrasse sous le ciel étoilé.
La grande dame de la maison, ancienne hôtesse de l'air
de la Lufthansa, qui a également conféré au jardin style et
noblesse grâce à plus de 50 espèces de plantes différentes,
y est pour beaucoup. La promenade matinale le long des
buissons de lavande, une séance de yoga intensive tout près
de la piscine et la pensée que les propriétaires apportent
leur très généreux soutien à une organisation turque pour
la défense des animaux rendent les vacances sur la côte
turquoise non seulement reposantes, mais réellement bien-
faisantes à tous égards.

Livres à emporter : « Le Yoga-Sûtra de Patañjali » de T. K. V.
Desikachar, « Le musée de l'innocence » d'Orhan Pamuk et
« Salman le solitaire » de Yaşar Kemal.

ANREISE	Im Norden der Halbinsel Bodrum gelegen. 45 km vom Flughafen Bodrum entfernt.
YOGA	Hatha, Jivamukti, Sivananda, Iyengar, Anusara, Energy.
GASTLEHRER	Durga Devi, Emma Henry, Lizzy Giles, Carin Zahn, Susan Desmarais.
ZIMMER	29 Zimmer für max. 58 Gäste.
KÜCHE	Mittelmeerküche. Japanische Salate, Lunch, Snacks. Vegetarisch und vegan möglich.
ANWENDUNGEN	Massage.
FREIZEIT	Schwimmen, Wandern, Ausflüge zu Basaren, Hamam und ins Nachtleben des türkischen St. Tropez Türkbükü.

ACCÈS	Situé au nord de la presqu'île de Bodrum, à 45 km de l'aéroport de Bodrum.
YOGA	Hatha, Jivamukti, Shivananda, Iyengar, Anusara, Energy.
PROFESSEURS	Durga Devi, Emma Henry, Lizzy Giles, Carin Zahn, Susan Desmarais.
CHAMBRES	29 chambres pour 58 personnes max.
RESTAURATION	Cuisine méditerranéenne. Salades japonaises, lunch, snacks. Option végétarienne / végétalienne.
TRAITEMENTS	Massages.
ACTIVITÉS	Natation, randonnées, visites de bazars, du hammam et du Saint-Tropez turc « by night », Türkbükü.

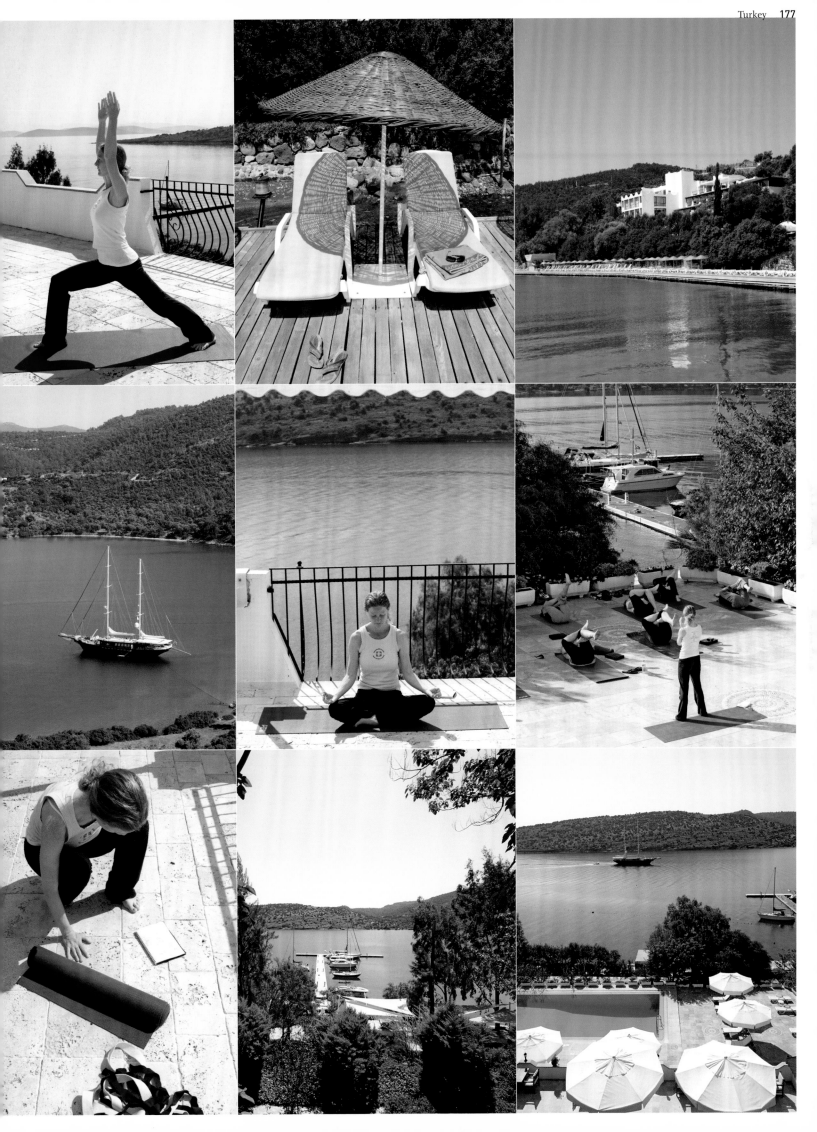

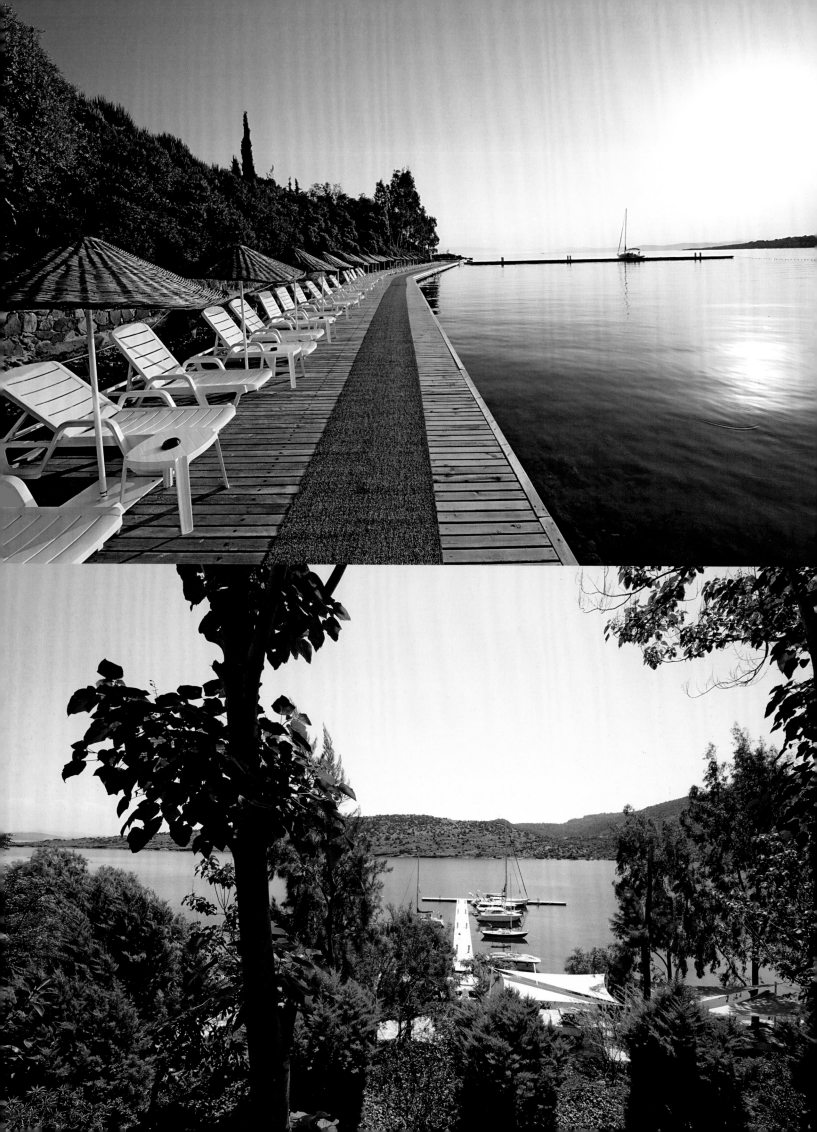

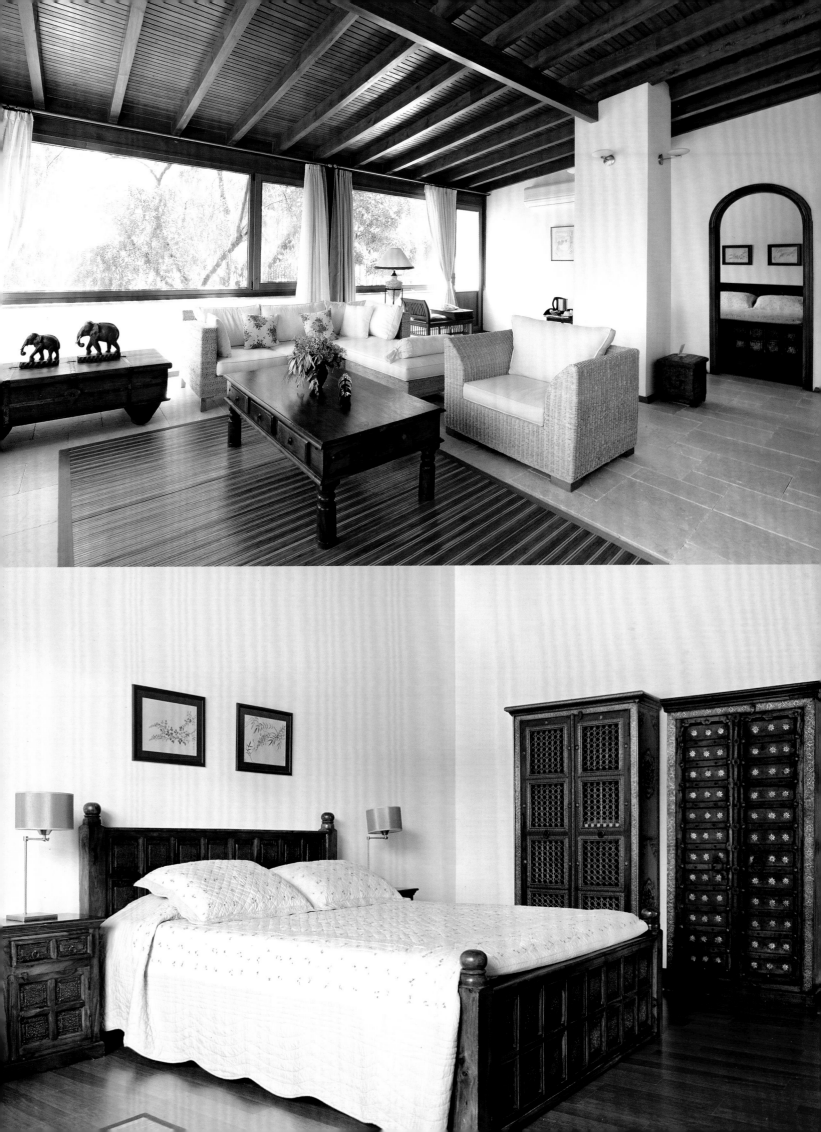

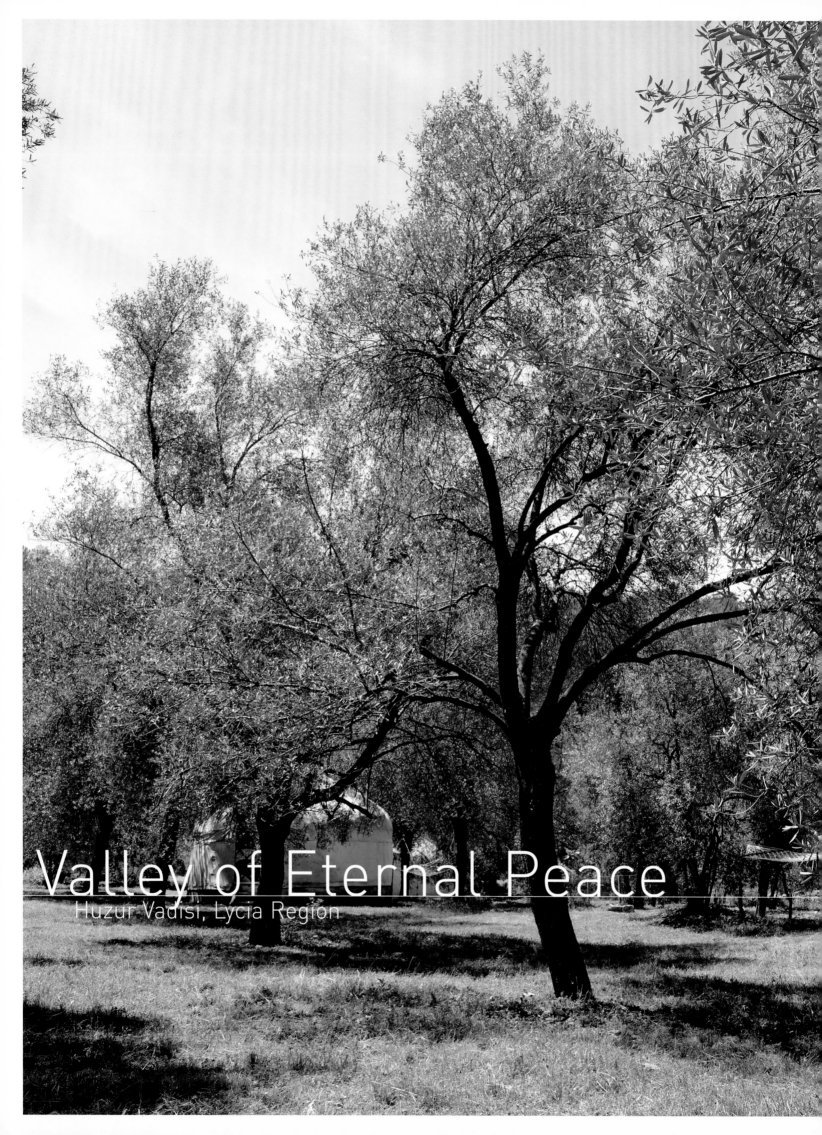

Valley of Eternal Peace
Huzur Vadisi, Lycia Region

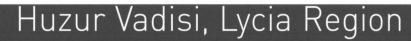

Huzur Vadisi, Lycia Region

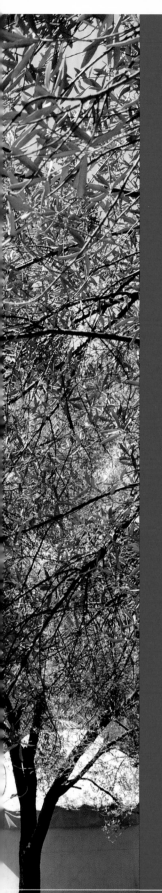

Valley of Eternal Peace

Ashtanga in the Mysore style is, as everybody knows, no picnic. By the tenth jump back into Chaturanga Dandasana at the latest, the arms are trembling, the thighs hurt and the Achilles tendon is sending distress signals. Or maybe not. Because those who are guided through Pattabhi Jois's Primary Series – as here by Joey Miles, one of Britain's leading Ashtanga teachers – will in the end love the köşk, as the wonderfully pretty wooden summer pavilion where the sessions take place is called. Indeed, this small, charming retreat, built in the midst of olive groves, is firmly in British hands. Almost all the teachers come from Triyoga, the famous Yoga school in London's Primrose Hill, and they have been coming for years. Is it because of the broad hammocks that invite you to take extended lunch breaks under the fig trees, or the delicious, lovingly prepared meals, attended by all at a long table in the open air, or the yurts, round, comfortable tents from which you can look at the stars in the sky whilst falling asleep under mosquito nets? Or is it just that in this peaceful valley, as the name Huzur Vadisi translates, with a view of the turquoise-coloured sea, a peace of mind sets in through which that slight ache in the legs and those tensed-up stomach muscles are – how do we put it in the rational world? – "transcended" in a general feeling of total bliss.

Books to pack: "Stillness Speaks: Whispers of Now" by Eckhart Tolle and "Memed, My Hawk" by Yaşar Kemal.

Huzur Vadisi
Gökçeovacık
Göcek 48310, Fethiye
Turkey
Tel. +90 252 644 0008 and +44 780 371 0574
huzvad@aol.com
www.huzurvadisi.com

DIRECTIONS	Located in the southwest of Turkey, 40 min from the next airport, Dalaman.
YOGA	Hatha, Bikram, Kundalini, Ashtanga.
TEACHERS	Simon Low, Louise Grime, Joey Miles.
ROOMS	10 yurts with 2 beds, 4 2-bed rooms for max. 30 guests.
FOOD	Predominantly vegetarian Turkish dishes, vegan, fish or meat on request.
TREATMENTS	Massage, Turkish bath.
RECREATION	Swimming pool, day trips, boat trips.

Tal des ewigen Friedens

Astanga im Mysore-Stil zu üben, ist, wie jeder weiß, kein
Zuckerschlecken. Spätestens beim zehnten Zurückspringen
in Chaturanga Dandasana zittern die Arme, schmerzen die
Oberschenkel, meldet sich die Achillessehne. Oder nicht.
Denn wer wie hier von Joey Miles, einem der führenden
Astanga-Lehrer Großbritanniens, durch Pattabhi Jois' Primary
Series begleitet wird, liebt am Ende den Köşk, wie der
wunderhübsche, aus Holz gebaute Sommerpavillon heißt,
in dem geübt wird. Überhaupt ist dieses kleine charmante
Retreat, mitten in einen Olivenhain gebaut, fest in britischer
Hand. Fast alle Lehrer kommen von Triyoga, der berühmten
Yogaschule in Primrose Hill, London, und sie kommen seit
Jahren. Liegt es an den breiten Hängematten, die unter
Feigenbäumen zu ausgedehnten Mittagspausen einladen,
an den köstlichen, liebevoll zubereiteten Mahlzeiten, zu
denen sich alle an einem langen Tisch im Freien einfinden,
an den Jurten, den runden komfortablen Zelten, in denen
man unter Moskitonetzen liegend die Sterne am Himmel
sehen kann? Oder einfach daran, dass sich in diesem fried-
lichen Tal wie Huzur Vadisi übersetzt heißt, mit Blick auf
die türkisfarbene türkische See, ein Seelenfrieden einstellt,
der das leichte Ziehen in den Beinen und die angekurbelten
Bauchmuskeln in ein generelles Summen der Glückseligkeit
– wie man in der rationalen Welt sagt – »transzendiert«.
**Buchtipps: »Stille spricht: Wahres Sein berühren« von Eckhart
Tolle und »Der Baum des Narren« von Yaşar Kemal.**

Vallée de la paix éternelle

Comme chacun sait, la pratique de l'Ashtânga dans le style
Mysore n'est vraiment pas du gâteau. Au plus tard au dixième
saut en arrière dans un Chaturanga Dandasana, les bras
tremblent, les cuisses sont douloureuses, le tendon d'Achille
se fait sentir. Ou non. Car celui qui, encadré ici par Joey
Miles, l'un des professeurs d'Ashtânga les plus éminents de
Grande-Bretagne, effectue les séries primaires de Pattabhi
Jois' finit par aimer le « köşk », comme on appelle le ravis-
sant pavillon d'été construit en bois dans lequel on s'entraîne.
Cette petite et charmante oasis bâtie au cœur d'un bosquet
d'oliviers est véritablement une petite « colonie » anglaise.
Presque tous les professeurs sont issus de Triyoga, la fameuse
école de yoga de la Primrose Hill à Londres, et viennent ici
depuis des années. Cela tient-il aux larges hamacs qui, sous
les figuiers, invitent à des siestes prolongées, aux succulents
repas concoctés avec amour, pour lesquels tout le monde se
réunit autour d'une longue table en plein air, aux yourtes,
ces confortables tentes rondes, où l'on peut, sous les mousti-
quaires, contempler la nuit les étoiles au firmament ? Ou
simplement à ce que, dans cette vallée paisible (traduction
littérale de Huzur Vadisi), les yeux posés sur la mer Egée de
couleur turquoise, la paix s'installe en vous qui – comme on
le dit dans le monde rationnel – « transcende » les petites
crampes dans les jambes et les muscles abdominaux stimu-
lés jusqu'à ce qu'il ne reste qu'un bruissement de béatitude.
**Livres à emporter : « Quiétude : A l'écoute de sa nature essen-
tielle » d'Eckhart Tolle et « Mémed le faucon » de Yaşar Kemal.**

ANREISE	Im Südwesten der Türkei, 40 min vom Flughafen Dalaman entfernt.
YOGA	Hatha, Bikram, Kundalini, Astanga.
GASTLEHRER	Simon Low, Louise Grime, Joey Miles.
ZIMMER	10 Jurten mit 2 Betten, 4 Zweibettzimmer für max. 30 Gäste.
KÜCHE	Überwiegend türkisch-vegetarisch, vegan, Fisch oder Fleisch auf Anfrage.
ANWENDUNGEN	Massage, türkisches Bad.
FREIZEIT	Schwimmbad, Ausflüge, Bootsfahrten.

ACCÈS	Situé au sud-ouest de la Turquie, à 40 min de l'aéroport le plus proche à Dalaman.
YOGA	Hatha, Bikram, Kundalinî, Ashtânga.
PROFESSEURS	Simon Low, Louise Grime, Joey Miles.
CHAMBRES	10 yourtes à 2 lits, 4 chambres à 2 lits pour 30 per- sonnes max.
RESTAURATION	Cuisine essentiellement turque et végétarienne, végétalienne, poisson ou viande sur demande.
TRAITEMENTS	Massages, bain turc.
ACTIVITÉS	Piscine, excursions, promenades en bateau.

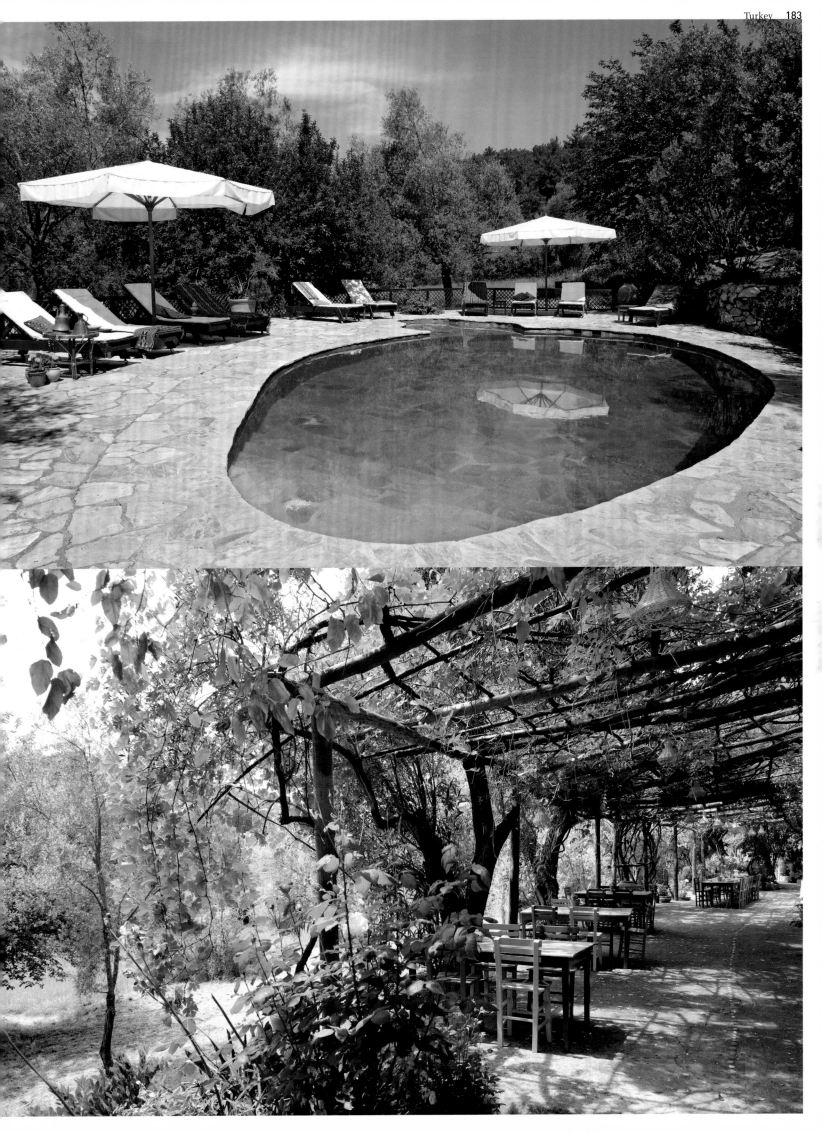

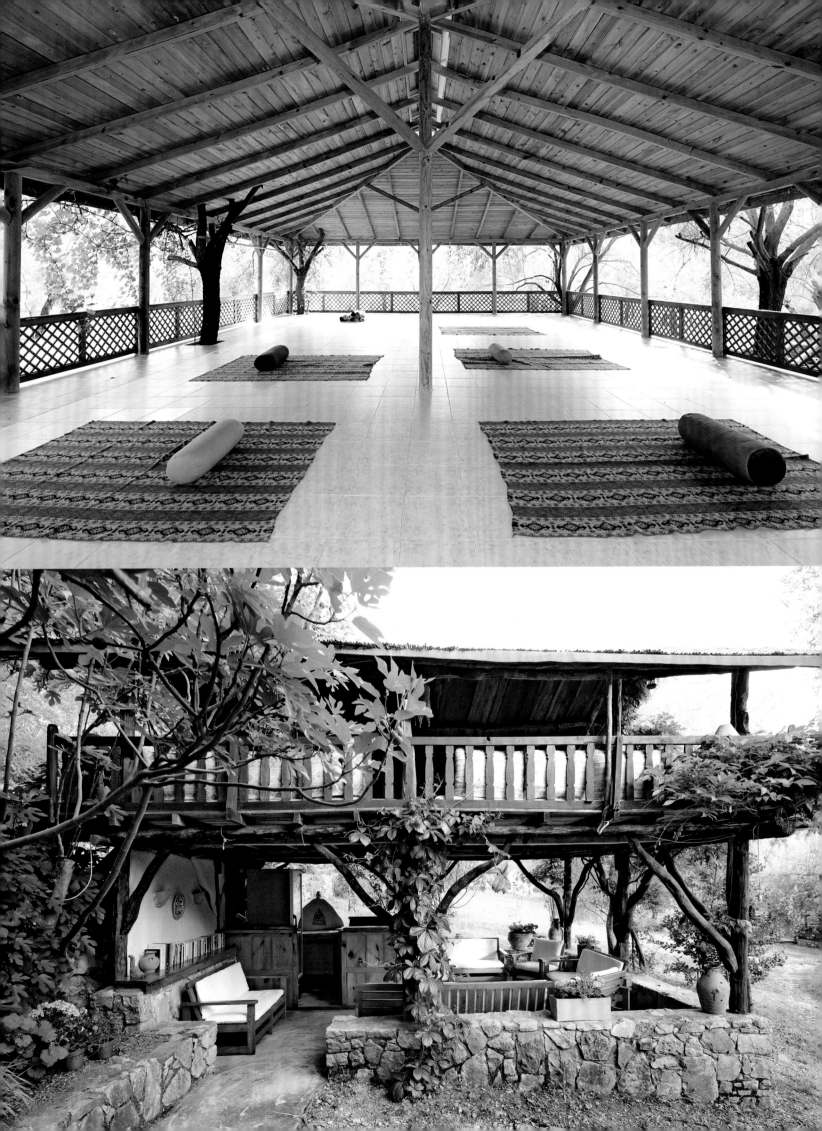

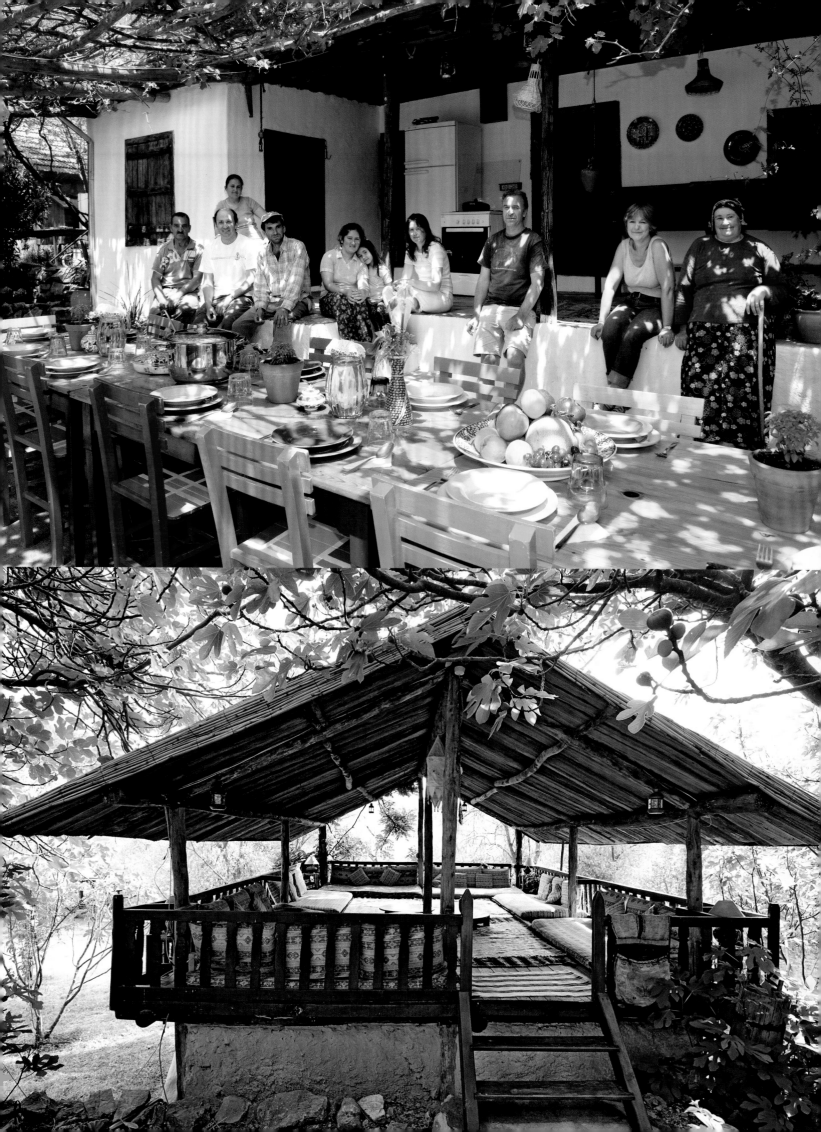

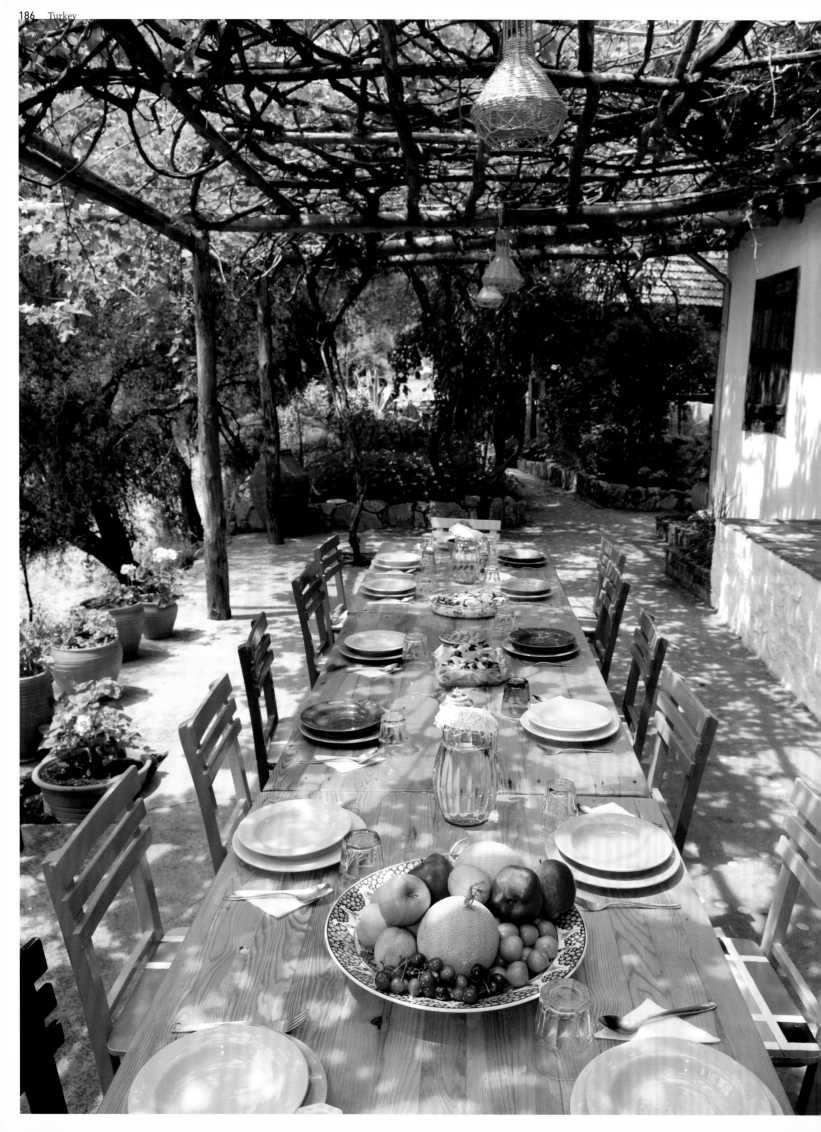

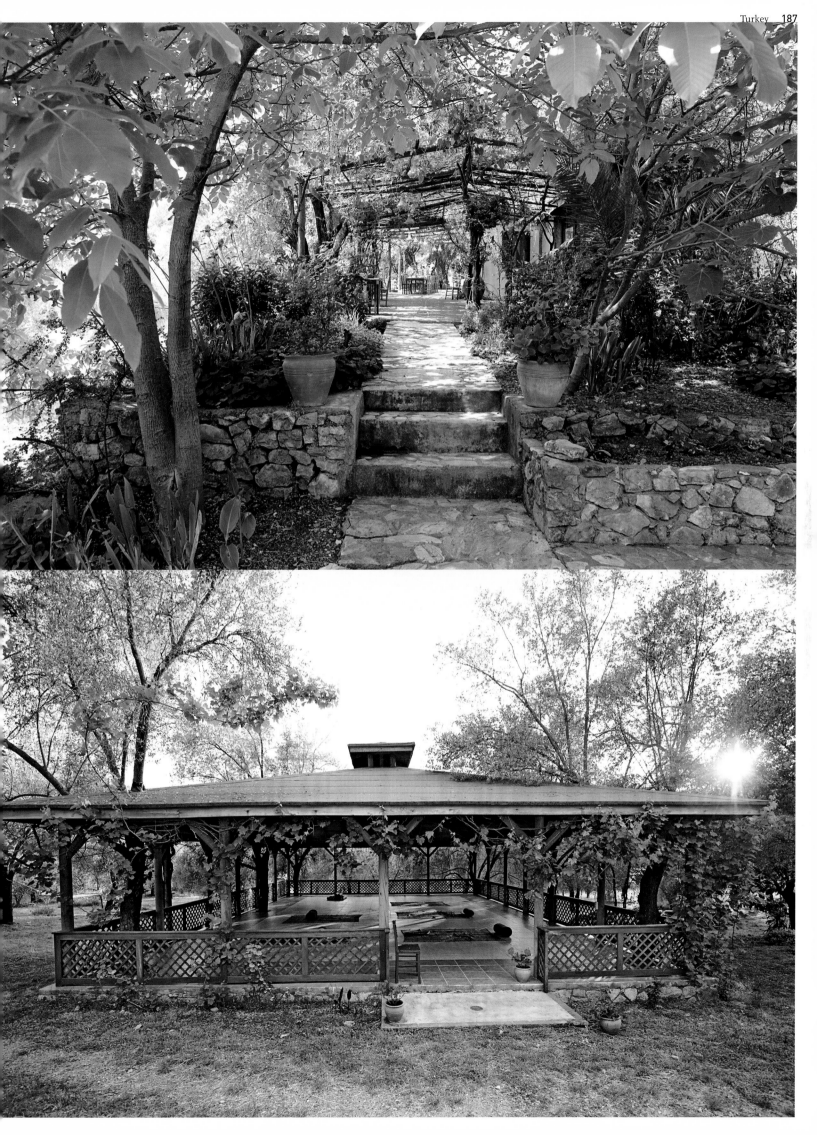

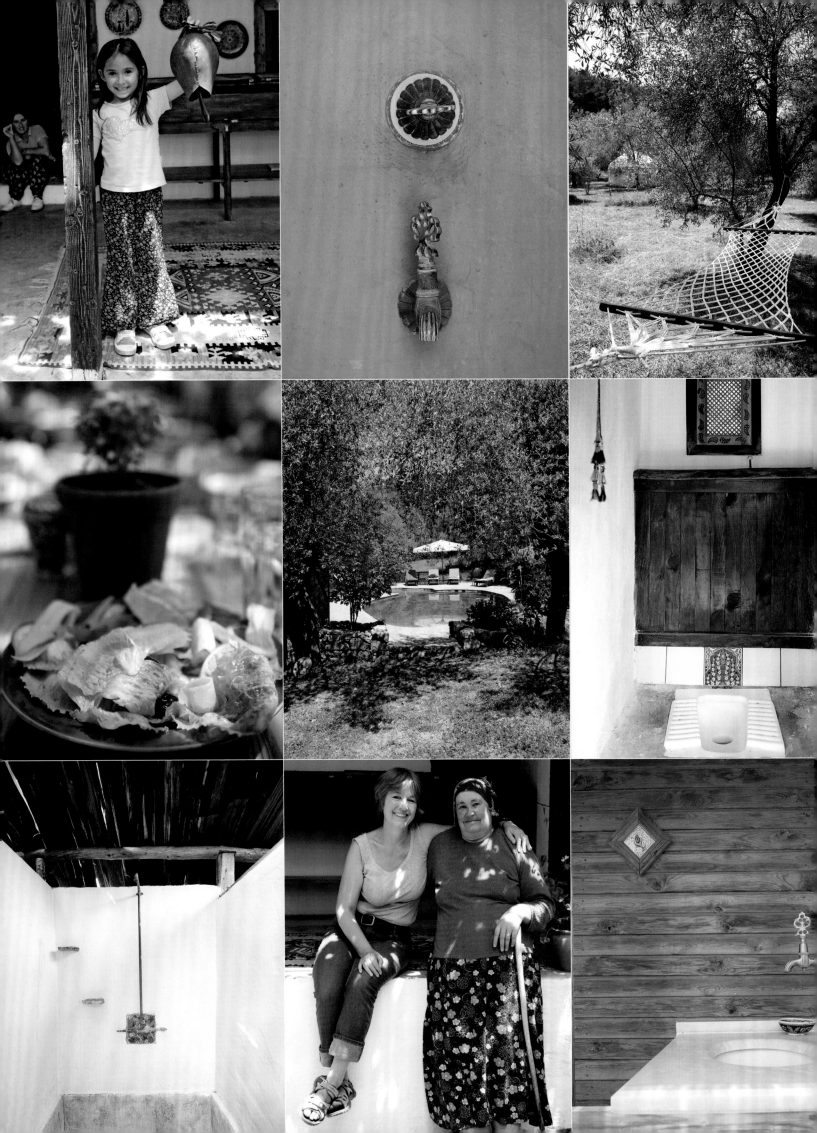

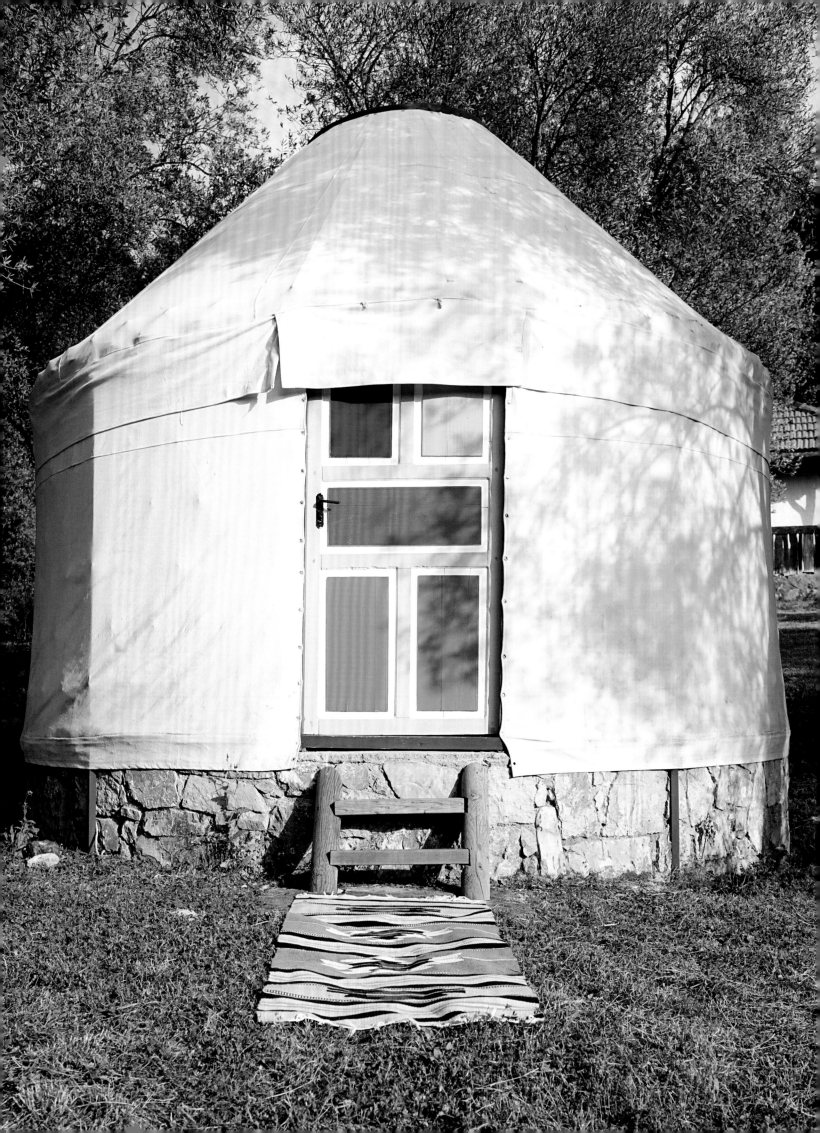

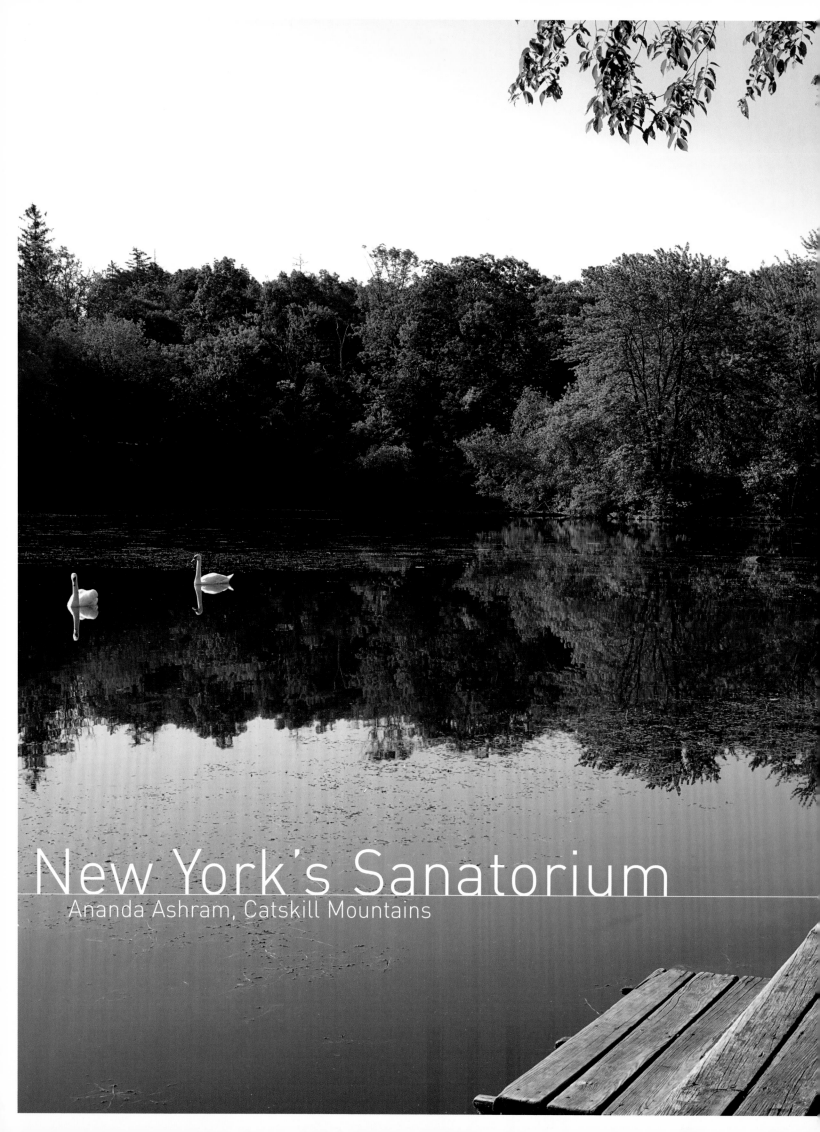

New York's Sanatorium
Ananda Ashram, Catskill Mountains

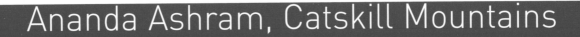

Ananda Ashram, Catskill Mountains

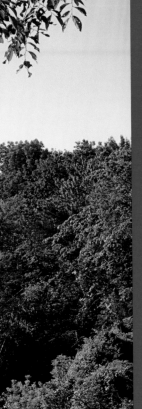

New York's Sanatorium

It is barely two hours from Park Avenue, but here at the foot of the Catskill Mountains even the leaves under your feet rustle more peacefully than they do in New York. It is easy to imagine that this ashram was once ultrafashionable, back in the days when girls in miniskirts and Timothy Leary himself sat in the grass between the pretty white wooden houses and learnt how to meditate from the Indian neurosurgeon and Sanskrit scholar Rammurti S. Mishra. Roe deer are still to be seen in the early-morning mist on the hill above the little lake, and the oddball old ladies who teach Sanskrit here and run the place wear little white dresses that swing when you dance. At least two daily sessions of Hatha Yoga and Sanskrit are included in the price. The weekend programme must be paid for separately, but it's worth it. When stars like Ruth Lauer-Manenti of Jivamukti, New York, are doing the teaching, the students, running with sweat, stagger afterwards with shining eyes down to the water. At other weekends, under the strict supervision of Joan Suval, no word may be spoken; a week later in Laraaji Nadananda's Laughter Workshop everyone is bent double in mirth for hours. The better end of the New York esoteric scene is regularly seen here, and people come from the entire East Coast to this idyllic mountain country to find themselves again amongst deep forests and hidden watercourses. Because, in spite of the ban on alcohol and tobacco and alongside a tender hint of nostalgia, one thing dominates here above all else: the spirit of enlightenment, which warmly welcomes every guest into the constantly self-renewing hippy community.

Books to pack: "The Textbook of Yoga Psychology" by Rammurti S. Mishra and "Glamorama" by Bret Easton Ellis.

Ananda Ashram,
Yoga Society of New York
13 Sapphire Road
Monroe, NY 10950
USA
Tel. +1 845 782 5575
Fax +1 845 774 7368
ananda@anandaashram.org
www.anandaashram.org

DIRECTIONS	About 1 1/2 hrs north of New York.
YOGA	Hatha, Kundalini, Jivamukti.
TEACHERS	Sharon Gannon, David Life, Dharma Mittra, Sharon Salzberg, Krishna Das, Jai Uttal.
ROOMS	Three guest houses with a total of 45 beds, 6-bed rooms and 2-bed rooms, camping possible in summer.
FOOD	Predominantly vegan, with a fantastic breakfast buffet.
TREATMENTS	Ayurvedic facial and massage, Swedish massage, Shiatsu, acupuncture, foot reflexology massage, aromatherapy, Raindrop Technique, relaxation training, sauna.
RECREATION	Meditation, Kathak dance, hiking, swimming, tabla and sitar lessons.

New Yorks Sanatorium

Es sind nicht mal zwei Stunden von der Park Avenue, aber hier am Fuße der Catskill Mountains raschelt selbst das Laub friedlicher unter den Füßen als in New York. Man kann es sich gut vorstellen, dass der Ashram früher tod-schick war, als Mädchen in Miniröcken und Timothy Leary im Gras zwischen den hübschen, weißen Holzhäusern saßen und von dem indischen Neurochirurgen und Sanskrit-gelehrten Rammurti S. Mishra lernten, wie man meditiert. Noch immer stehen morgens Rehe im Frühnebel auf dem Hügel oberhalb des kleinen Sees, und auch die schrulligen älteren Damen, die hier Sanskrit unterrichten und den Laden schmeißen, tragen weiße Kleidchen, die beim Tanzen schwingen. Täglich mindestens zweimal Hatha Yoga und Sanskrit sind im Preis inbegriffen. Das Wochenendpro-gramm muss extra bezahlt werden, lohnt sich aber. Wenn Stars wie Ruth Lauer-Manenti von Jivamukti New York, unterrichten, taumeln die Schüler hinterher schweißüber-strömt mit glänzenden Augen hinunter zum Wasser. An anderen Wochenenden darf unter der strengen Aufsicht von Joan Suval kein Wort geredet werden, eine Woche später biegen sich im Lach-Workshop von Laraaji Nadananda alle stundenlang vor Lachen. Die bessere New Yorker Esoterik-szene lässt sich regelmäßig sehen, und von der ganzen Ostküste kommen Menschen, um in der idyllischen Berg-landschaft zwischen tiefen Wäldern und versteckten Wasser-läufen wieder zu sich zu finden. Denn trotz Alkohol- und Tabakverbot herrscht hier neben einem zärtlichen Hauch von Nostalgie vor allem eins: der Geist der Aufklärung, der jeden Gast herzlich in die immer nachwachsende Hippiegemeinde aufnimmt.

Buchtipps: »The Textbook of Yoga Psychology« von Rammurti S. Mishra und »Glamorama« von Bret Easton Ellis.

Le sanatorium de New York

Park Avenue n'est qu'à deux heures à peine, mais ici, au pied des montagnes Catskill, même le feuillage bruisse plus doucement sous les pas qu'à New York. Il est aisé d'imaginer que l'âshram fut, à une époque, du dernier chic, lorsque des filles en minijupe et Timothy Leary, assis dans l'herbe entre les jolies maisons de bois blanc, apprenaient la méditation de Rammurti S. Mishra, neurochirugien indien et spécialiste du sanskrit. Comme autrefois, sur la colline dominant le petit lac, les biches se promènent dans la brume matinale et même les vieilles dames excentriques qui enseignent ici le sanskrit et tiennent boutique, portent des petites robes blanches qui volent quand elles dansent. Au moins deux séances d'Hatha-yoga et de sanskrit par jour sont inclues dans le prix. Le programme du week-end doit être payé en sus, mais il en vaut la peine. Quand des stars, comme Ruth Lauer-Manenti du centre new-yorkais Jivamukti, enseignent, les élèves, en nage et les yeux brillants, la suivent en titubant jusque dans l'eau. Pendant d'autres week-ends, sous la sur-veillance rigoureuse de Joan Suval, il est interdit de parler et, une semaine plus tard, tous se tordent de rire des heures durant dans l'atelier du rire de Laraaji Nadananda. La fine fleur de la scène ésotérique new-yorkaise fait régulièrement irruption ici, et les adeptes viennent de toute la côte est pour se retrouver avec eux-mêmes dans ce cadre idyllique de montagnes entre forêts profondes et torrents sauvages. Car, malgré l'interdiction d'alcool et de tabac, et teinté de nostalgie, règne surtout le souffle de la révélation et chaque hôte est accueilli chaleureusement dans la communauté hippie sans cesse renouvelée.

Livres à emporter : « The Textbook of Yoga Psychology » de Rammurti S. Mishra et « Glamorama » de Bret Easton Ellis.

ANREISE	Etwa 1,5 Std. nördlich von New York.		ACCÈS	Situé à environ 1 h 30 au nord de New York.
YOGA	Hatha, Kundalini, Jivamukti.		YOGA	Hatha, Kundalini, Jivamukti.
GASTLEHRER	Sharon Gannon, David Life, Dharma Mittra, Sharon Salzberg, Krishna Das, Jai Uttal.		PROFESSEURS	Sharon Gannon, David Life, Dharma Mittra, Sharon Salzberg, Krishna Das, Jai Uttal.
ZIMMER	3 Gästehäuser mit insgesamt 45 Betten.		CHAMBRES	3 maisons d'hôtes avec en tout 45 lits.
KÜCHE	Überwiegend vegan, fantastisches Frühstücksbüfett.		RESTAURATION	Essentiellement végétalienne, fantastique buffet de petit-déjeuner avec papaye fraîche, porridge de fenouil.
ANWENDUNGEN	Ayurvedische Facials und Massagen, Schwedische Massage, Shiatsu, Akupunktur, Fußreflexzonen-Massage, Aromatherapie, Raindrop Technique, Entspannungstraining, Eukalyptus-Sauna.		TRAITEMENTS	Soins du visage et massage ayurvédiques, massage suédois, shiatsu, acupuncture, aromathérapie, Raindrop Technique, sauna à l'eucalyptus.
FREIZEIT	Meditation, Kathak-Tanz, Wandern, Schwimmen, Unterricht in Tabla und Sitar.		ACTIVITÉS	Méditation, danse kathak, randonnées, natation, cours de tablâ et de sitar.

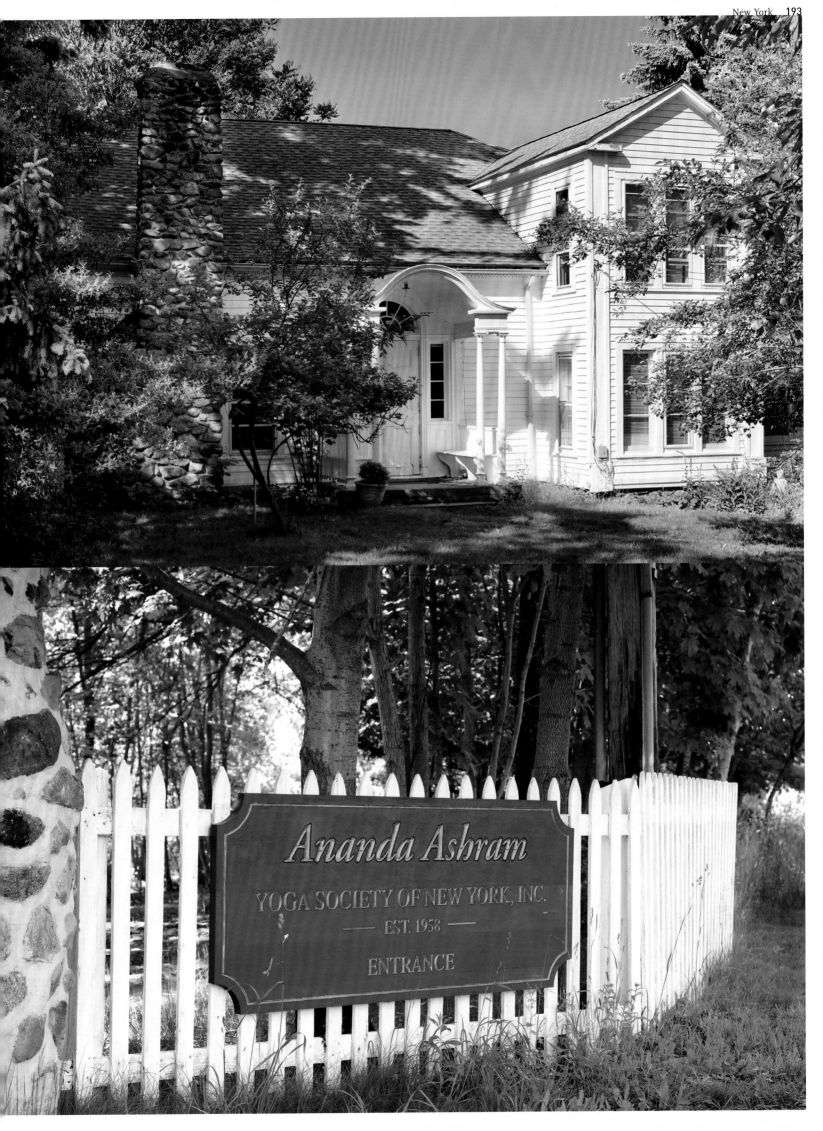

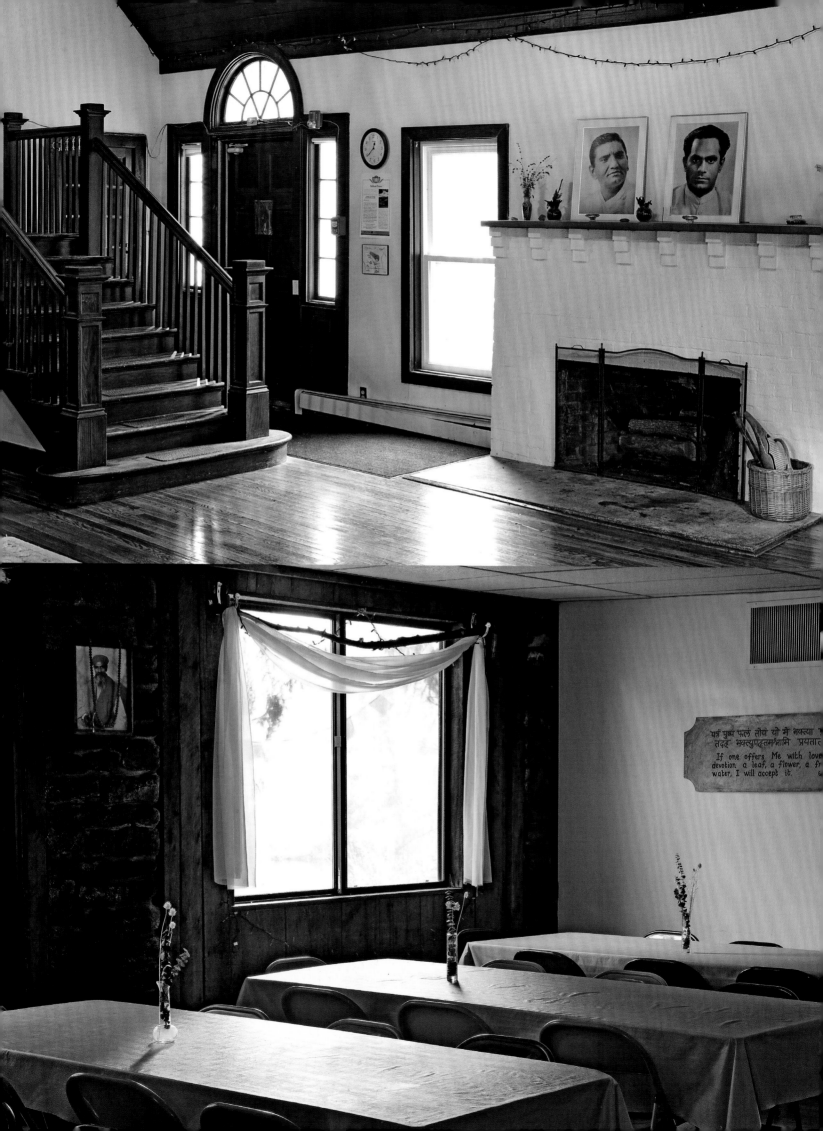

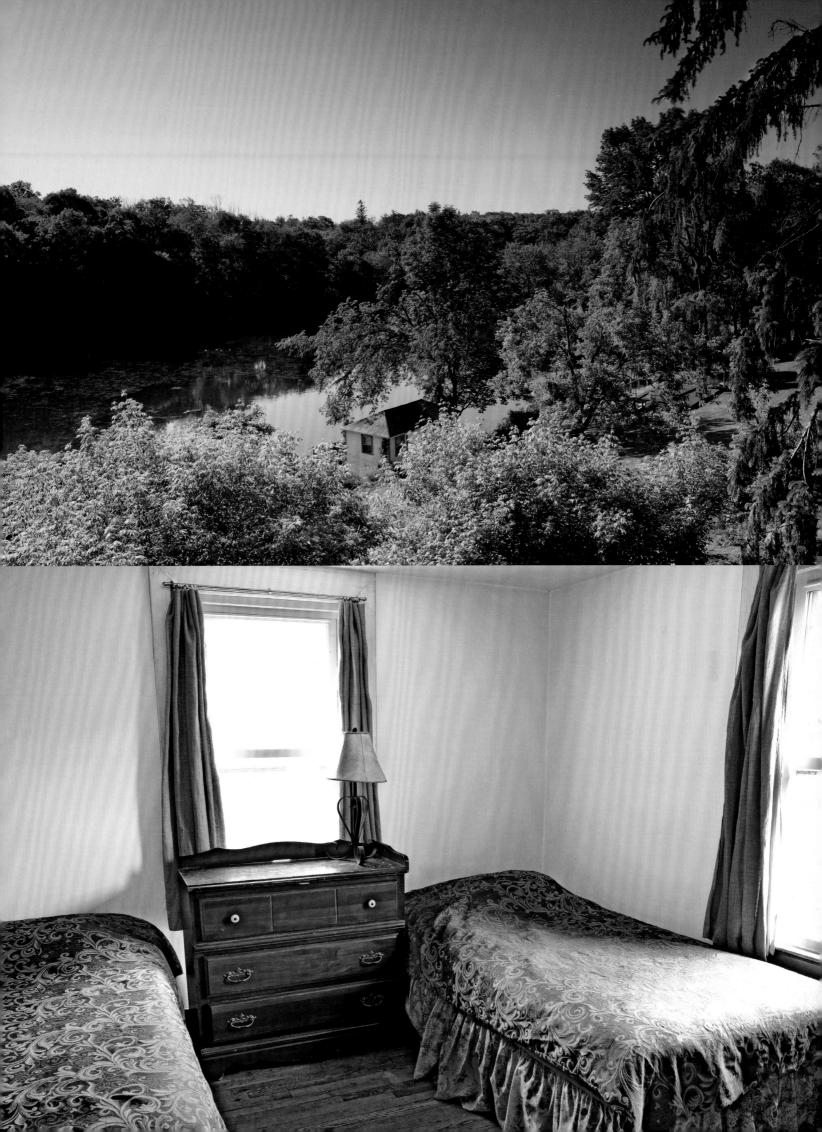

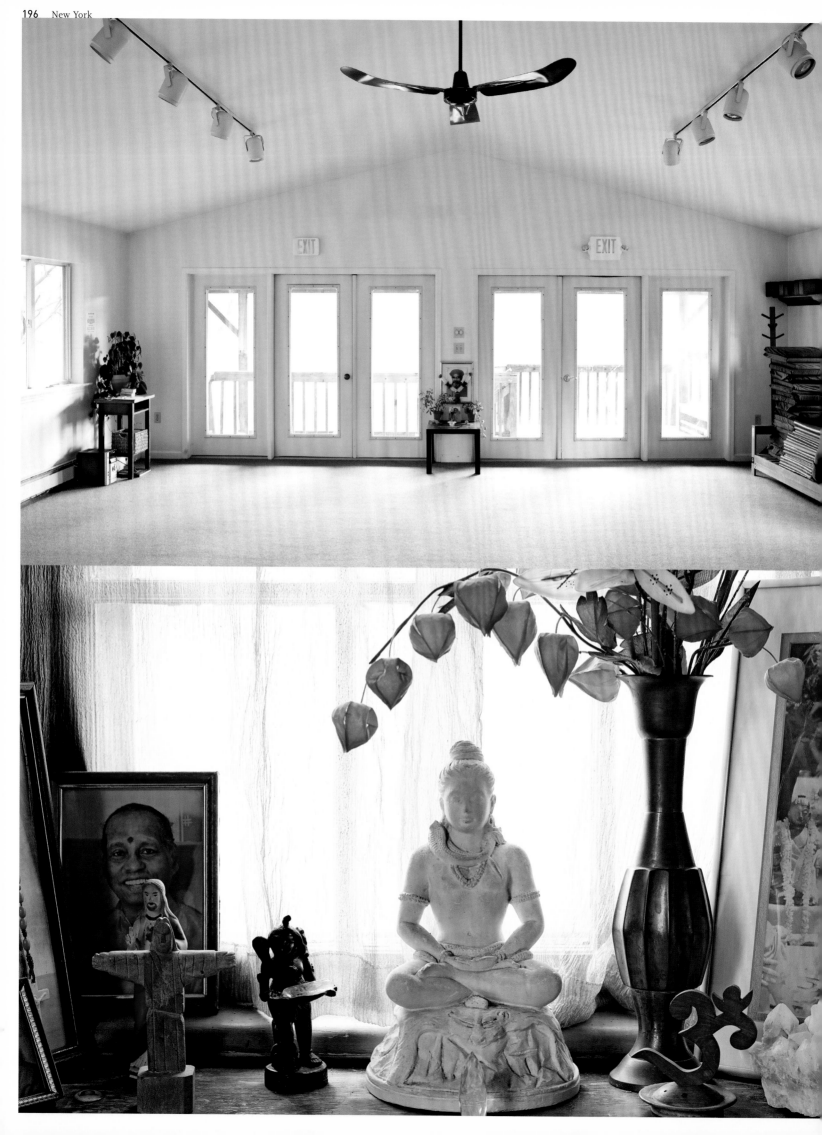

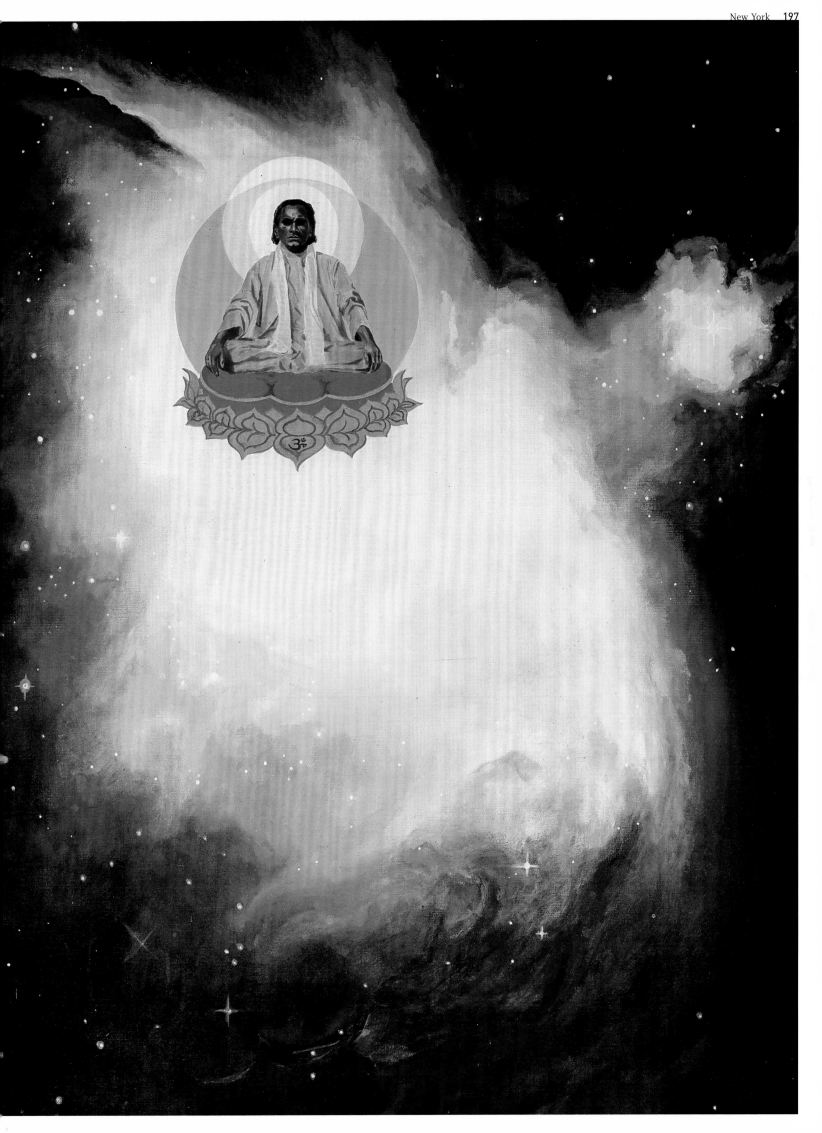

Yoga on the Ponderosa

Heathen Hill Yoga, Catskill Mountains

Heathen Hill Yoga, Catskill Mountains

Yoga on the Ponderosa

What happens when a former revue girl from Las Vegas, in her own opinion too old to become a cowgirl or an astronaut, becomes a Yoga teacher just doesn't bear thinking about. After her legendary morning sessions in New York's "OM" Yoga centre Susan "Lip" Orem decided to go freelance, painted a house in the country lilac and invited her teachers. Since then, stars of the New York Yoga scene like Genny Kapuler and Rodney Yee have been holding highly sought-after, familial workshops here, in which the "Susan Sarandon of Yoga" still serves her own blueberry pancakes with bacon on a Sunday and likes to open a bottle of red wine in the evenings. Delightful little rooms with names such as "Ponderosa", "Westwing" or "Betty Ford Clinic", a wild garden with a maze and a pond that has been left to nature serve to underline the individual understatement of this retreat. Only the excellently appointed Yoga room gives away something about the outstanding quality of the Yoga taught here without the customary pathos but instead with plenty of dry humour. Where else can you spend a weekend hidden away in Delaware County practising Yoga and tasting wine with characters straight out of a Woody Allen film?

Books to pack: "When Things Fall Apart" by Pema Chödrön and "The Art of Happiness" by the Dalai Lama.

Heathen Hill Yoga	
810 Heathen Hill Road	
Franklin, NY 13775	
USA	
Tel. +1 607 829 5328	
info@heathenhillyoga.net	
www.heathenhillyoga.net	

DIRECTIONS	About 150 miles northwest of Manhattan, in the heart of the northern Catskill Mountains. A 3-hr drive from Manhattan; next airport Albany.
YOGA	Hatha, Ashtanga, Vinyasa, Iyengar.
TEACHERS	Rodney Yee, Genny Kapuler.
ROOMS	2 single rooms, 5 2-bed rooms, camping.
FOOD	Grown on site; eggs from Heathen Hill hens.
RECREATION	Hot tub, swimming, badminton, bocce, hula hoops, hiking.

Yoga auf der Ponderosa

Nicht auszudenken, was passiert, wenn ein ehemaliges
Revue-Girl aus Las Vegas, nach eigenen Aussagen zu alt,
um Cowgirl oder Astronaut zu werden, Yogalehrerin wird.
Nach ihren legendären Vormittagsstunden im New Yorker
Yogacenter »OM« beschloss Susan »Lip« Orem, sich selbst-
ständig zu machen, strich ein Haus auf dem Land lila an
und lud ihre Lehrer ein. Seitdem halten hier Stars der New
Yorker Yogaszene wie Genny Kapuler und Rodney Yee heiß
begehrte, familiäre Workshops ab, bei denen die »Susan
Sarandon des Yoga« sonntags noch immer eigenhändig
Blaubeerpfannkuchen mit Speck serviert und abends gerne
eine Flasche Rotwein öffnet. Entzückende kleine Zimmer
mit dem Namen »Ponderosa«, »Westwing« oder »Betty Ford
Clinic«, ein wilder Labyrinthgarten und ein naturbelassener
Teich unterstreichen das individuelle Understatement dieses
Retreats. Nur der erstklassig ausgerüstete Yogaraum verrät
etwas über die herausragende Qualität des Yoga, das hier
ohne das übliche Pathos, dafür mit viel trockenem Humor
unterrichtet wird. Wo sonst kann man an einem Wochen-
ende versteckt in Delaware County mit Charakteren wie aus
einem Woody-Allen-Film »Yoga und Wine Tasting« machen?
Buchtipps: »Wenn alles zusammenbricht« von Pema Chödrön
und »Die Regeln des Glücks« des Dalai Lama.

Faire du yoga à Ponderosa

Que croyez-vous qu'il arrive lorsqu'une ancienne danseuse
de revue de Las Vegas, se jugeant trop vieille pour devenir
cow-girl ou astronaute, devient professeur de yoga ? Après
avoir donné les légendaires séances du matin au centre de
yoga new-yorkais « OM », Susan « Lip » Orem décida de se
mettre à son compte, repeignit une maison de campagne en
violet et invita ses professeurs. Depuis, des stars du yoga
new-yorkais comme Genny Kapuler und Rodney Yee organi-
sent des stages conviviaux et fort prisés au cours desquels la
« Susan Sarandon du yoga » sert en personne, le dimanche,
ses crêpes aux myrtilles et lardons, débouchant volontiers une
bouteille de vin rouge le soir. D'adorables petites chambres
aux noms de « Ponderosa », « Westwing » ou encore « Betty
Ford Clinic », un jardin-labyrinthe romantique et un étang
laissé dans son état naturel soulignent le caractère individuel
de ce lieu de méditation. Seule la salle de yoga, dotée d'un
équipement haut de gamme, laisse deviner la qualité excep-
tionnelle du yoga enseigné ici, sans le pathos habituel mais
avec une bonne portion d'humour pince-sans-rire. Où sinon
ici peut-on le temps d'un week-end, bien caché, s'adonner au
« Yoga and Wine Tasting » (yoga et dégustation de vin) avec
des personnages tout droit sortis d'un film de Woody Allen ?
Livres à emporter : « Quand tout s'effondre » de Pema Chödrön
et « L'Art du bonheur » du Dalaï Lama.

ANREISE	Etwa 250 km nordwestlich von Manhattan im Herzen der nördlichen Catskill Mountains. 3 Std. Fahrzeit von Manhattan, nächster Flugplatz Albany.
YOGA	Hatha, Astanga, Vinyasa, Iyengar.
GASTLEHRER	Rodney Yee, Genny Kapuler.
ZIMMER	2 Einzelzimmer, 5 Zweibettzimmer, Camping.
KÜCHE	Aus eigenem Anbau, Eier von Heathen-Hill-Hühnern.
FREIZEIT	Hot Tub, Schwimmen, Badminton, Boccia, Hula-Hoops, Wandern.

ACCÈS	Situé à environ 250 km au nord-ouest de Manhattan au cœur des montagnes Catskill. A 3 h de route de Manhattan, l'aéroport le plus proche est Albany.
YOGA	Hatha, Ashtânga, Vinyasa, Iyengar.
PROFESSEURS	Rodney Yee, Genny Kapuler.
CHAMBRES	2 chambres simples, 5 chambres à deux lits, camping.
RESTAURATION	Produits cultivés sur place, œufs des poules d'Heathen Hill.
ACTIVITÉS	Bain tourbillon, natation, badminton, boules, hula hoop, randonnées.

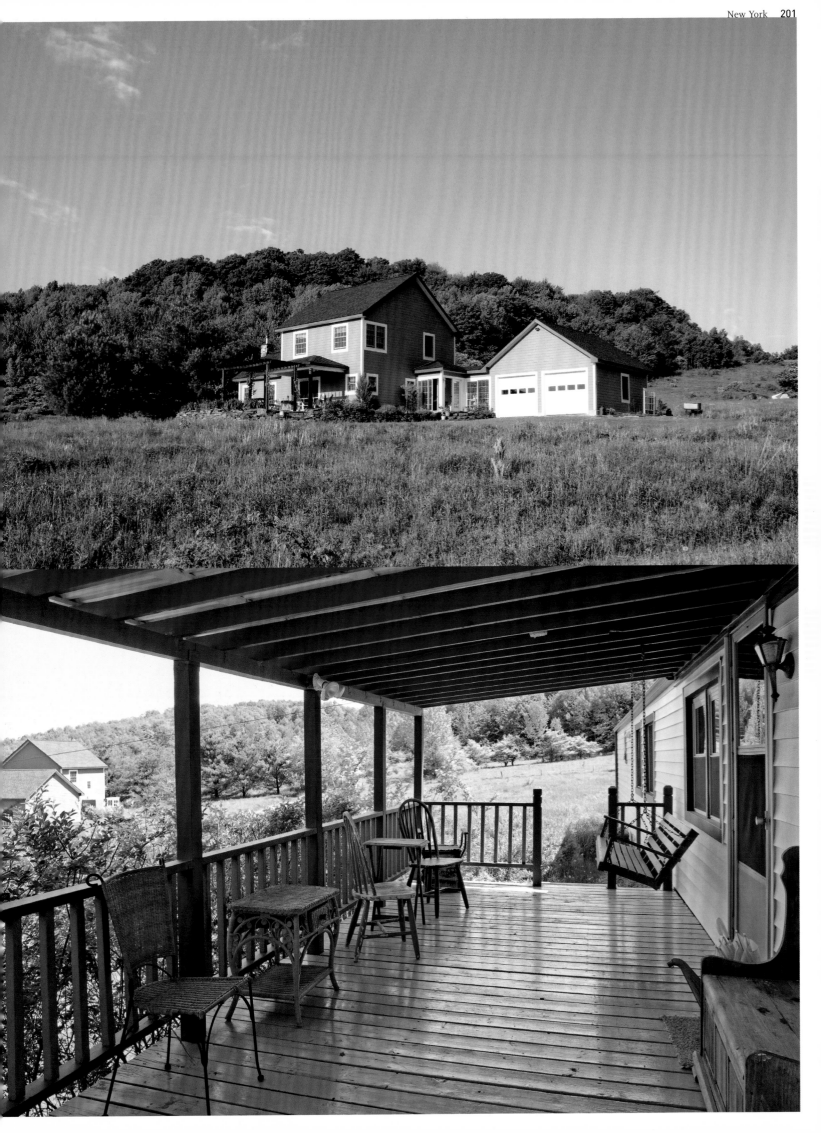

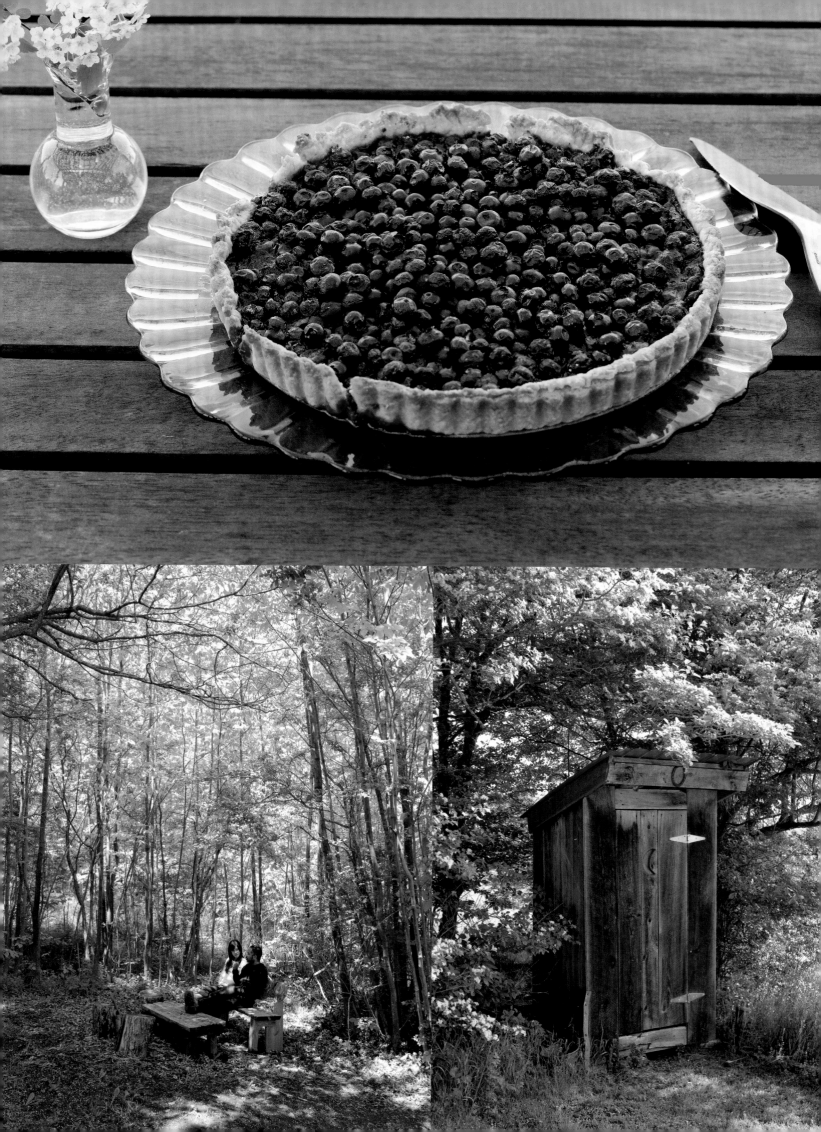

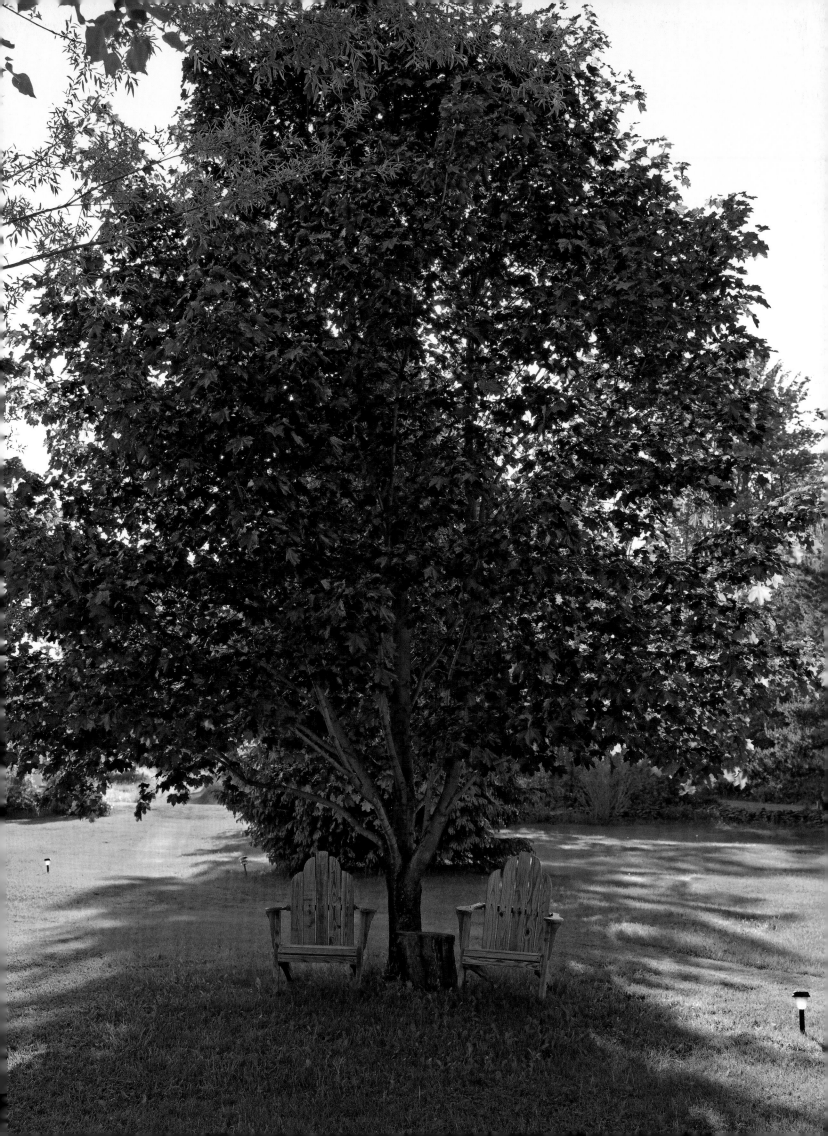

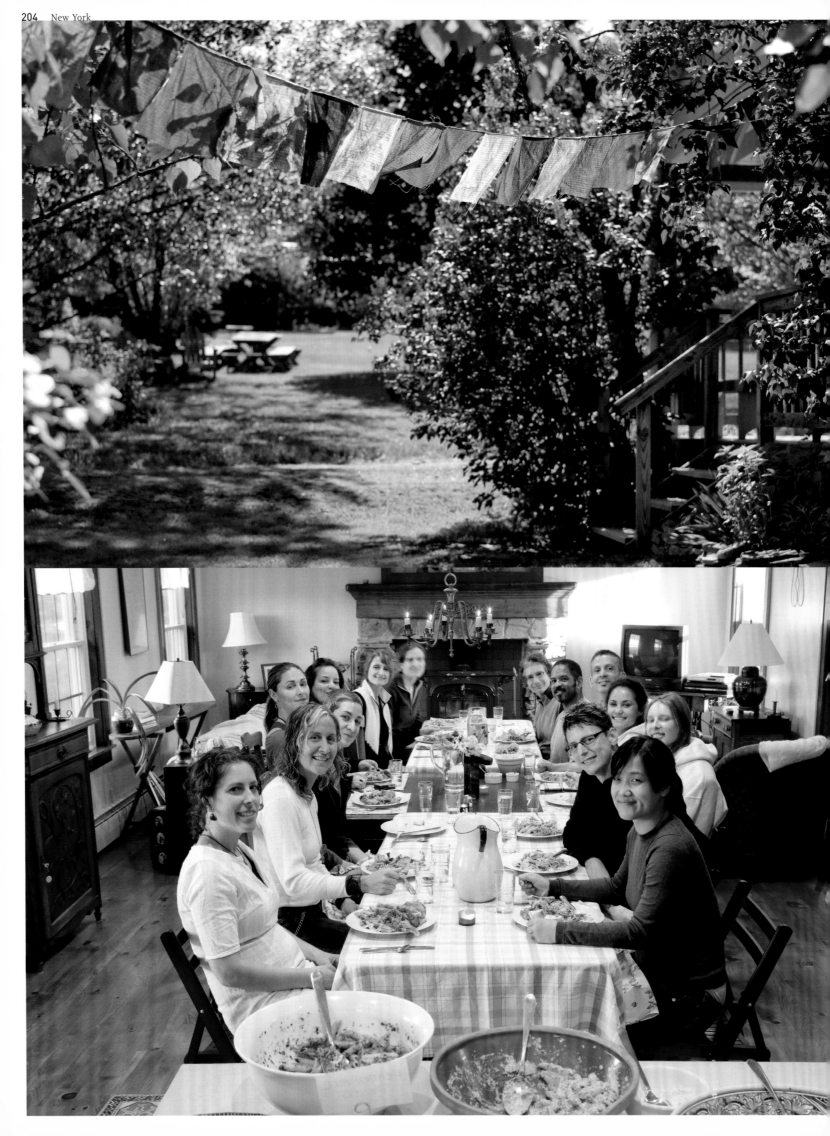

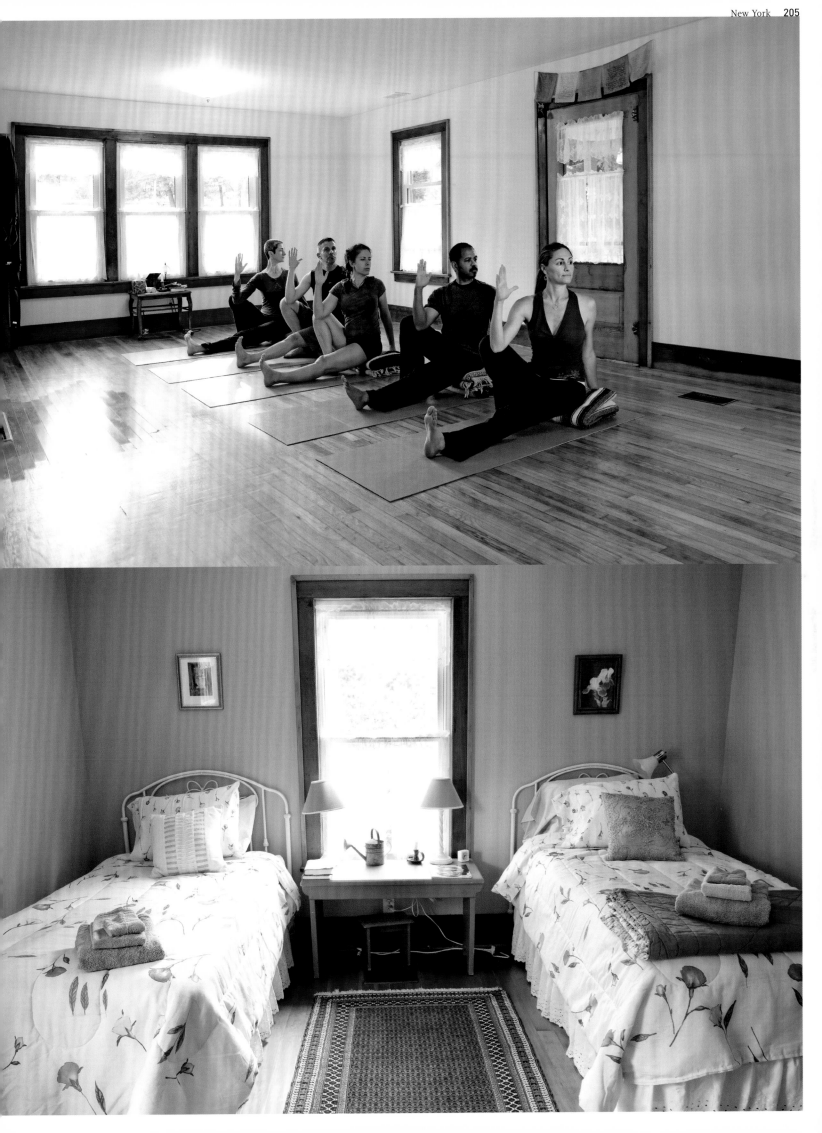

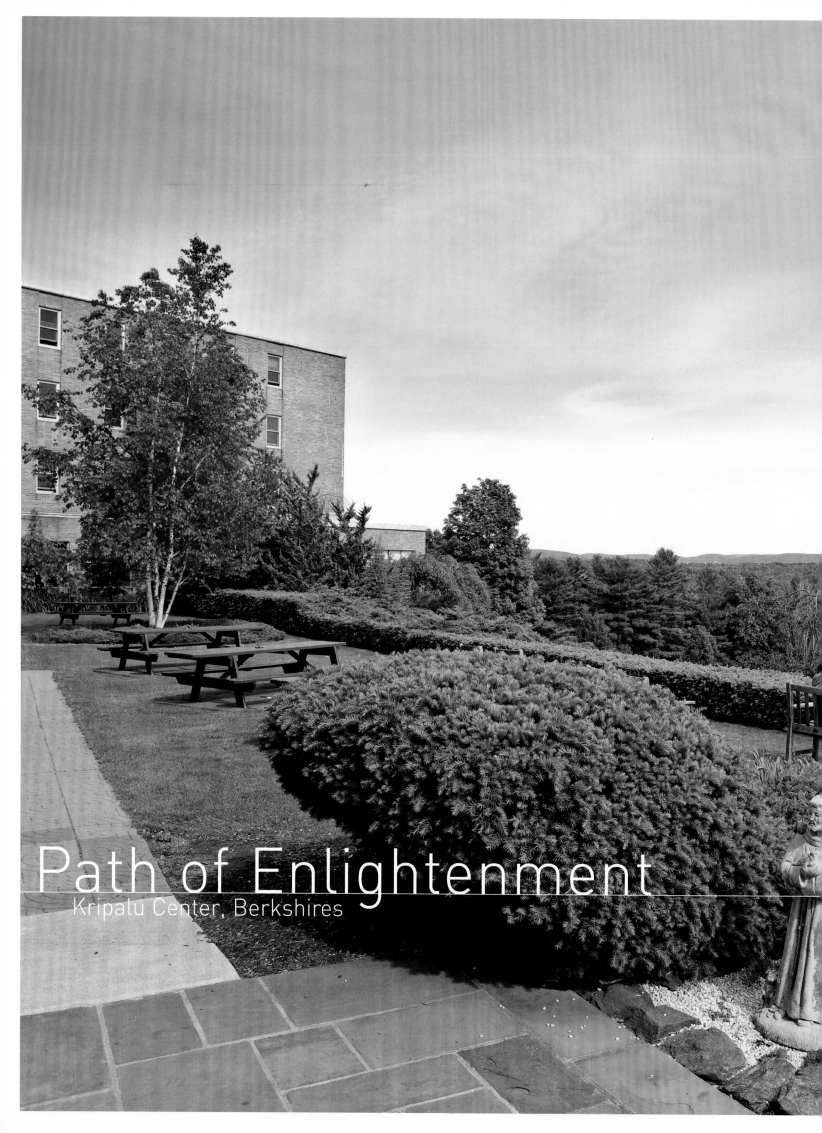

Path of Enlightenment

Kripalu Center, Berkshires

Kripalu Center, Berkshires

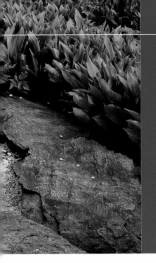

Path of Enlightenment
In Sanskrit, Kripalu means compassionate, and you can indeed feel some sympathy for those who have to choose just one of the countless workshops in the Center for Yoga and Health. Every year over 10,000 guests come to this brick complex, built by Jesuits in the charming meadows of the Berkshires. It may not be easy to decide upon the right path to enlightenment, but at this New Age university you can at least be sure that the courses on offer undergo careful scrutiny. Almost 90 per cent of those who wish to teach here are turned down. Yogi Amrit Desai, who founded the institution in 1966, failed spectacularly to live up to his own requirement for celibacy and had to take his leave of the campus; but his successors are distinctly more tolerant of worldly weaknesses and even allow the use of laptops in the café. The rich breakfast buffet, on the other hand, is so heavenly that it is a real pleasure to abide by the rules to the letter, and enjoy it in total silence.
Books to pack: "On Love and Loneliness" by Jiddu Krishnamurti and "The Road to Wellville" by T. C. Boyle.

Kripalu Center	
P.O. Box 309	
Stockbridge, MA 01262	
USA	
Tel. +1 866 200 5203	
Fax +1 413 448 3384	
guestservices@kripalu.org	
www.kripalu.org	

DIRECTIONS	About 150 miles north of New York, 45 min away from Albany Airport. Airport transfer by arrangement. Charter buses from Penn Station New York City.
YOGA	Hatha, Ashtanga, Sivananda, Iyengar, Anusara, Vinyasa, Kripalu.
TEACHERS	Edward Clark, Krishna Das, Ana Forrest, David Frawley, Amy Ippoliti, Tias Little, Ethan Nichtern, Sarah Powers, Shiva Rea, Robert Thurman, Patricia Walden.
ROOMS	Dormitory, double and single rooms for max. 475 guests.
FOOD	Regional, organic whole foods.
TREATMENTS	More than 30 different healing therapies.
RECREATION	Swimming, hiking, Yoga training courses, massage courses.

Pfad der Erleuchtung

Kripalu bedeutet auf Sanskrit barmherzig, und Mitleid kann man tatsächlich mit denen bekommen, die eine Wahl unter den unzähligen Workshops des Center für Yoga und Gesundheit treffen müssen. Über 10.000 Gäste kommen pro Jahr in diesen Backsteinkomplex, den Jesuiten 1957 in die lieblichen Wiesen der Berkshires bauten. Es ist nicht einfach, sich für den richtigen Weg zur Erleuchtung zu entscheiden, aber an dieser New-Age-Universität darf man zumindest sicher sein, dass das Angebot sorgfältig überprüft wird. Fast 90 Prozent derer, die hier unterrichten wollen, werden abgelehnt. Yogi Amrit Desai, der die Einrichtung 1966 gründete, scheiterte spektakulär am eigenen Anspruch aufs Zölibat und musste den Campus verlassen, dafür sind die Nachfolger nun deutlich toleranter gegenüber weltlichen Schwächen und erlauben sogar die Benutzung von Laptops im Café. Das reichhaltige Frühstücksbüfett ist dagegen so himmlisch, dass es geradezu ein Vergnügen ist, es ganz nach Vorschrift schweigend einzunehmen.

Buchtipps: »Über die Liebe« von Jiddu Krishnamurti und »Willkommen in Wellville« von T. C. Boyle.

La voie de la révélation

Kripalu signifie « charitable » en sanskrit et l'on peut, en effet, être pris de pitié pour ceux qui doivent choisir l'un des innombrables stages de ce centre yoga-santé. Plus de 10 000 visiteurs viennent chaque année dans ce complexe construit en briques par des jésuites, en 1957, dans les prairies ondoyantes du Berkshire. Il n'est certes pas aisé de choisir la voie qui mène à la révélation, mais à cette université du New Age l'on peut être au moins certain que le choix proposé fait l'objet d'un examen minutieux. Presque 90 pour cent des personnes désirant enseigner ici sont refusées. Le yogi Amrit Desai, fondateur de cette institution en 1966, se heurta avec fracas à sa propre exigence de célibat et dut quitter le campus, alors que ses successeurs, eux, font preuve d'une tolérance manifeste vis-à-vis des faiblesses humaines et autorisent même l'utilisation d'ordinateurs portables au café. En revanche, le buffet du petit-déjeuner est si divin que c'est un réel plaisir de le prendre en silence, comme le veut la règle.

Livres à emporter : « De l'amour et de la solitude » de Jiddu Krishnamurti et « Aux bons soins du docteur Kellogg » de T. C. Boyle.

ANREISE	Etwa 250 km nördlich von New York, 45 min vom Flughafen Albany.	ACCÈS	Situé à environ 250 km au nord de New York. A 45 min de l'aéroport d'Albany.
YOGA	Hatha, Astanga, Sivananda, Iyengar, Anusara, Vinyasa, Kripalu.	YOGA	Hatha, Ashtânga, Shivananda, Iyengar, Anusara, Vinyasa, Kripalu.
GASTLEHRER	Edward Clark, Krishna Das, Ana Forrest, David Frawley, Amy Ippoliti, Tias Little, Ethan Nichtern, Sarah Powers, Shiva Rea, Robert Thurman, Patricia Walden.	PROFESSEURS	Edward Clark, Krishna Das, Ana Forrest, David Frawley, Amy Ippoliti, Tias Little, Ethan Nichtern, Sarah Powers, Shiva Rea, Robert Thurman, Patricia Walden.
ZIMMER	Schlafsaal, Doppel- und Einzelzimmer für max. 475 Gäste.	CHAMBRES	Dortoirs, chambres doubles et simples pour 475 personnes max.
KÜCHE	Regional-biologische Vollwertküche.	RESTAURATION	Cuisine bio et régionale aux aliments complets.
ANWENDUNGEN	Mehr als 30 verschiedene Heiltherapien.	TRAITEMENTS	Plus de 30 soins thérapeutiques différents.
FREIZEIT	Schwimmen, Wandern, Massagekurse.	ACTIVITÉS	Natation, randonnées, cours de massage.

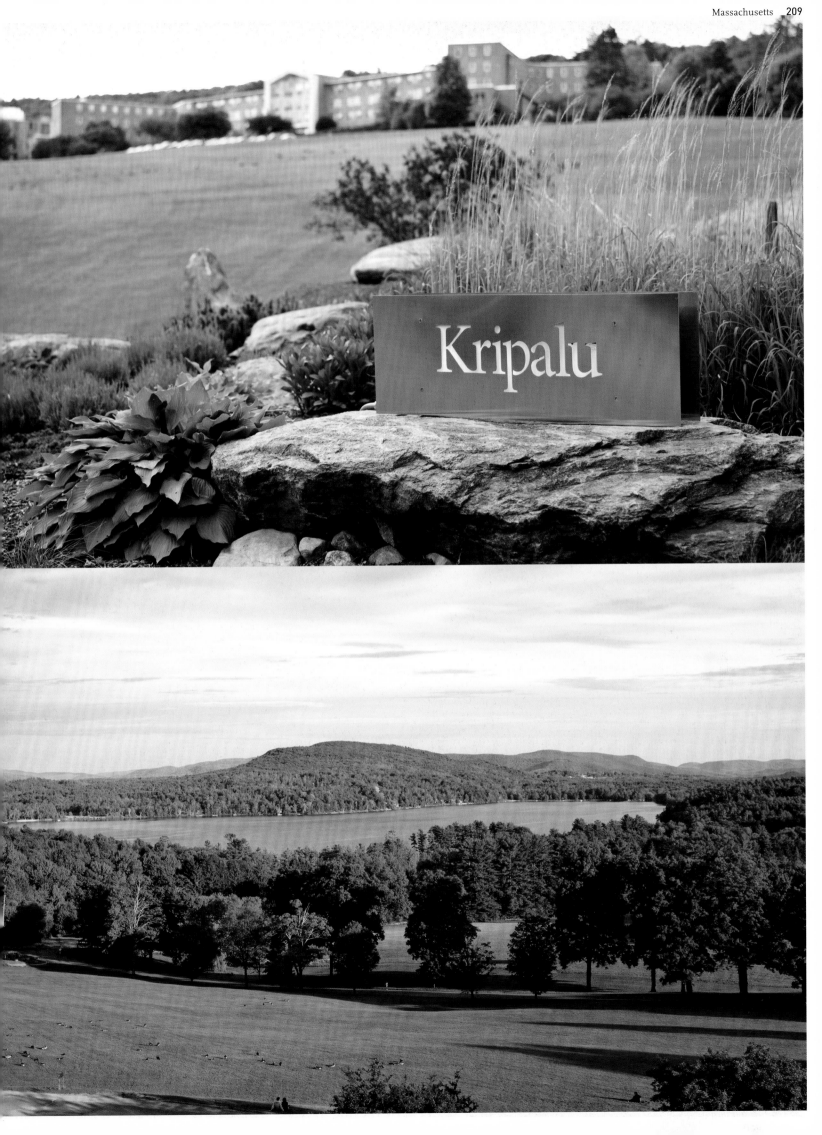

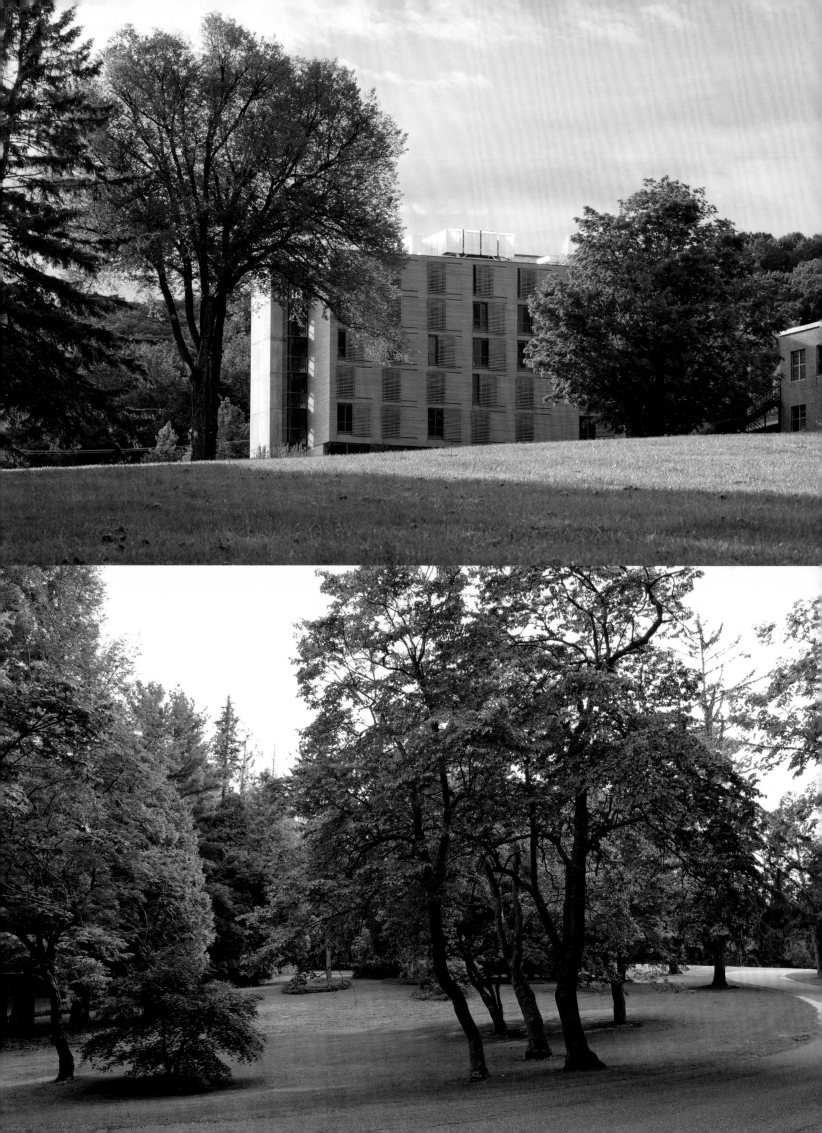

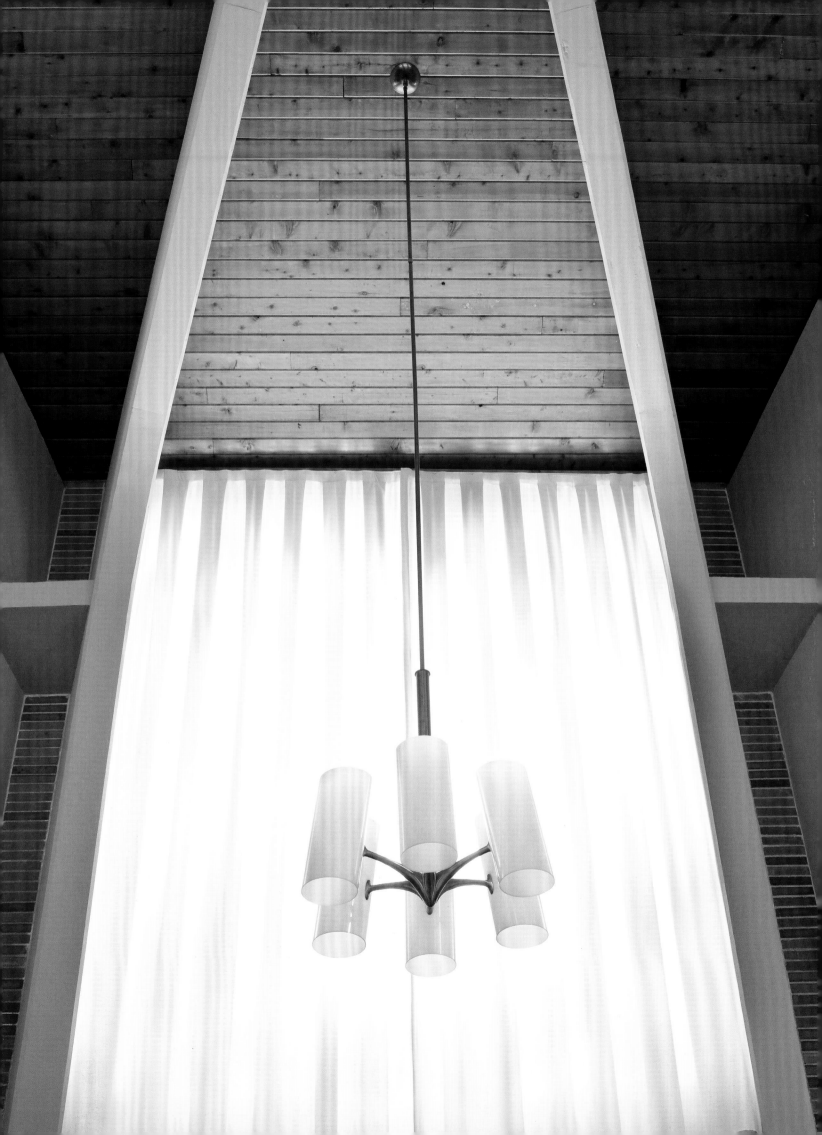

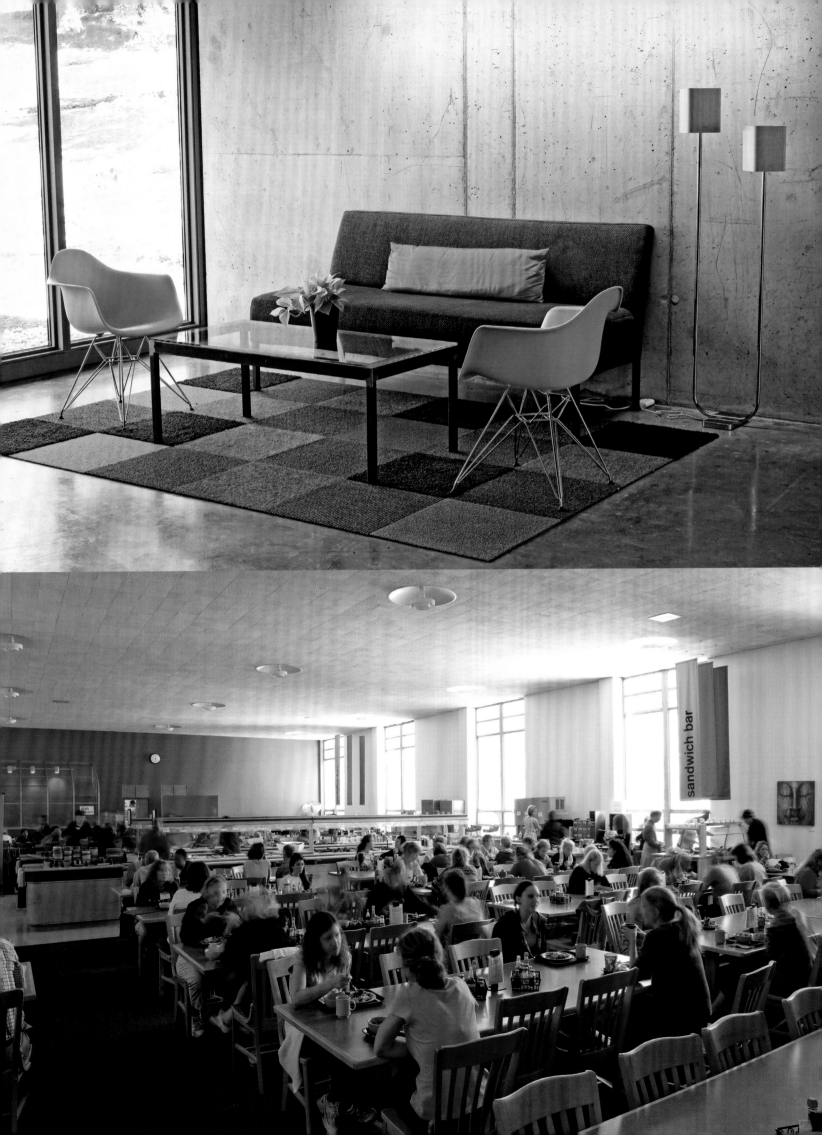

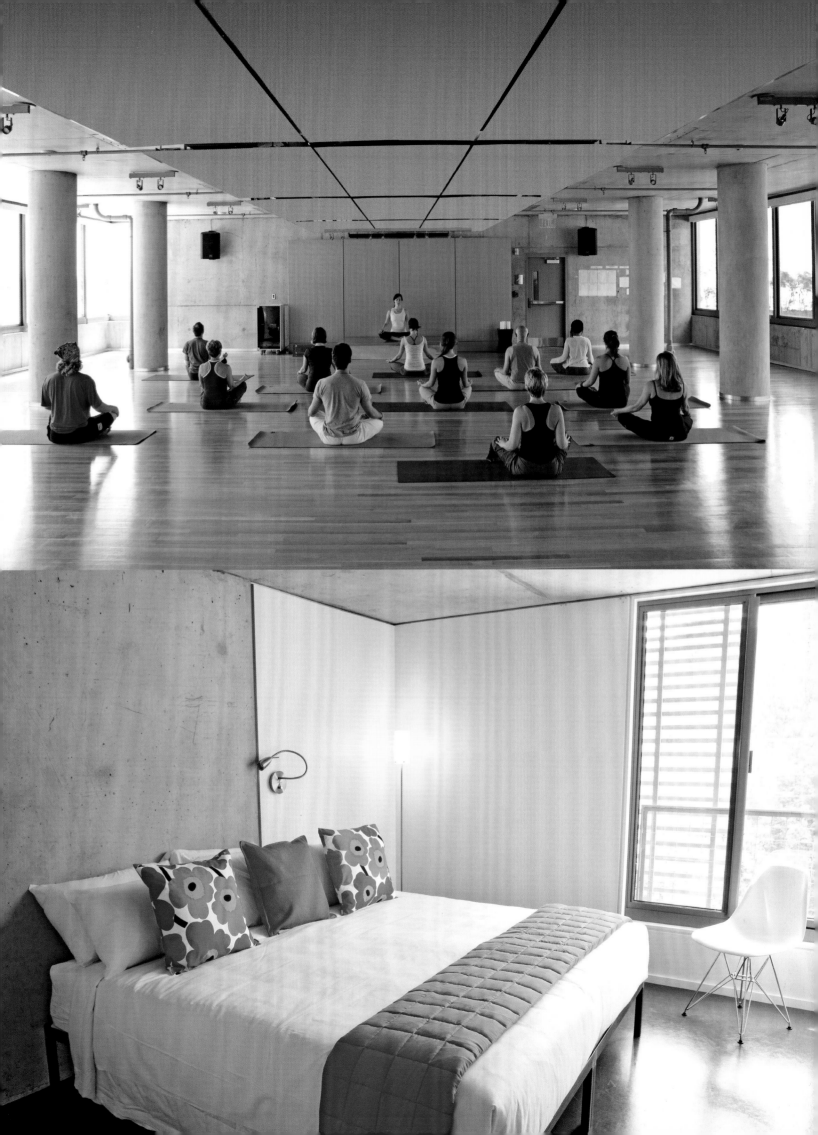

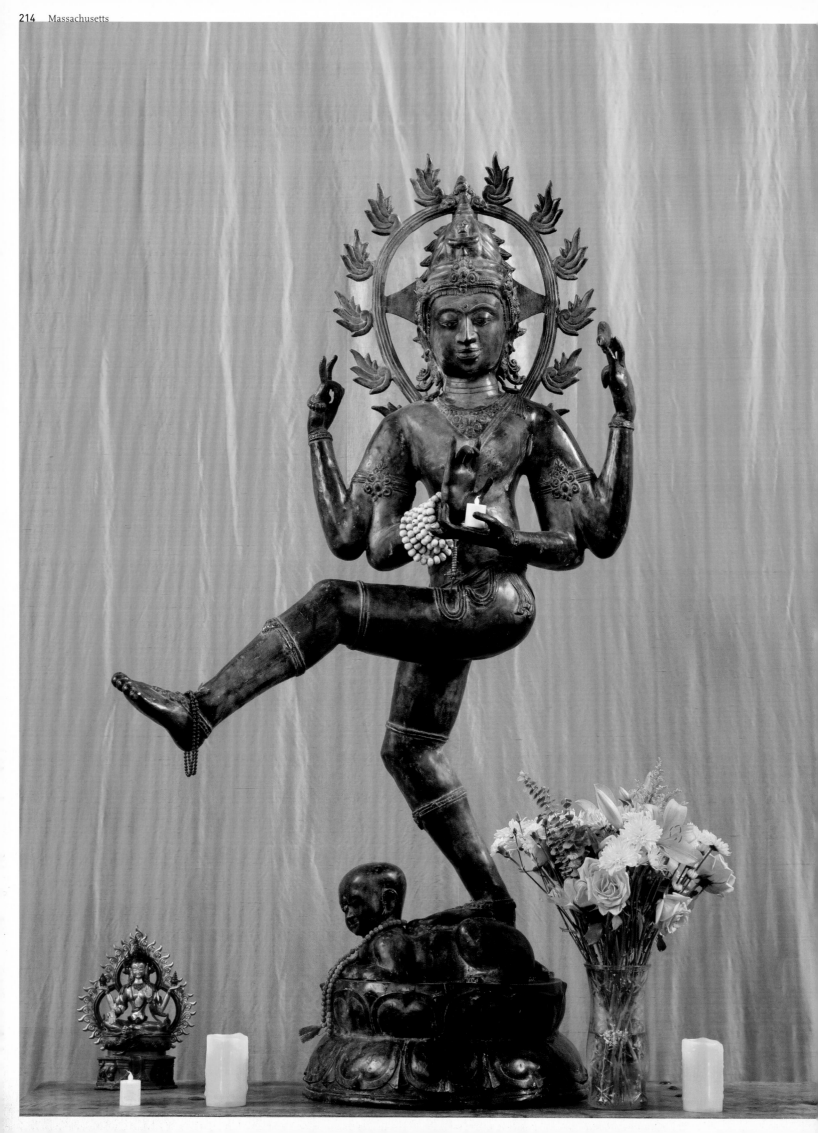

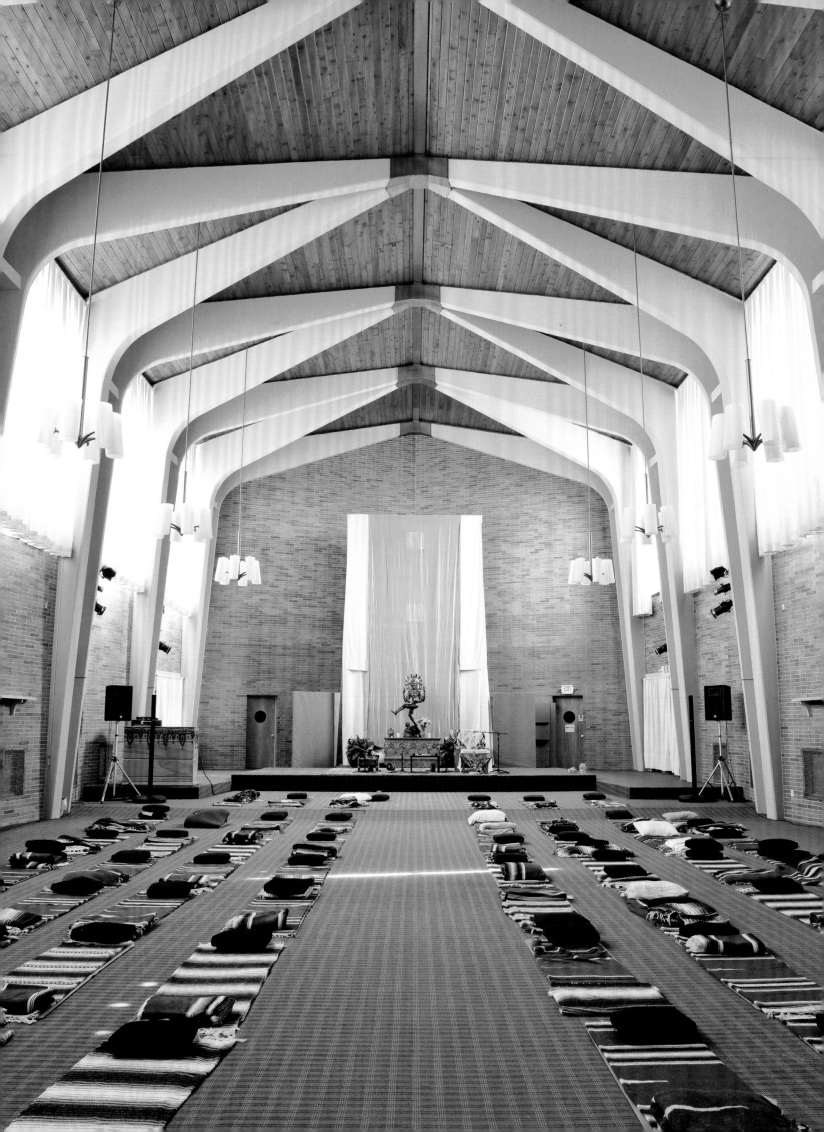

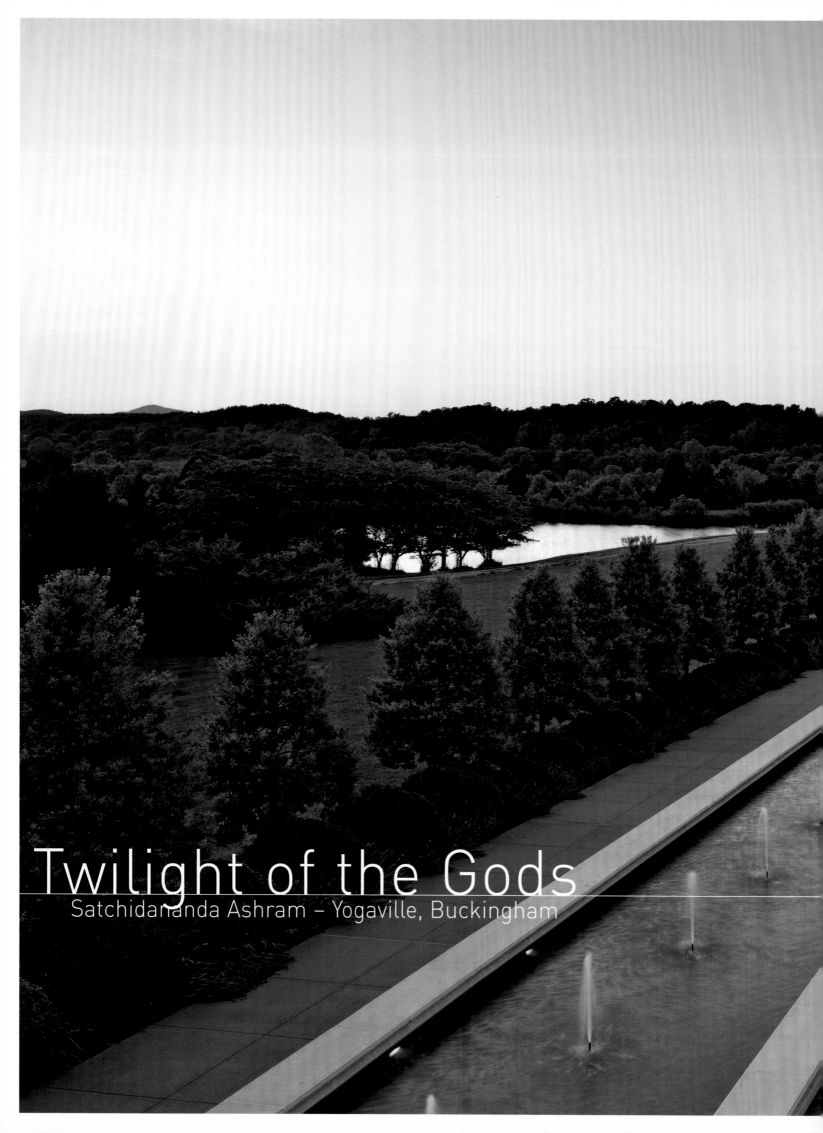

Twilight of the Gods
Satchidananda Ashram – Yogaville, Buckingham

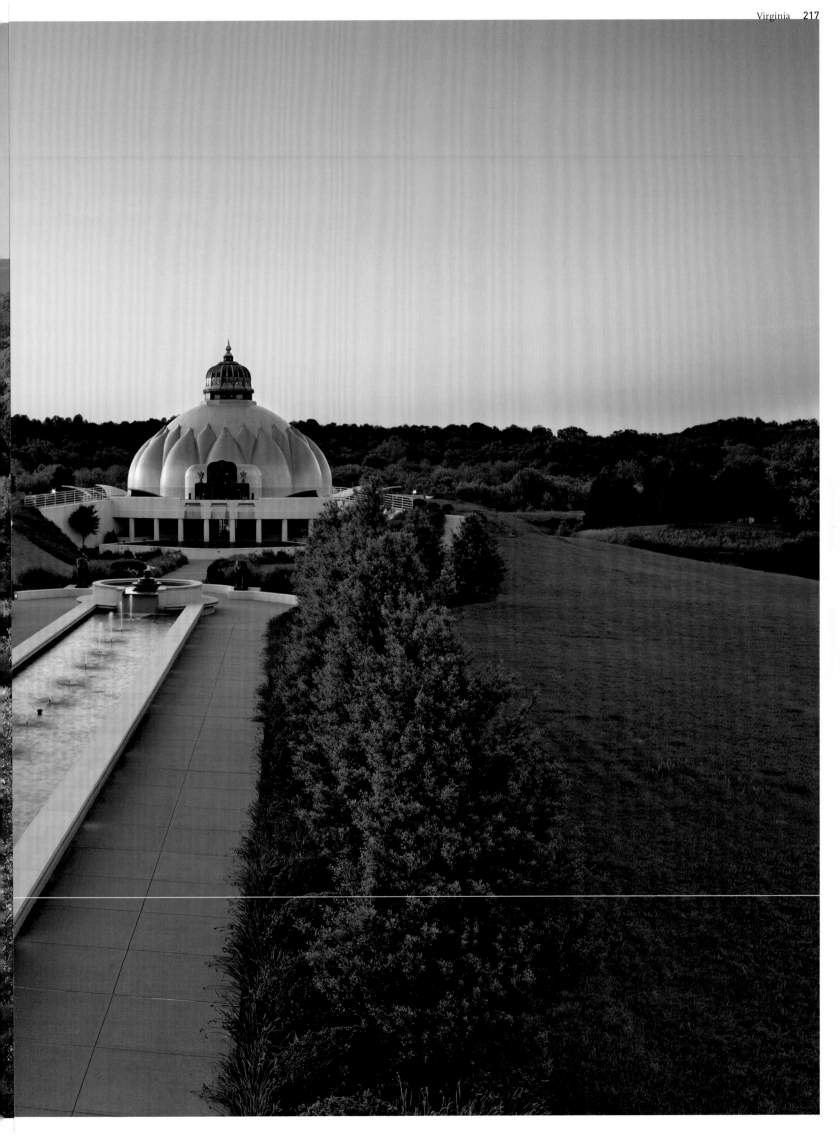

Götterdämmerung

Die bewährte Mischung verschiedener Yoga-Methoden, Integral Yoga genannt, hat sich ein Mann ausgedacht: Swami Satchidananda, der damit in kürzester Zeit ein Star in der New Yorker Hippieszene wurde. 1969 flog man ihn mit einem Helikopter nach Woodstock, damit er das Festival segnete. Später spendierten ihm prominente Schüler wie Carole King, Jeff Goldblum, das Model Lauren Hutton und der Diät-Experte Dean Ornish sogar Land für seinen Ashram, in dessen Mitte ein ziemlicher Angebertempel in Form einer Lotosblüte thront. Neben einer Ausbildung zum Integral-Yogalehrer, kann man hier Workshops zum Thema Stressmanagement, Yoga und Skoliose, Tantrische Massage oder Freie Hüften buchen, einfach nur die täglichen Hatha-Yogaklassen besuchen oder am Memorial Weekend mit Krishna Das singen. Swami Satchidananda, von seinen Anhängern als heilig verehrt, mag einen wertvollen Cadillac und einen kirschroten Rolls Royce gefahren und die Verehrung blütenbehängter Schülerinnen nur zu gern zugelassen haben: Yogaville ist dennoch der Eiffelturm unter den Ashrams in den USA. Die Integrität und der weltweite Erfolg von Integral Yoga lassen Beschwerden außerdem kleinlich erscheinen. Mick Jagger wirft ja auch niemand vor, Lippenstift zu benutzen.

Buchtipps: »Sei, was du bist!« von Ramana Maharshi und »Zehn Wahrheiten« von Miranda July.

Le crépuscule des dieux

C'est un certain Swami Satchidananda qui a imaginé l'association très probante de différentes méthodes de yoga, portant aussi le nom de yoga intégral, et devint ainsi en peu de temps une star de la scène hippie new-yorkaise. En 1969, on l'envoya par hélicoptère à Woodstock afin qu'il donne sa bénédiction au festival. Plus tard, des élèves très connus comme Carole King, Jeff Goldblum, le top-model Lauren Hutton et l'expert en diététique Dean Ornish lui offrirent même du terrain pour son âshram, au centre duquel trône, assez prétentieusement, un temple en forme de fleur de lotus. En plus d'une formation de professeur de yoga intégral, il est possible de s'inscrire à des stages aux thèmes tels que la maîtrise du stress, le yoga et la scoliose, les massages tantriques ou les hanches sans douleurs, de fréquenter simplement chaque jour les classes de Hatha-yoga ou de chanter avec Krishna Das pour célébrer le Memorial Day. Swami Satchidananda, qui est vénéré comme un saint par ses adeptes, peut bien avoir roulé en Cadillac de luxe et en Rolls Royce rouge cerise, avoir laissé avec un peu trop de complaisance ses admiratrices couvertes de fleurs exprimer leur adoration : Yogaville n'en est pas moins la tour Eiffel des âshrams américains. En outre, les plaintes semblent bien mesquines face à l'intégrité et au succès planétaire du yoga intégral. Après tout, on ne reproche pas à Mick Jagger de se mettre du rouge à lèvres.

Livres à emporter : « Sois ce que tu es ! » de Ramana Maharshi et « Un bref instant de romantisme » de Miranda July.

ANREISE	85 km südwestlich von Charlottesville und 300 km südwestlich von Washington, D.C.	
YOGA	Hatha, Restorative, Meditation, Yoga-Philosophie.	
GASTLEHRER	David Newman, Swami Karunananda, Swami Vidyananda, Manorama.	
ZIMMER	207 Betten in Doppel- und Mehrbettzimmern sowie Schlafsäle und 12 Zelte.	
KÜCHE	Überwiegend vegan, auf Wunsch Käse und Joghurt.	
ANWENDUNGEN	Ayurveda, Panchakarma, Alexander-Technik, Thai-Yoga-Massage, Myofascial Release, Shamanen-Heilung.	
FREIZEIT	Schwimmen, Wandern.	

ACCÈS	Situé à 85 km au sud-ouest de Charlottesville et à 300 km au sud-ouest de Washington D.C.
YOGA	Hatha, yoga restoratif, méditation, philosophie du yoga.
PROFESSEURS	David Newman, Swami Karunananda, Swami Vidyananda, Manorama.
CHAMBRES	207 lits dans des chambres doubles et à plusieurs lits, ainsi que des dortoirs et 12 tentes.
RESTAURATION	Essentiellement végétalienne, laitages sur demande.
TRAITEMENTS	Ayurveda, panchakarma, technique Alexander, massage de yoga thaïlandais, myofascial release, guérison de chaman.
ACTIVITÉS	Natation, randonnées.

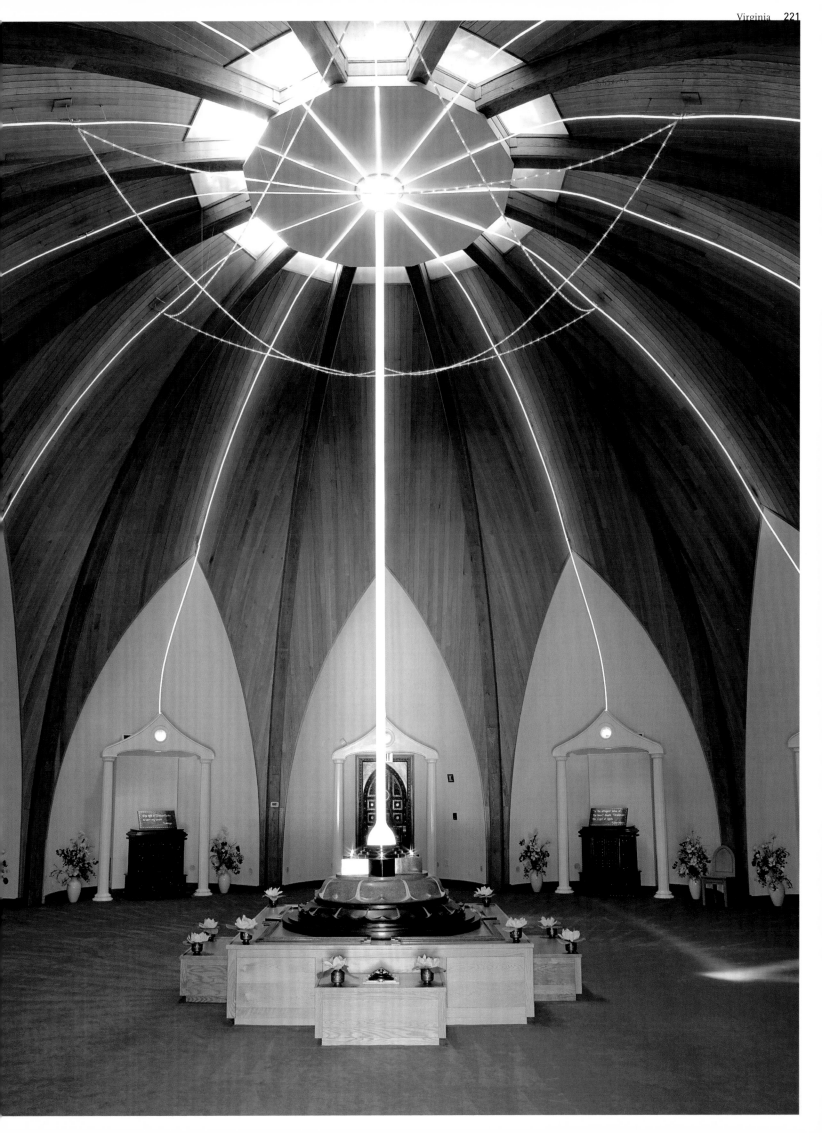

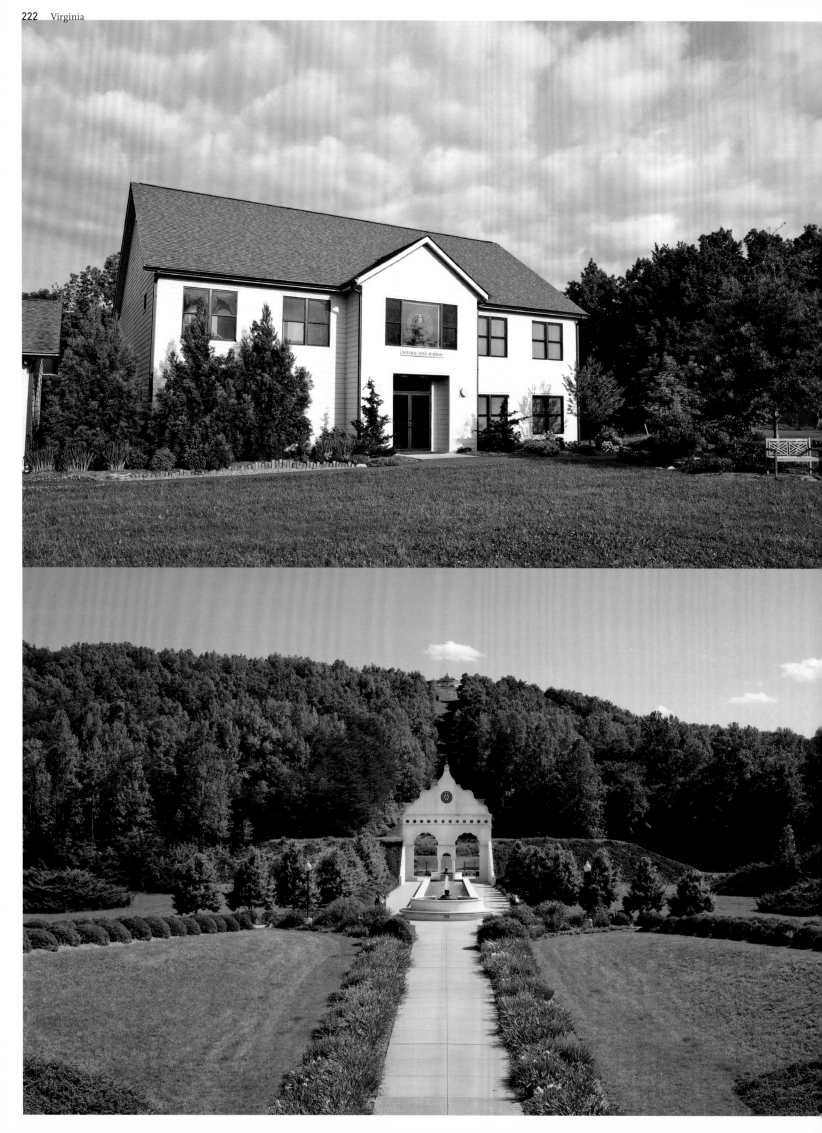

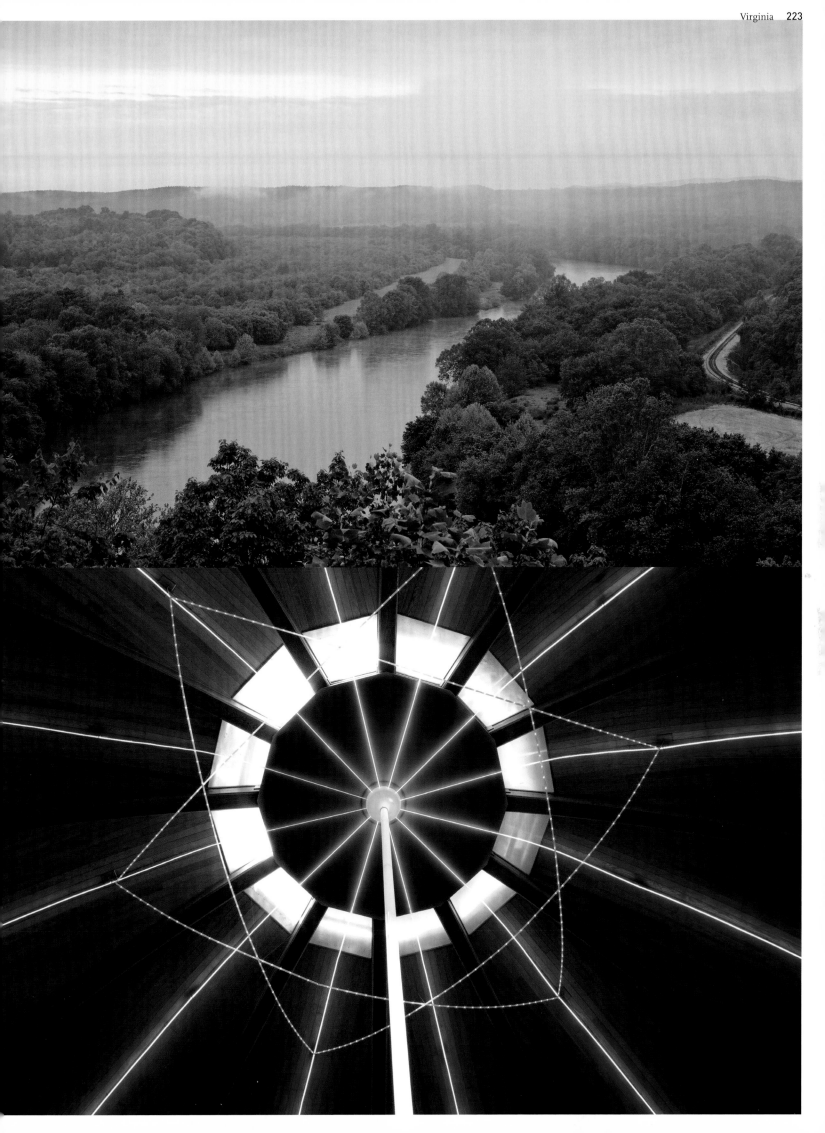

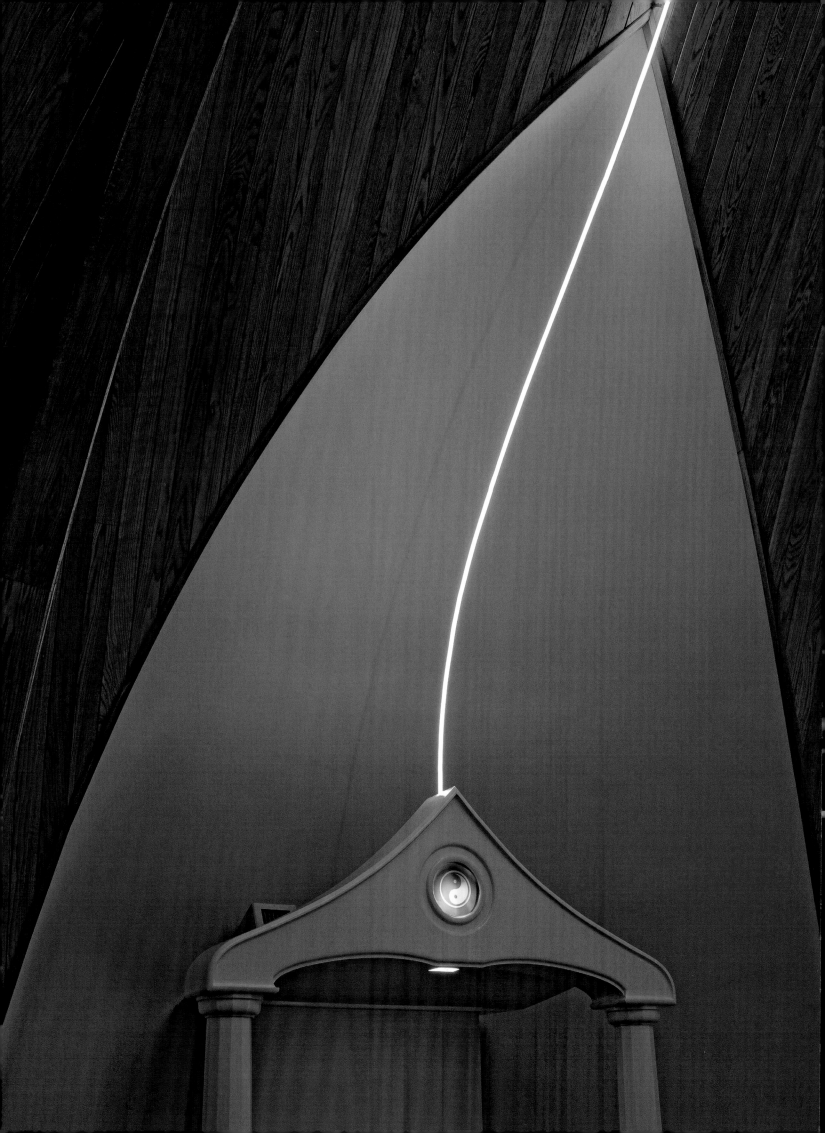

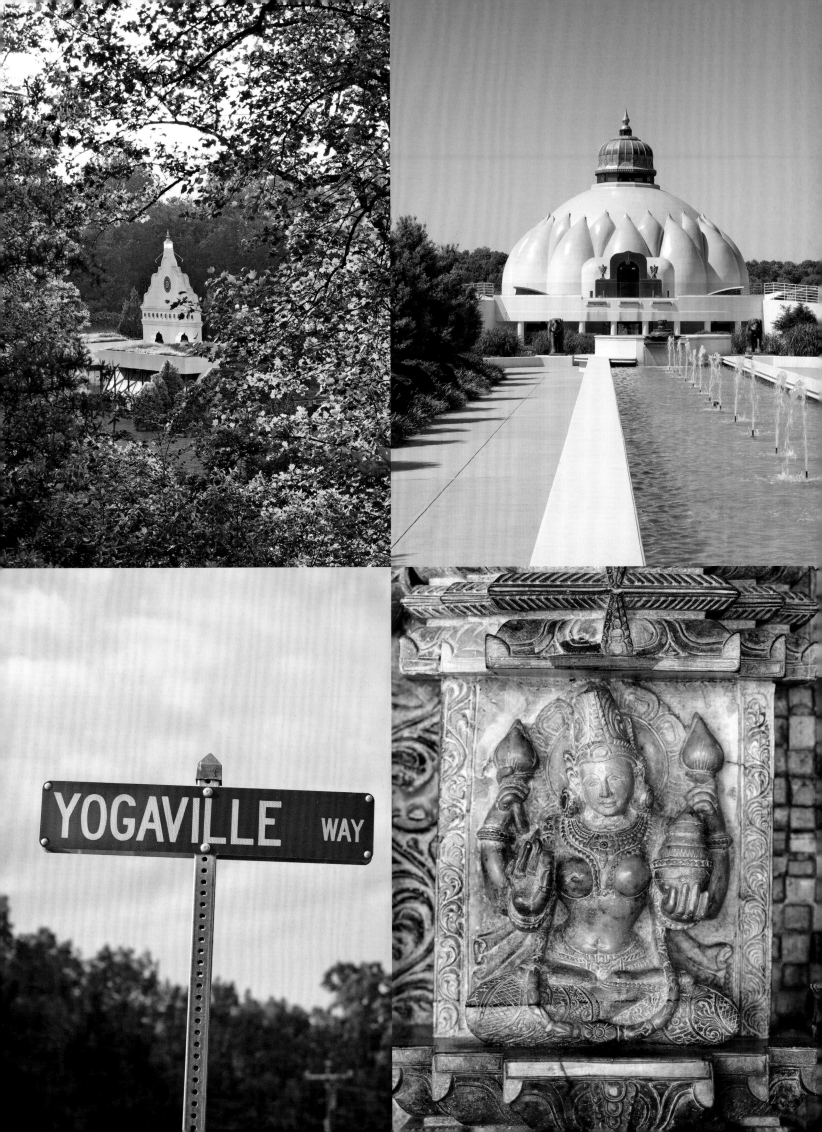

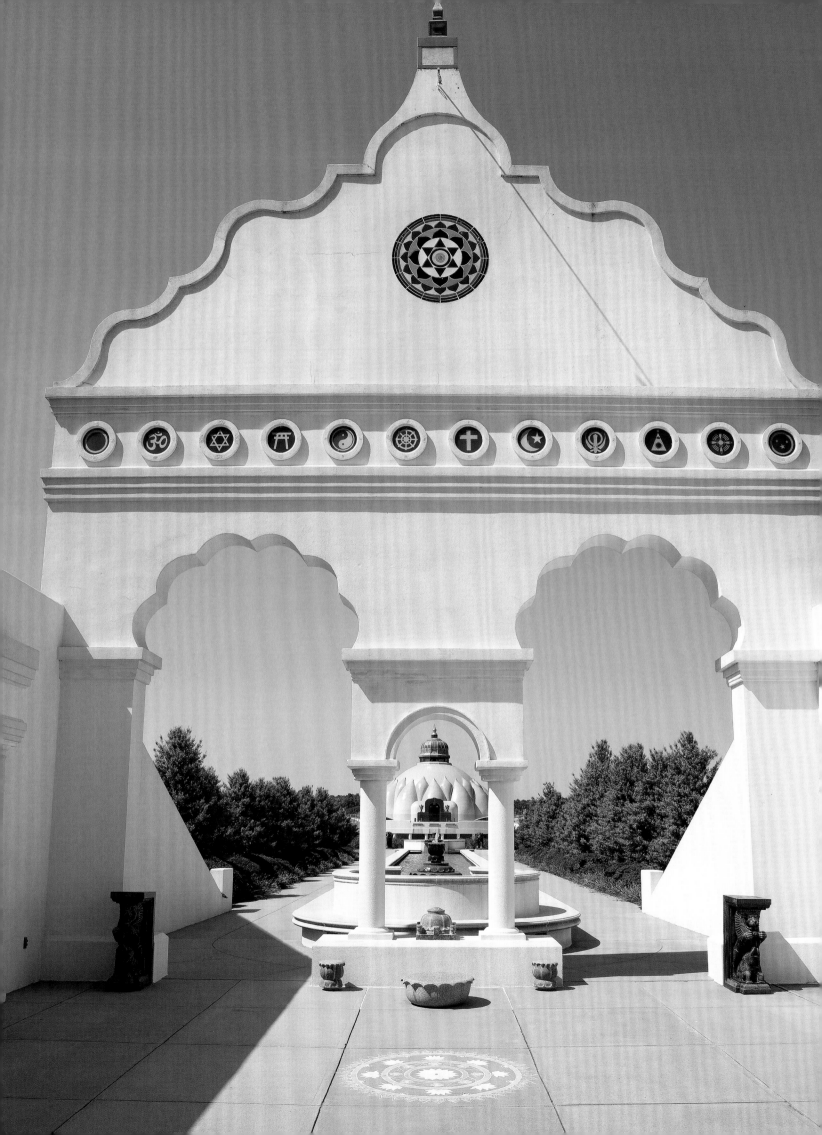

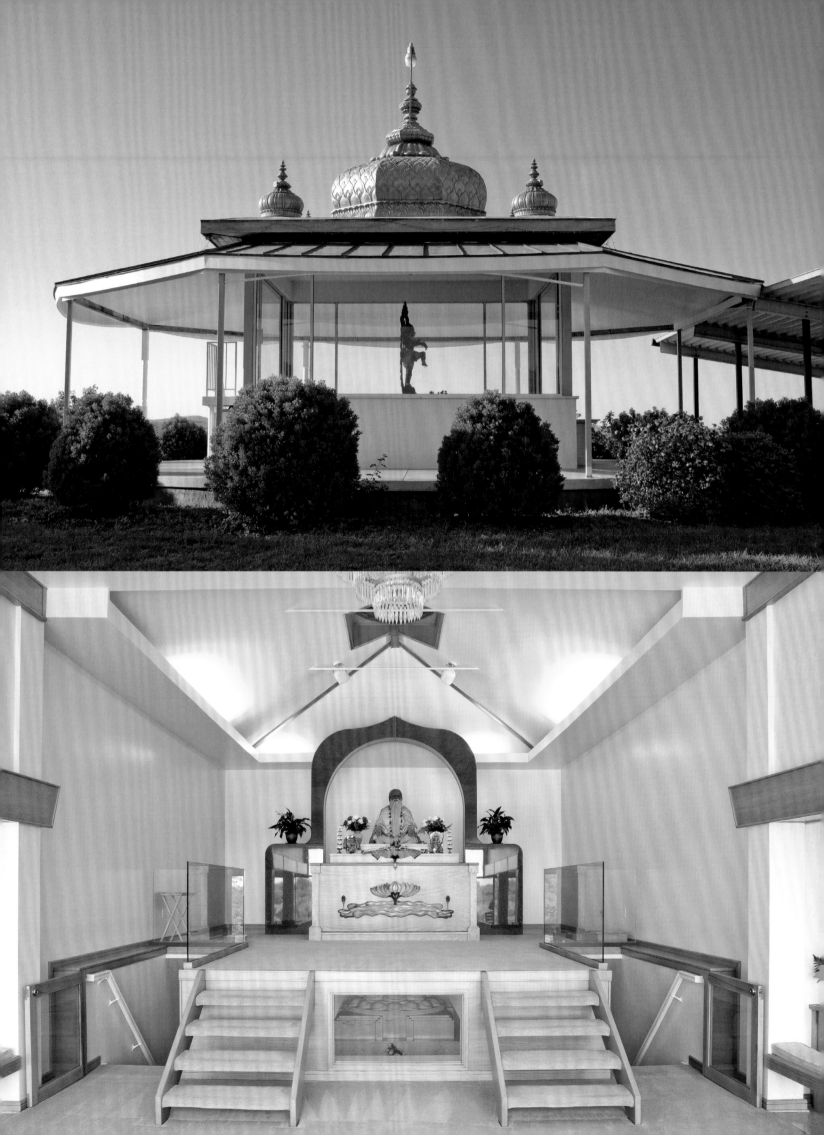

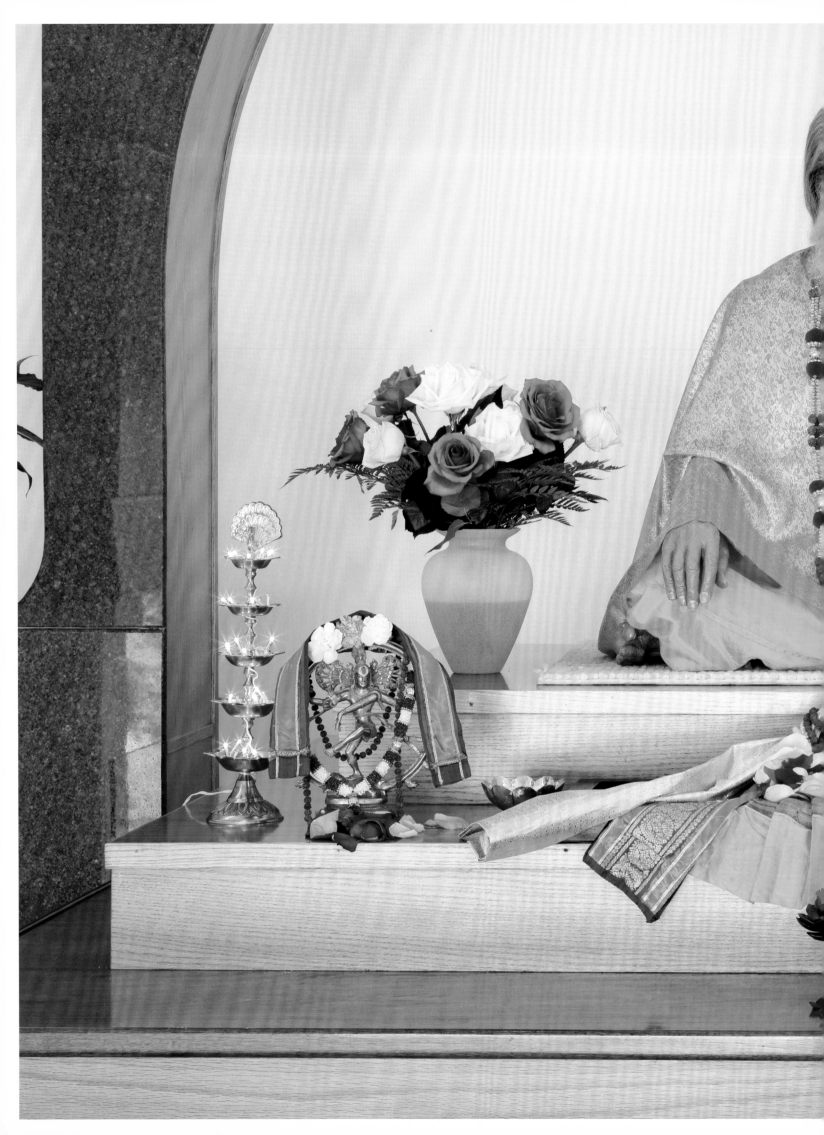

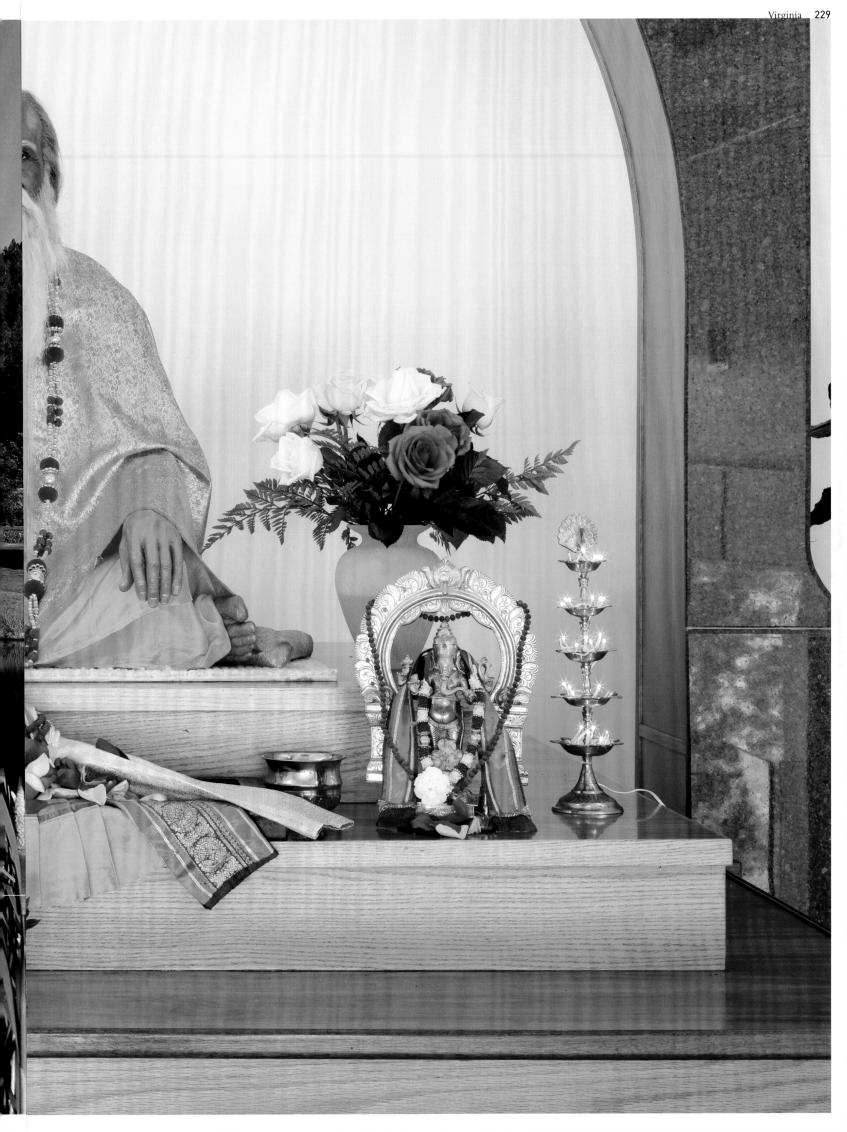

Yoga Bonanza

Yogastudios mögen mittlerweile so allgegenwärtig und etwa so exotisch sein wie Starbucks. Aber Adressen wie die Feathered Pipe Ranch, wo Yoga schon unterrichtet wurde, bevor es in Mode kam, erinnern daran, worauf es eigentlich ankommt. Man schläft in einfachen Blockhäusern, in gemütlich eingerichteten Tipis, Zelten oder Jurten, als Belohnung mag es eine tüchtige Massage geben oder ein Bad im Hot Tub. Aber die Hauptattraktion liegt in den intensiven Yogaklassen, die von den Besten des Landes unterrichtet werden, für Anfänger ebenso wie für Fortgeschrittene. Wenn sich nach einer Stunde Schwitzen im Chippewa-Cree-Wigwam gegen Abend Stille senkt auf die Wildwiesen zwischen den Montana Rockies, der Himmel sich bewölkt und ein kühler Wind aufweht, versteht man, was India Supera vor sich sah, als sie das alte Haus im Adirondack-Stil, von dem die Wiesen sanft zum See abfallen, 1975 von einem Hippiefreund erbte: einen Platz, der einen gestärkt, ruhig und klar wieder entlässt. Außerdem ist das Yogastudio mit seinen hohen Wänden und dem Kamin vermutlich das einzige in der Welt, das ein Elchkopf ziert.

Buchtipps: »Das Glück, einen Baum zu umarmen« von Thich Nhat Hanh und »Fresh Air Fiend« von Paul Theroux.

Yoga Bonanza

Même si les instituts de yoga sont maintenant aussi omniprésents et à peu près aussi exotiques que les cafés Starbucks, des adresses telles que le Feathered Pipe Ranch, où l'on enseignait le yoga bien avant qu'il devienne une mode, rappellent ce qui compte vraiment. On dort dans de simples fustes, dans des tipis, tentes ou yourtes agréablement aménagés et, comme récompense, il peut y avoir un bon massage ou un bain tourbillon. Mais l'attraction majeure, ce sont les cours intensifs de yoga, donnés par les meilleurs professeurs du pays, pour les débutants comme pour les yogis chevronnés. Lorsque, vers le soir, après avoir transpiré une heure durant dans un wigwam Chippewa-Cri, on voit la paix descendre sur les plaines sauvages qui se déploient entre les Rocheuses, le ciel se couvrir de nuages et une brise fraîche se lever, on comprend ce qu'India Supera découvrit quand, en 1975, elle hérita de la vieille maison de style Adirondack, d'où les prairies descendent en pente douce vers le lac : un endroit qui vous rend fort, calme et serein. De plus, l'institut de yoga, avec ses hauts murs et sa cheminée, est sans doute le seul au monde à être décoré d'une tête d'élan.

Livres à emporter : « La plénitude de l'instant » de Thich Nhat Hanh et « Fresh Air Fiend » de Paul Theroux.

ANREISE	Im Herzen der Montana Rockies, 25 km westlich vom Flughafen in Helena gelegen.
YOGA	Vinyasa, Iyengar, Anusara, Power Yoga, Restorative.
GASTLEHRER	Cora Wen, Cyndi Lee, David Nichtern, Marla Apt, Erich Schiffmann, Lilias Folan.
ZIMMER	4 Vierbettzimmer, 9 Doppelzimmer, 5 Jurten, 5 Tipis, 10 Zelte für max. 60 Gäste.
KÜCHE	Überwiegend biologisch-vegetarisch, gelegentlich Huhn und Fisch.
ANWENDUNGEN	Massage.
FREIZEIT	Schwimmen, Wandern, Kanu und Rudern.

ACCÈS	Situé au cœur des Rocheuses, à 25 km à l'ouest de l'aéroport de Helena.
YOGA	Vinyasa, Iyengar, Anusara, Power Yoga, yoga restoratif.
PROFESSEURS	Cora Wen, Cyndi Lee, David Nichtern, Marla Apt, Erich Schiffmann, Lilias Folan.
CHAMBRES	4 chambres à 4 lits, 9 chambres doubles, 5 yourtes, 5 tipis, 10 tentes pour 60 personnes max.
RESTAURATION	Essentiellement bio et végétarienne, occasionnellement poulet et poisson.
TRAITEMENTS	Massages.
ACTIVITÉS	Natation, randonnées, canoë et aviron.

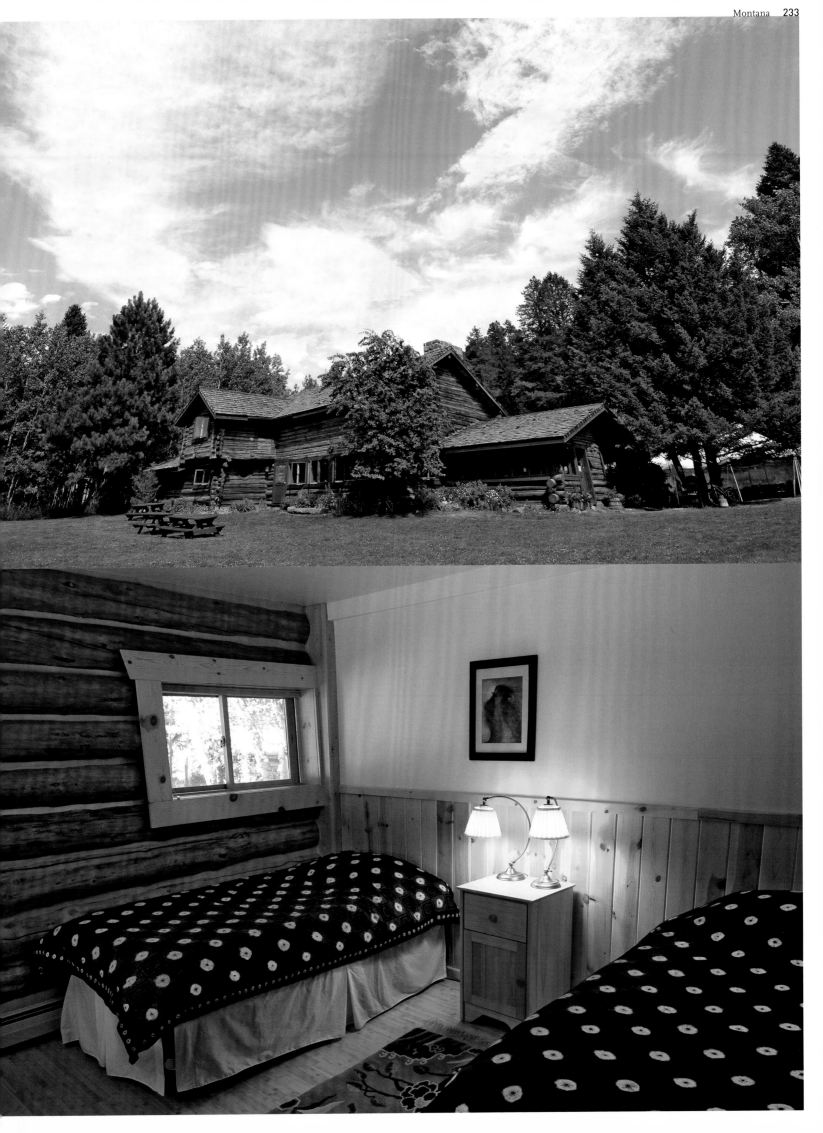

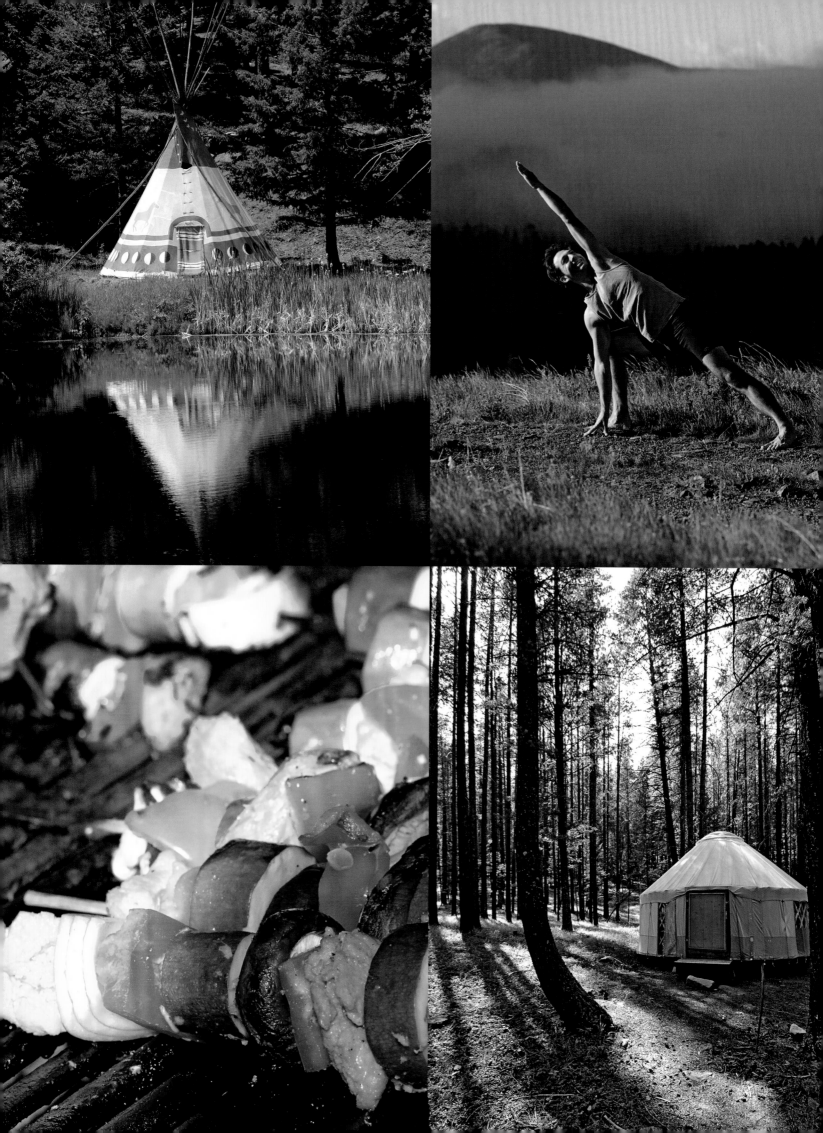

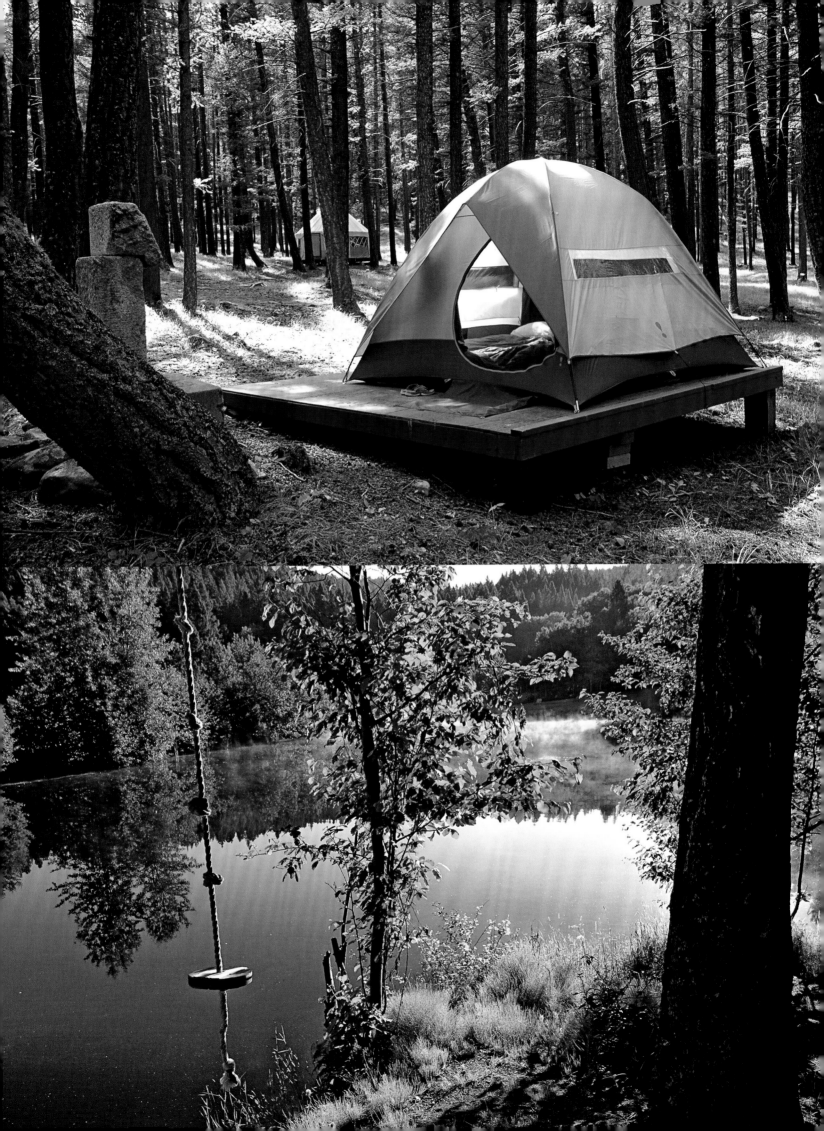

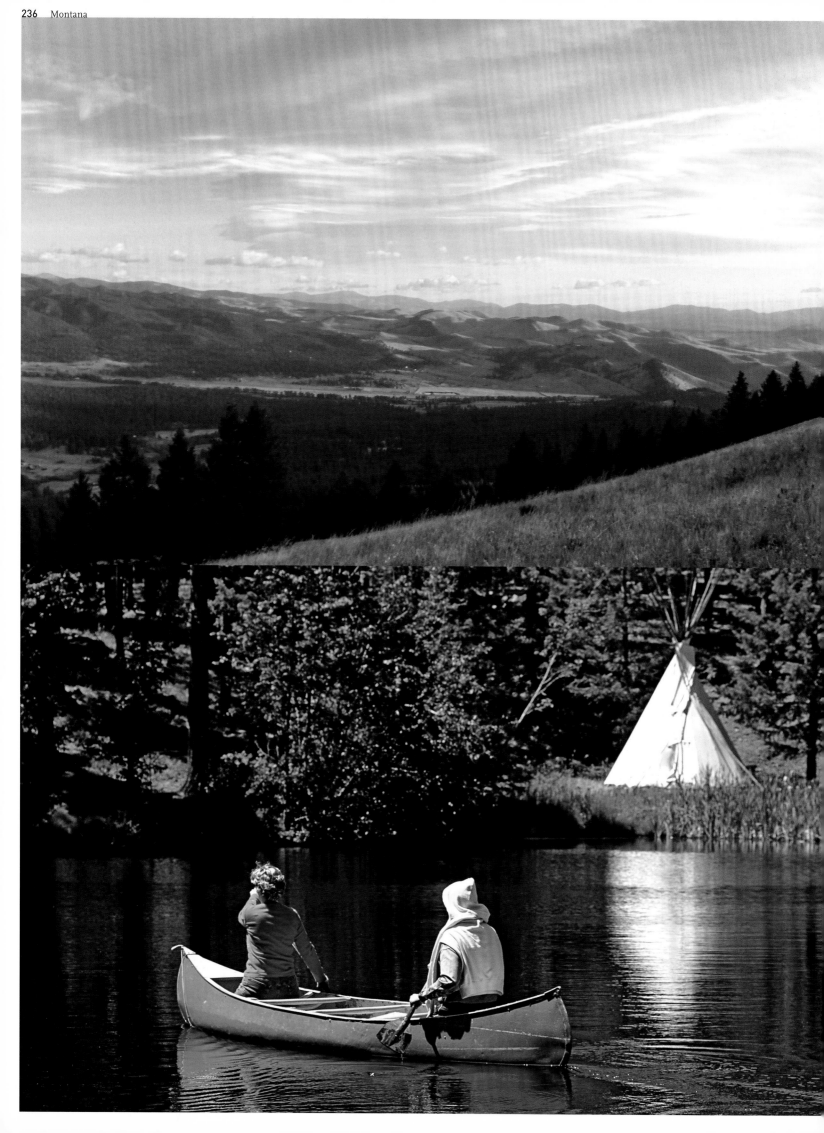

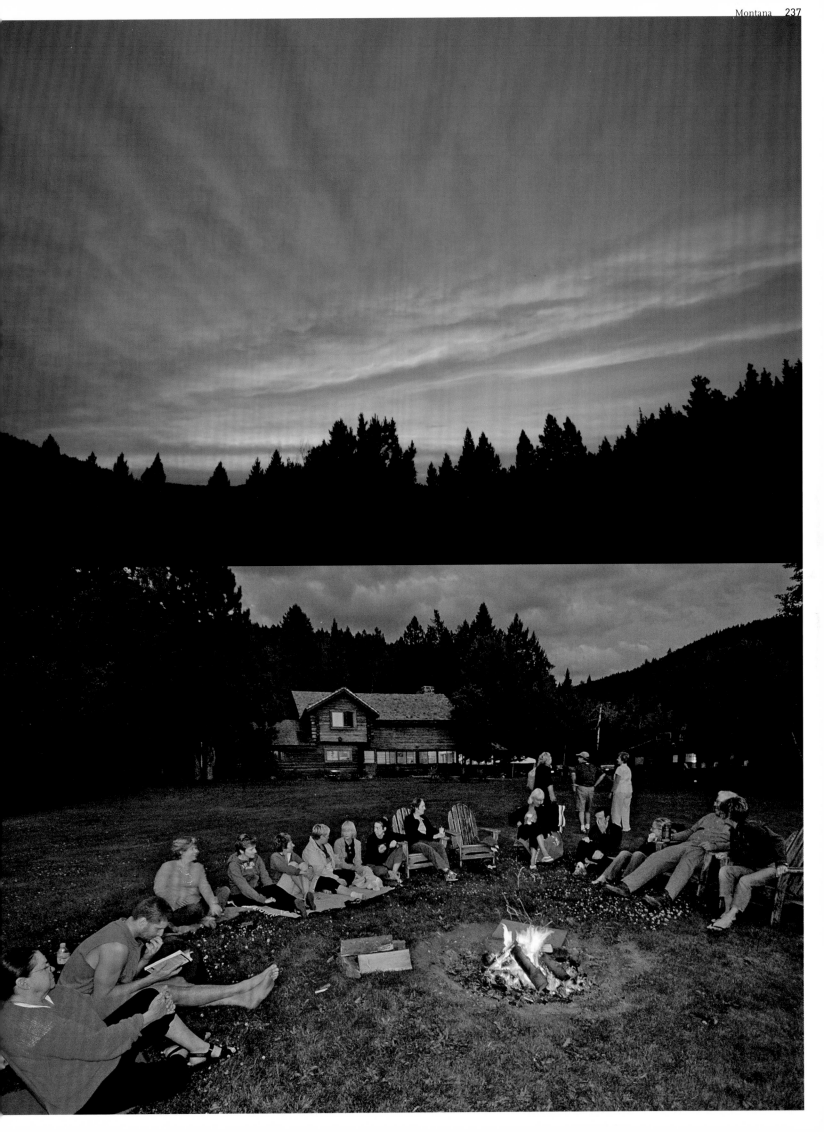

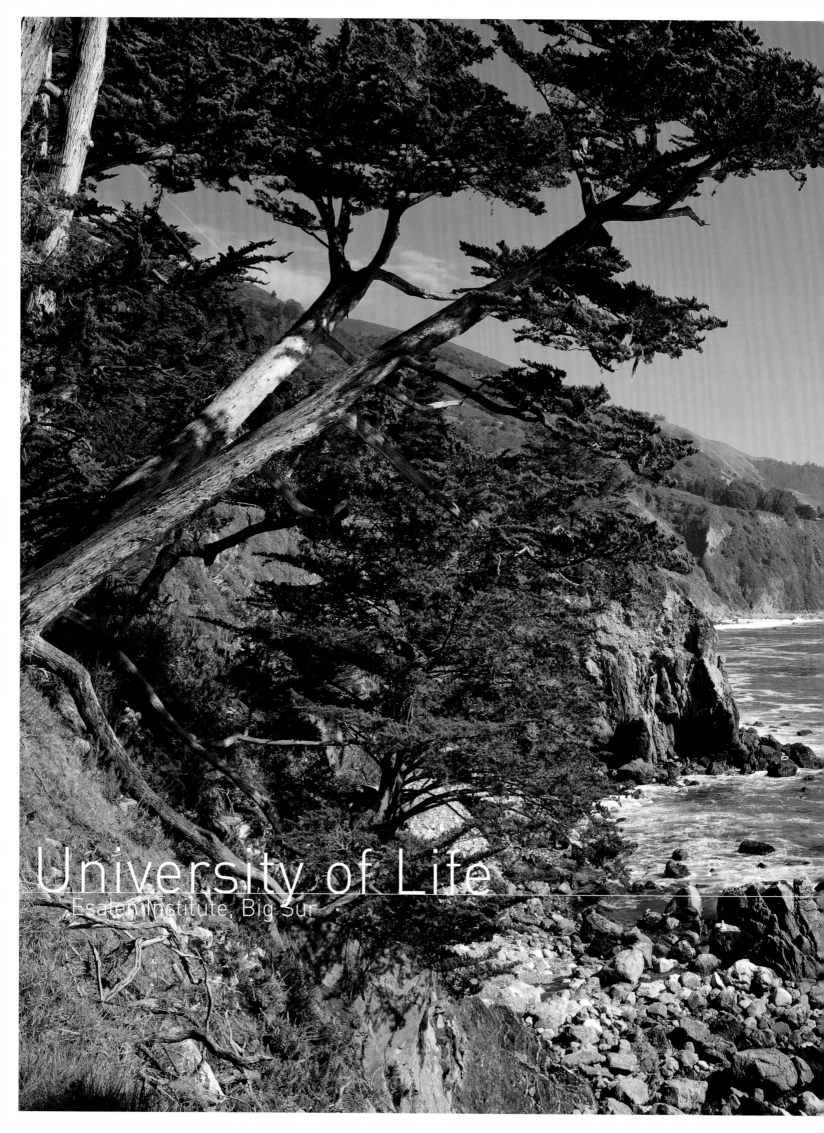

University of Life
Esalen Institute, Big Sur

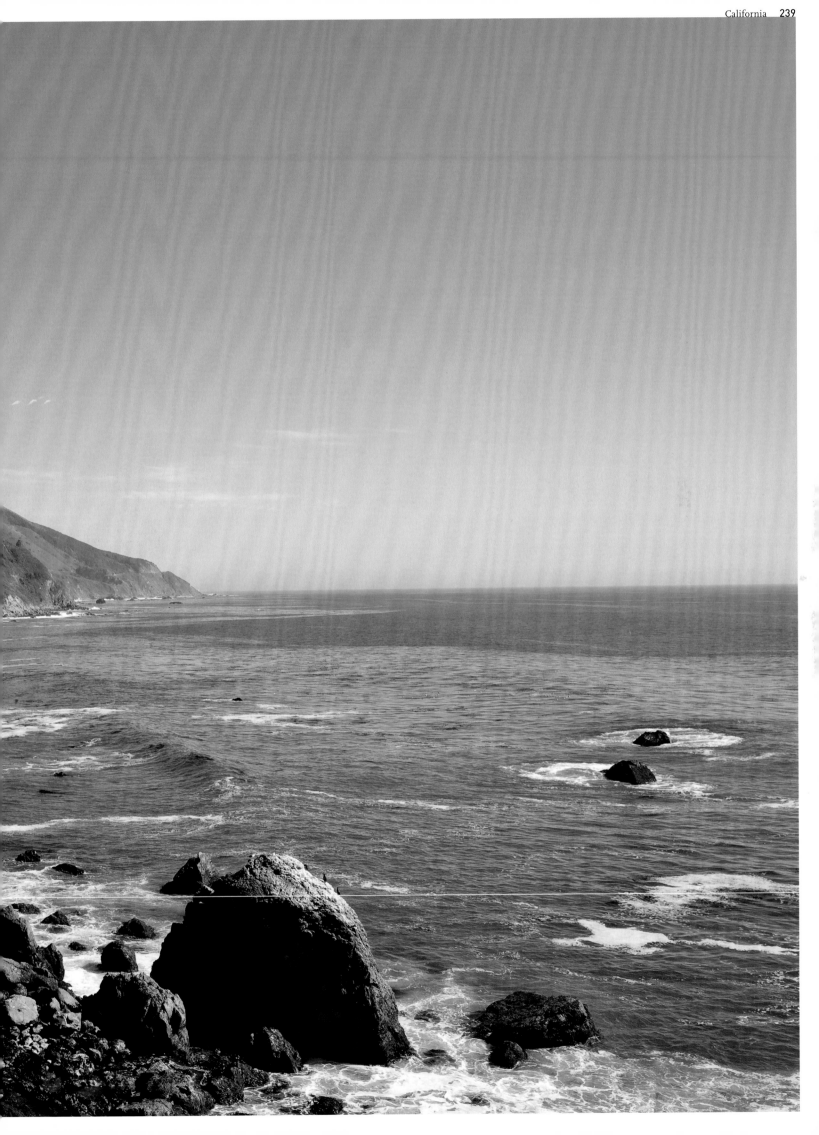

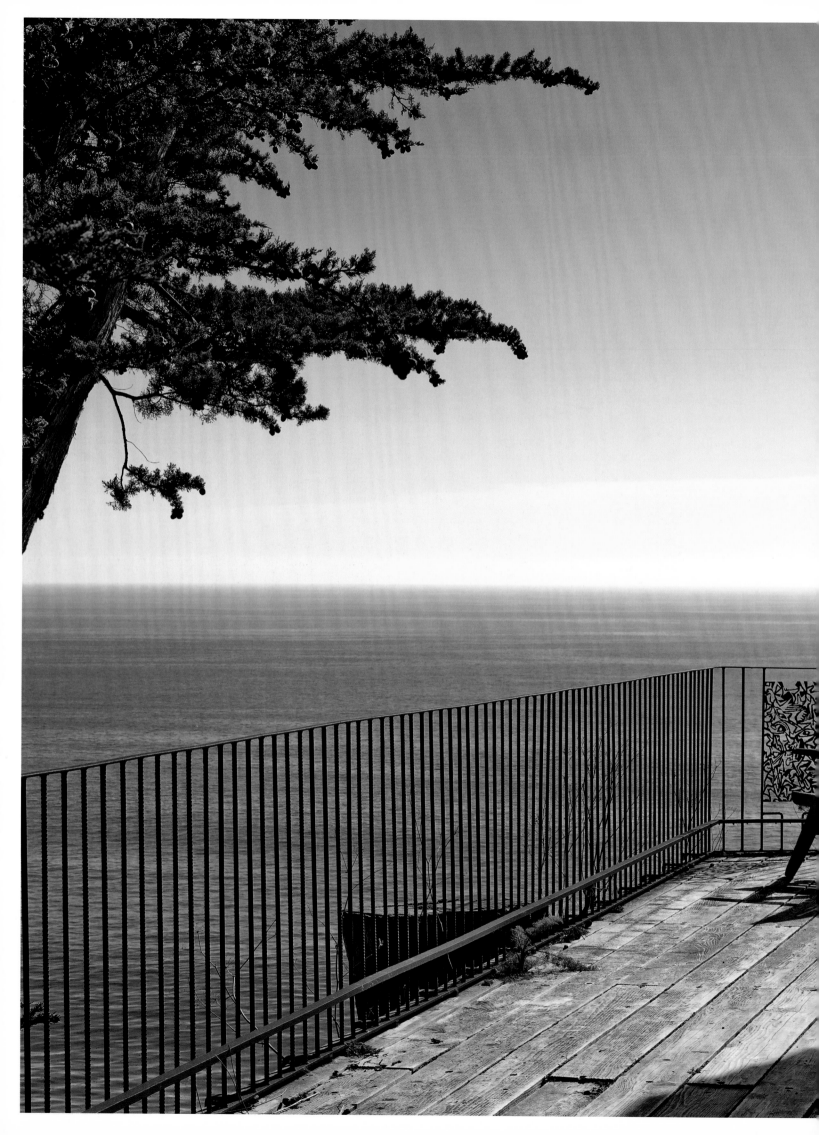

Esalen Institute, Big Sur

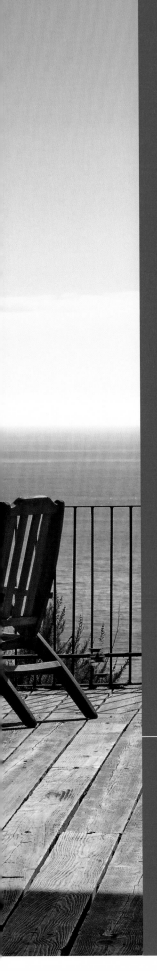

University of Life

Esalen stands on the edge. In Big Sur, just behind the legendary Highway 1, it perches on a cliff high above the crashing surf. The institute, part think tank, part refuge, devotes itself to research into "human potential", as Aldous Huxley put it. How a sequence is formed from single Asanas can be learned here from Srivatsa Ramaswami, as well as Chinese Yoga, also known as Qigong, Tantric alchemy from Darren Rhodes or, from the beautiful and intelligent Seane Corn, how you combine Yoga and your actions. Even without visiting the excellent workshops you can, if there is room, take part in stimulating Yoga sessions with an ensuing dip in the hot springs. The spectacular cliffs, the Santa Lucia Mountains behind, the hot springs and equally heated discussions attracted Joan Baez, Hunter S. Thompson and Henry Miller to Esalen back in the 1960s. The spiritual revolution, which at that time rather shook up the American soul, would have looked meagre without Esalen's thinkers. The thinkers themselves have the hot mineral springs, which bubble powerfully from deep beneath the earth at 119 degrees Fahrenheit, to thank for their cool heads.

Books to pack: "Confessions of an English Opium Eater" by Thomas de Quincey and "Fear and Loathing in Las Vegas" by Hunter S. Thompson.

Esalen Institute		
55000 Highway 1	DIRECTIONS	A 3-hr drive south of San Francisco.
Big Sur, CA 93920	YOGA	Hatha, Anusara, Raja, Tantra, Chinese Yoga, Tibetan Buddhist meditation, Ashtanga, Sivananda, Iyengar.
USA	TEACHERS	Seane Corn, Sianna Sherman, Daniel Brown, Srivatsa Ramaswami, Shiva Rea.
Tel. +1 831 667 3000	ROOMS	2–3-bed rooms, single rooms, single-family house, rooms with bunk beds. Places to sleep with sleeping bags.
info@esalen.org	FOOD	Vegan, vegetarian and meat cuisine, mainly organic, much grown on site.
www.esalen.org	TREATMENTS	Swedish massage, wellness/stress management massage.
	RECREATION	Arts centre, Big Sur National Park, hot springs, night swimming, massage training.

Universität des Lebens

Esalen steht am äußersten Rande. In Big Sur, gleich hinter dem legendären Highway 1, thront es auf einem Kliff, hoch über der krachenden Brandung. Das Institut ist teils Denkfabrik, teils Refugium für die Erforschung des »menschlichen Potenzials«, wie Aldous Huxley schrieb. Wie man aus einzelnen Asanas eine Sequenz formt, kann man hier von Srivatsa Ramaswami lernen, chinesisches Yoga, auch bekannt als Qigong, tantrische Alchemie bei Darren Rhodes oder von der schönen und klugen Seane Corn, wie man Yoga und Handeln zusammenbringt. Auch ohne die exzellenten Workshops zu besuchen, kann man, wenn Platz ist, anregende Yogastunden und ein anschließendes Bad in den heißen Quellen nehmen. Die spektakuläre Steilküste, das Santa-Lucia-Gebirge im Rücken, die heißen Quellen und ebenso heißen Diskussionen haben in den 1960ern schon Joan Baez, Hunter S. Thompson und Henry Miller nach Esalen gelockt. Die spirituelle Revolution, die die amerikanische Seele damals ziemlich umgekrempelt hat, hätte ohne Esalens Denker mager ausgesehen. Die Denker selber verdanken bis heute ihre kühlen Köpfe den heißen Mineralquellen, die mit großer Kraft mit 48 Grad Celcius tief aus der Erde sprudeln.

Buchtipps: »Bekenntnisse eines englischen Opiumessers« von Thomas de Quincey und »Angst und Schrecken in Las Vegas« von Hunter S. Thompson.

L'université de la vie

Esalen est situé à l'extrême limite. A Big Sur, juste derrière la légendaire Highway 1, surplombant les vagues déferlantes, il se dresse majestueusement sur une haute falaise. Dans cet institut qui, à la fois fabrique intellectuelle et refuge, se consacre à la recherche du « potentiel humain », selon l'expression d'Aldous Huxley, on peut apprendre de Srivatsa Ramaswami comment faire de plusieurs Âsanas une série complète, ou le yoga chinois connu sous le nom de qigong, ou l'alchimie tantrique auprès de Darren Rhodes ou enfin avec la belle et subtile Seane Corn comment associer yoga et action. Même sans assister aux excellents stages, on peut, s'il y a encore des places, suivre des séances inspiratrices de yoga et, ensuite, prendre un bain aux sources chaudes. Déjà dans les années 1960, l'imposante côte escarpée, le massif de Santa-Lucia à l'arrière-plan, les sources chaudes et les discussions également bouillonnantes ont attiré Joan Baez, Hunter S. Thompson et Henry Miller à Esalen. Sans les penseurs d'Esalen, la révolution spirituelle qui, à l'époque, a sensiblement bouleversé l'âme américaine aurait fait piètre figure. Aujourd'hui encore, ces penseurs ont gardé la tête froide grâce aux sources thermales qui, à 48 degrés Celcius, jaillissent puissamment de la terre.

Livres à emporter : « Les Confessions d'un mangeur d'opium anglais » de Thomas de Quincey et « Las Vegas Parano » de Hunter S. Thompson.

ANREISE	3 Std. Autofahrt südlich von San Francisco.
YOGA	Hatha, Anusara, Raja, Tantra, chinesisches Yoga, Tibetan Buddhist Meditation, Astanga, Sivananda, Iyengar.
GASTLEHRER	Seane Corn, Sianna Sherman, Daniel Brown, Srivatsa Ramaswami, Shiva Rea.
ZIMMER	2–3-Bettzimmer, Einzel- und Stockbettzimmer, Einfamilienhäuser, Schlafsackschlafplätze.
KÜCHE	Vegan, vegetarisch und Fleischküche.
ANWENDUNGEN	Schwedische Massage, Wellness-Stressmanagement-Massage.
FREIZEIT	Arts Center, Big Sur National Park, heiße Quellen, Nachtbaden, Massagetraining.

ACCÈS	Situé à 3 h de voiture au sud de San Francisco.
YOGA	Hatha, Anusara, Râja, Tantra, yoga chinois, méditation bouddhiste tibétaine, Ashtânga, Shivananda, Iyengar.
PROFESSEURS	Seane Corn, Sianna Sherman, Daniel Brown, Srivatsa Ramaswami, Shiva Rea.
CHAMBRES	Chambres à 2–3 lits, chambres simples, maisons familiales, chambres avec lits à étages. Places pour dormir avec sacs de couchage.
RESTAURATION	Cuisine végétalienne et végétarienne et avec viande.
TRAITEMENTS	Massages suédois, de bien-être et anti-stress.
ACTIVITÉS	Centre artistique, Parc national de Big Sur, sources chaudes, bains nocturnes, entraînement au massage.

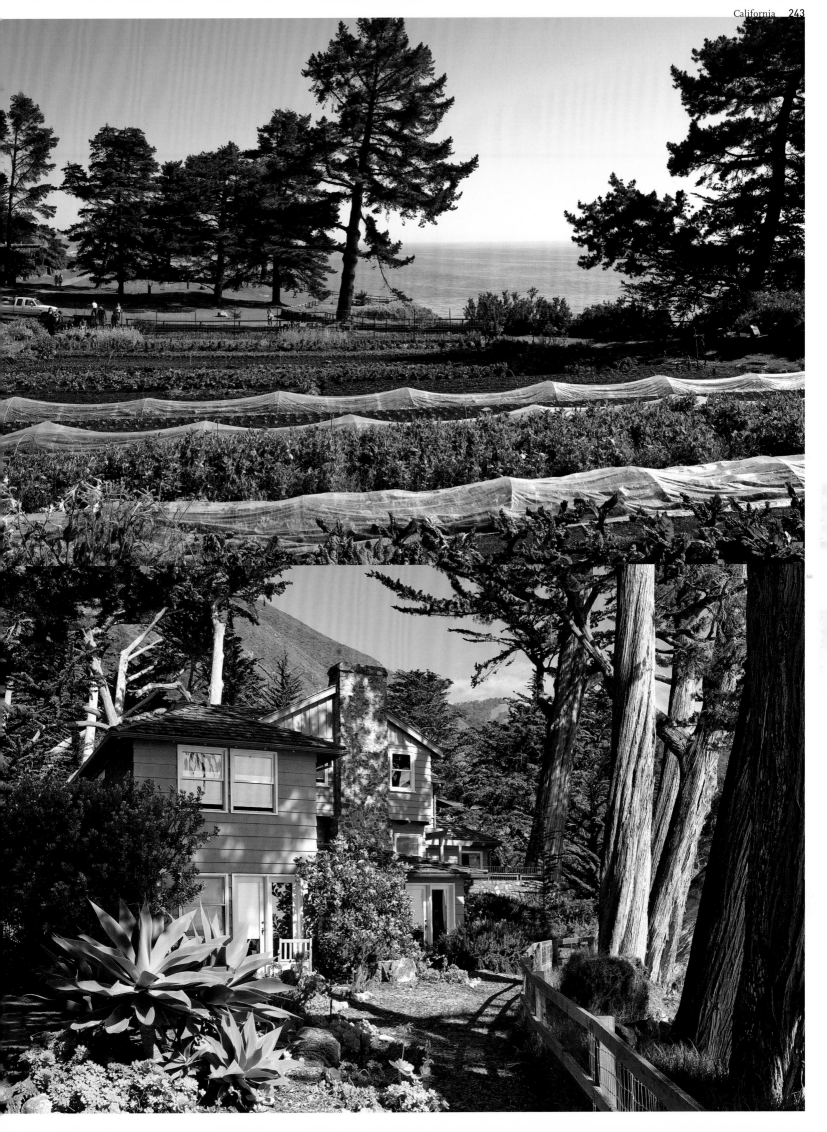

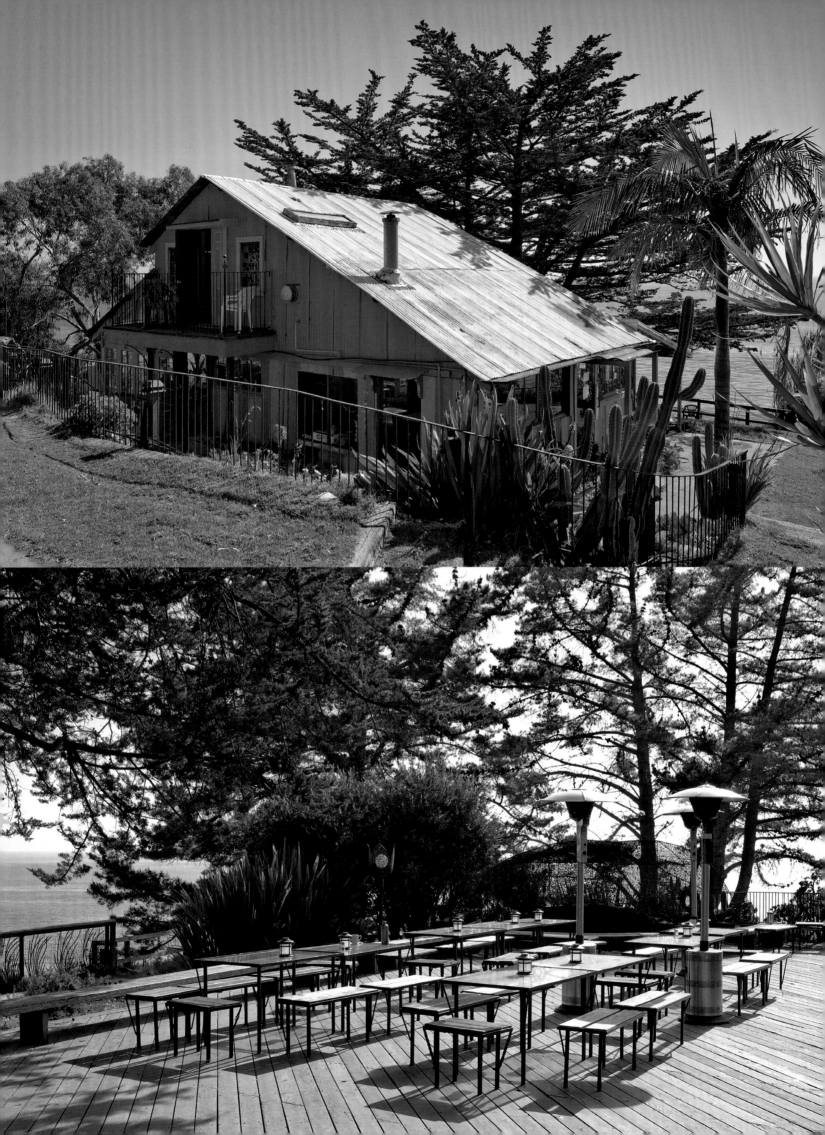

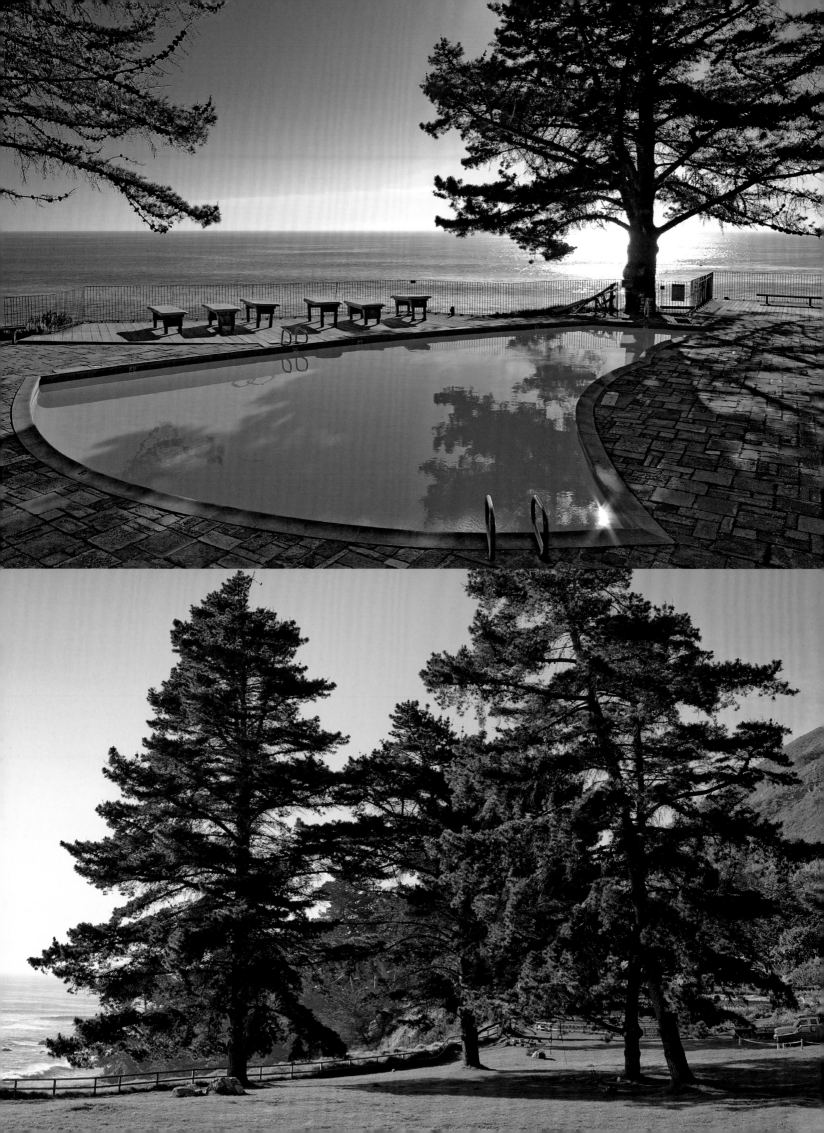

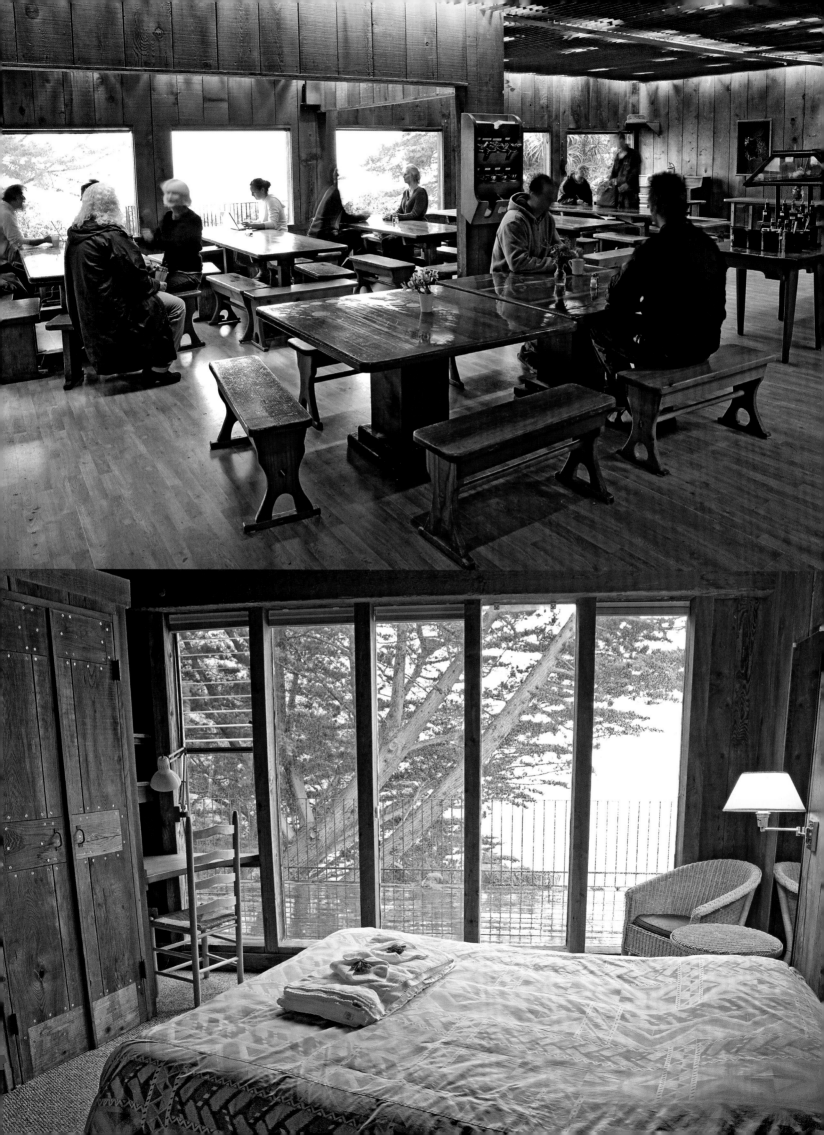

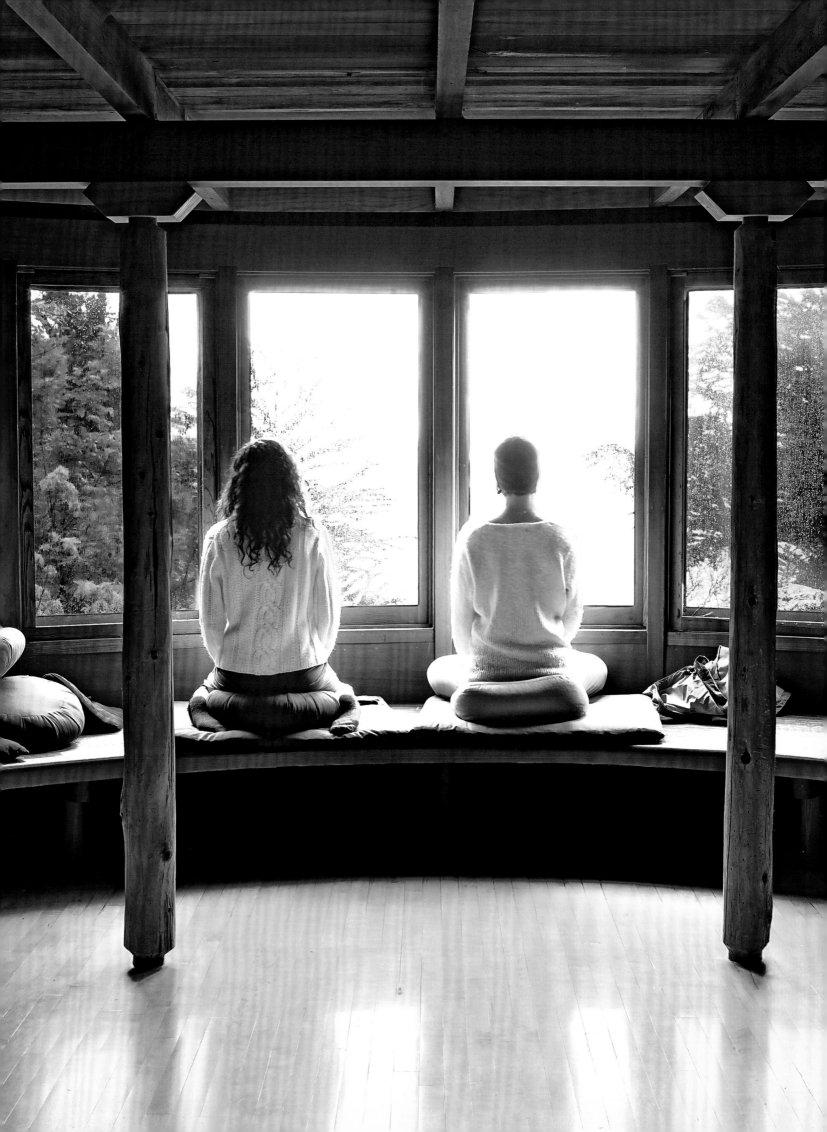

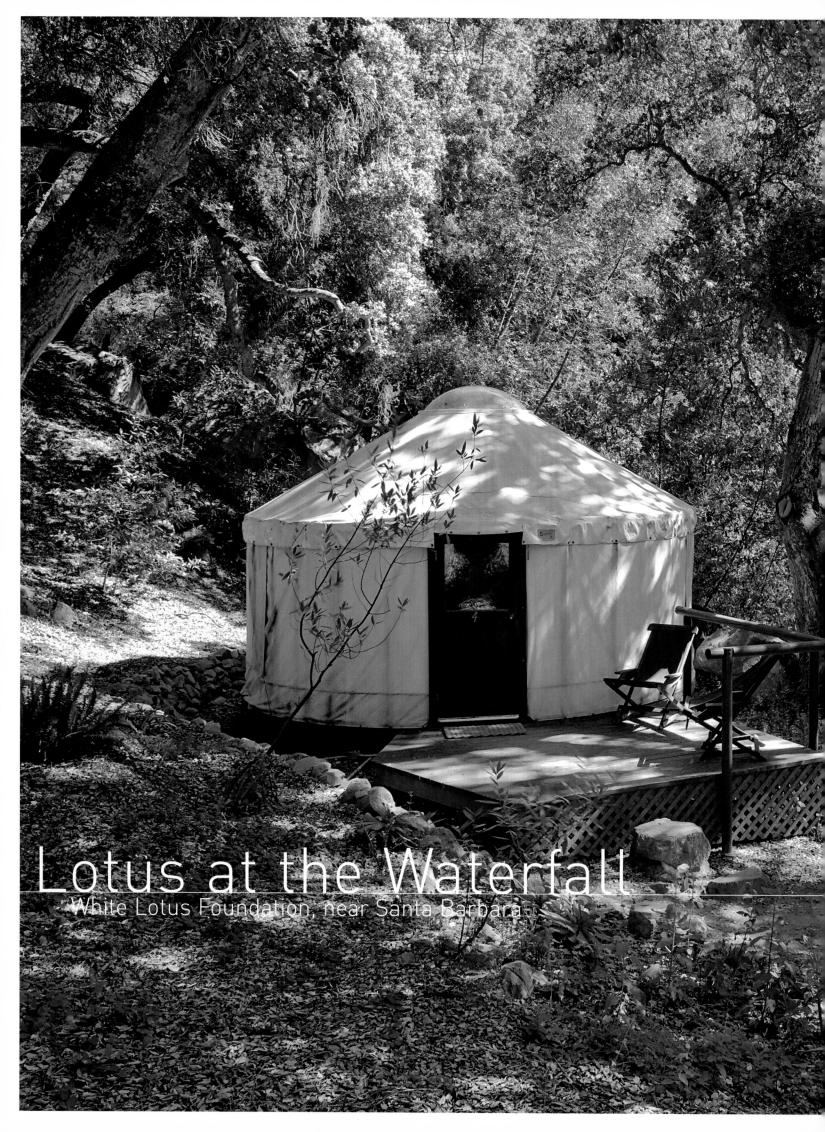

Lotus at the Waterfall
White Lotus Foundation, near Santa Barbara

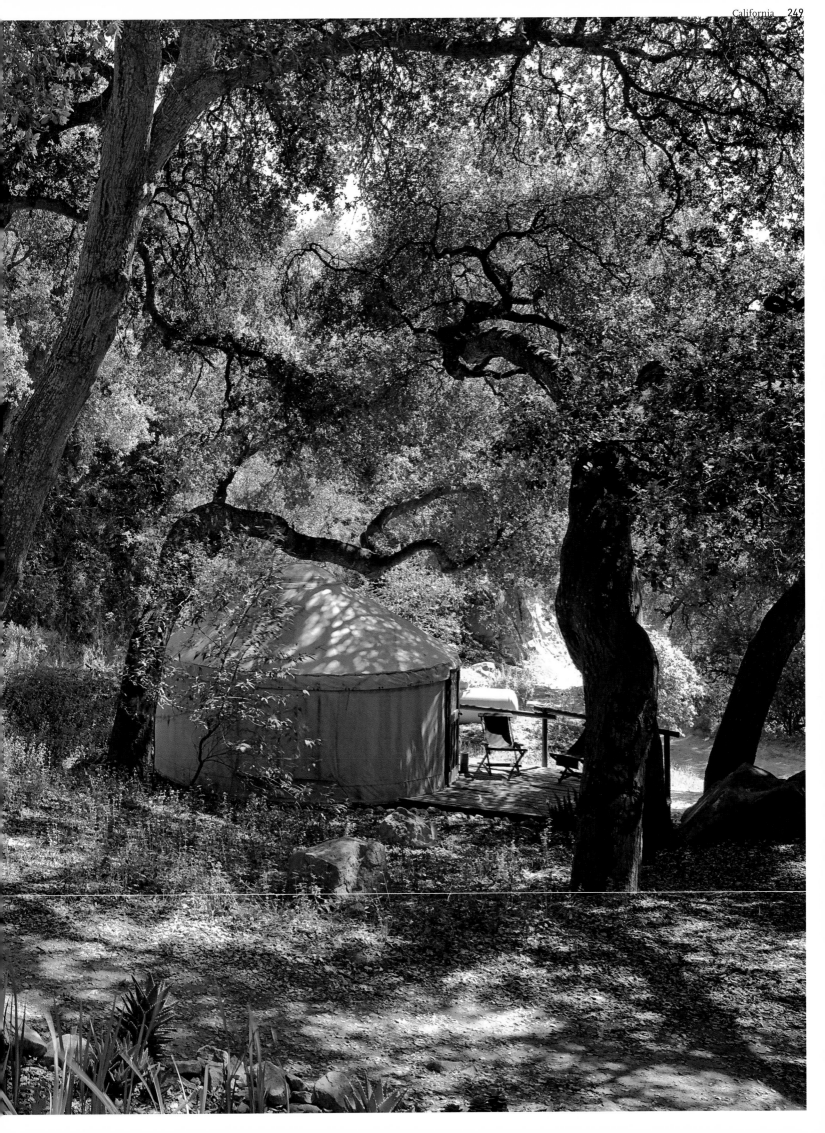

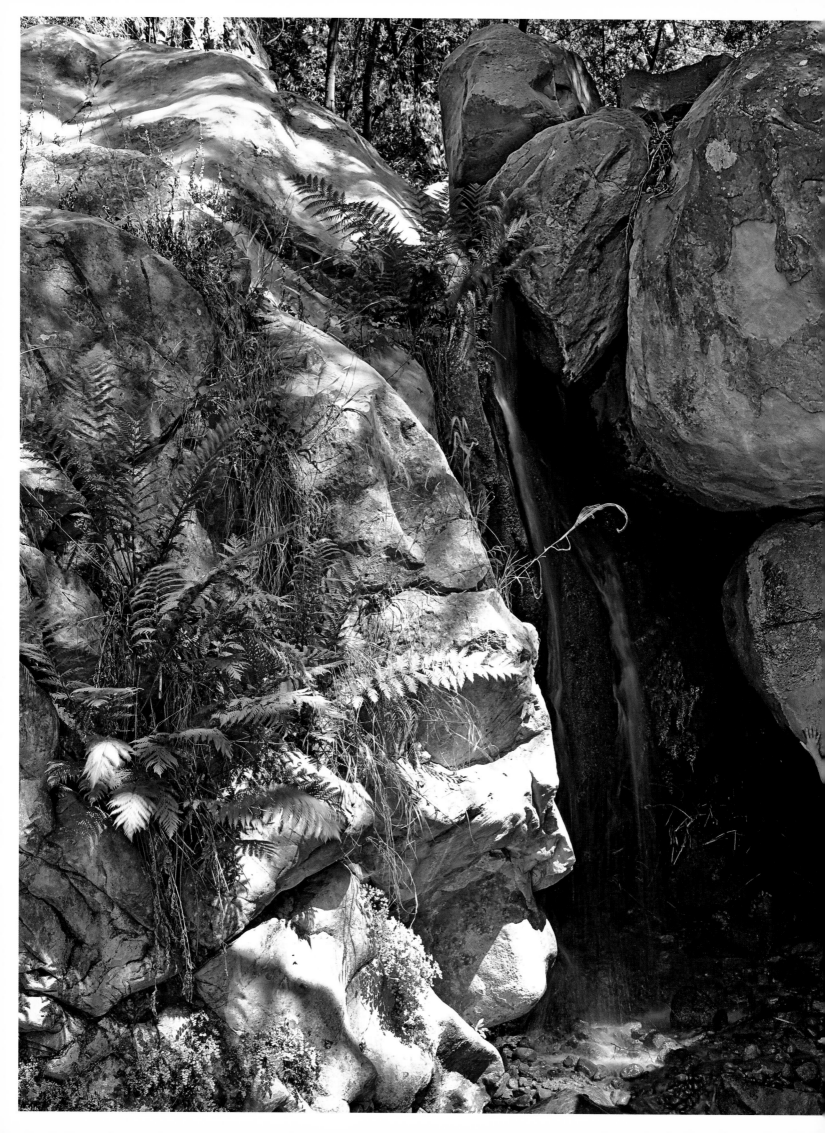

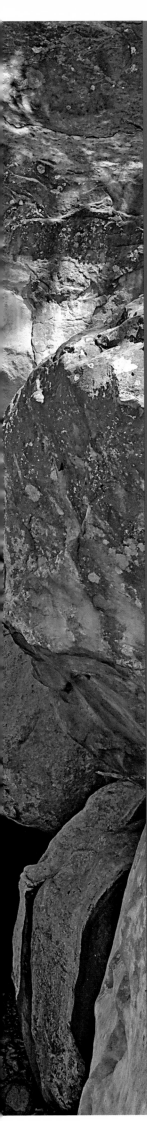

White Lotus Foundation, near Santa Barbara

Lotus at the Waterfall

It goes without saying that you would have liked flying over the War Memorial in 1967 during the anti-Vietnam War demonstration in San Francisco with Ganga White in Swami Vishnu's "Peace Plane", throwing flowers and flyers into the air, or watching with curiosity alongside Vietnam War protestor Muhammad Ali as Ganga demonstrated a perfect Dhanurasana (bow pose), but an intensive Yoga session with him today is nothing to be sniffed at either. From the tiny beauty salon on Sunset Boulevard in Los Angeles, in which White Lotus began as a Yoga school, to the retreat in the mountains above Santa Barbara, the founder has seen a lot of water flow down the San José river. B. K. S Iyengar and Pattabhi Jois were his guests before they became world famous. With its waterfalls, the Indian trails that lead through the steep canyon, the pond full of water lilies, the pretty sandstone bays ideal for bathing, the meditation caves and the enchantingly appointed sleeping tents, the retreat he runs with the impressive Yogini Tracey Rich is a classic like Muhammad Ali's left hook: convincing, clear, a direct hit – without the knock-out.

Books to pack: "Love, Freedom and Aloneness" by Osho and "Budding Prospects" by T. C. Boyle.

White Lotus Foundation
2500 San Marcos Pass
Santa Barbara, CA 93105
USA
Tel. +1 805 964 1944
Fax +1 805 964 9617
info@whitelotus.org
www.whitelotus.org

DIRECTIONS	106 miles north of Los Angeles and 12 miles north of Santa Barbara Airport.
YOGA	Undogmatic, Vinyasa Flow.
TEACHERS	Phoebe Diftler, Cheri Clampett, James Morrison.
ROOMS	7 yurts for max. 3 people, 7 1-2-bed rooms. Max. 30 guests.
FOOD	Lacto-ovo-vegetarian, vegan alternatives.
TREATMENTS	Hot tub, sauna, bodywork, Thai Yoga therapy.
RECREATION	Private hiking trails, waterfalls, swimming.

Lotus am Wasserfall

Natürlich wäre man gerne mit Ganga White in Swami Vishnus »Peace Plane« 1967 während der Anti-Vietnam-Demonstration über das War Memorial in San Francisco geflogen, um Blumen und Flugblätter in die Luft zu werfen, oder hätte mit Vietnam-Gegner Muhammad Ali neugierig zugesehen, wie Ganga eine perfekte Dhanurasana (Bogen) vorführt, aber eine intensive Yogasession mit ihm heutzutage ist auch nicht übel. Von dem winzigen Schönheitssalon auf dem Sunset Boulevard in Los Angeles, in dem White Lotus als Yogaschule anfing, bis zum Retreat in den Bergen oberhalb Santa Barbaras hat der Gründer eine Menge Wasser den San-José-Fluss hinunterfließen sehen. B. K. S Iyengar und Pattabhi Jois waren schon seine Gäste, bevor sie weltberühmt wurden. Mit seinen Wasserfällen, den indianischen Wanderwegen, die durch den steilen Canyon führen, dem Teich voller Seerosen, hübschen Schwimmbuchten aus Sandstein, den Meditationshöhlen und den bezaubernd eingerichteten Schlafzelten ist das Retreat, das er zusammen mit der beeindruckenden Yogini Tracey Rich führt, ein Klassiker wie die Linke von Muhammad Ali: überzeugend, klar, ein Volltreffer. Nur eben ohne K. o.

Buchtipps: »Liebe, Freiheit, Alleinsein« von Osho und »Grün ist die Hoffnung« von T. C. Boyle.

Le lotus près de la cascade

Bien sûr, on aurait aimé accompagner Ganga White dans le « Peace Plane » de Swami Vishnu, en 1967, pendant la manifestation contre la guerre du Vietnam et survoler le War Memorial de San Francisco pour lancer des fleurs et des tracts ou encore avec Muhammad Ali, opposant à la guerre du Vietnam, observer avec intérêt Ganga en train d'effectuer une parfaite Dhanurasana (posture d'extension), mais une séance intensive de yoga avec lui, de nos jours, n'est pas mal non plus. Du petit institut de beauté sur le Sunset Boulevard de Los Angeles, où White Lotus fut d'abord une école de yoga, au domaine retiré dans les montagnes au-dessus de Santa Barbara, le fondateur a vu beaucoup d'eau couler sous les ponts du fleuve San José. B. K. S Iyengar et Pattabhi Jois comptaient déjà parmi ses hôtes avant de devenir mondialement célèbres. Avec ses cascades, ses sentiers de randonnée indiens qui sillonnent le canyon escarpé, l'étang aux nénuphars, les jolies criques aux roches de grès, les cavernes de méditation et les tentes-dortoirs délicieusement aménagées, le domaine qu'il codirige avec l'extraordinaire yogini Tracey Rich est un classique, au même titre que le gauche de Muhammad Ali : convaincant, clair, droit au but. Mais sans K.O.

Livres à emporter : « Amour, liberté et solitude » d'Osho et « La belle affaire » de T. C. Boyle.

ANREISE	170 km nördlich von Los Angeles und 20 km nördlich vom Flughafen Santa Barbara gelegen.
YOGA	Undogmatisch, Vinyasa Flow.
GASTLEHRER	Phoebe Diftler, Cheri Clampett, James Morrison.
ZIMMER	7 Jurten für max. 3 Leute, 7 1–2-Bettzimmer. Max. 30 Gäste.
KÜCHE	Lacto-ovo-vegetarisch, vegane Alternativen.
ANWENDUNGEN	Hot Tub, Sauna, Bodywork, Thai-Yoga-Therapie.
FREIZEIT	Private Wanderwege, Wasserfälle, Schwimmen.

ACCÈS	Situé à 170 km au nord de Los Angeles et à 20 km au nord de l'aéroport de Santa Barbara.
YOGA	Hors dogme, Vinyasa Flow.
PROFESSEURS	Phoebe Diftler, Cheri Clampett, James Morrison.
CHAMBRES	7 yourtes pour 3 personnes max., 7 chambres à 1 et 2 lits. 30 personnes max.
RESTAURATION	Cuisine lacto-ovo-végétarienne, alternatives végétaliennes.
TRAITEMENTS	Bain tourbillon, sauna, bodywork, thérapie de yoga thailandais.
ACTIVITÉS	Chemins de randonnée privés, cascades, natation.

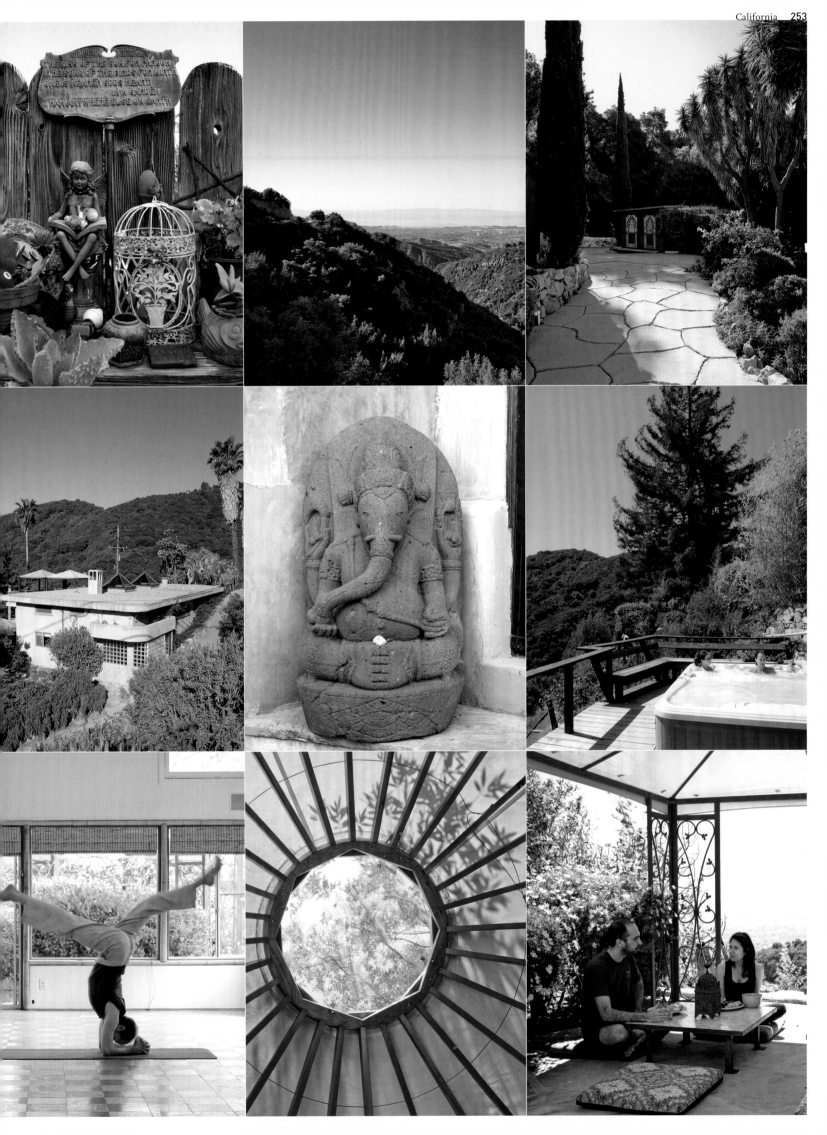

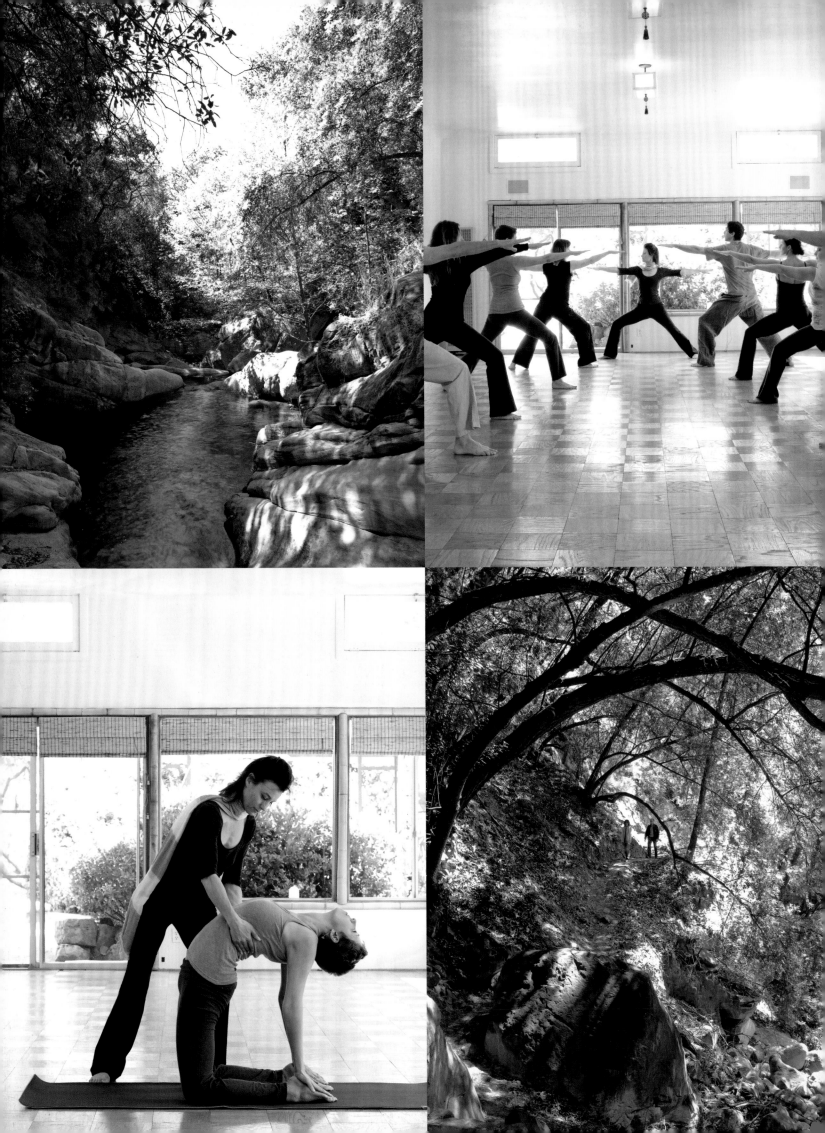

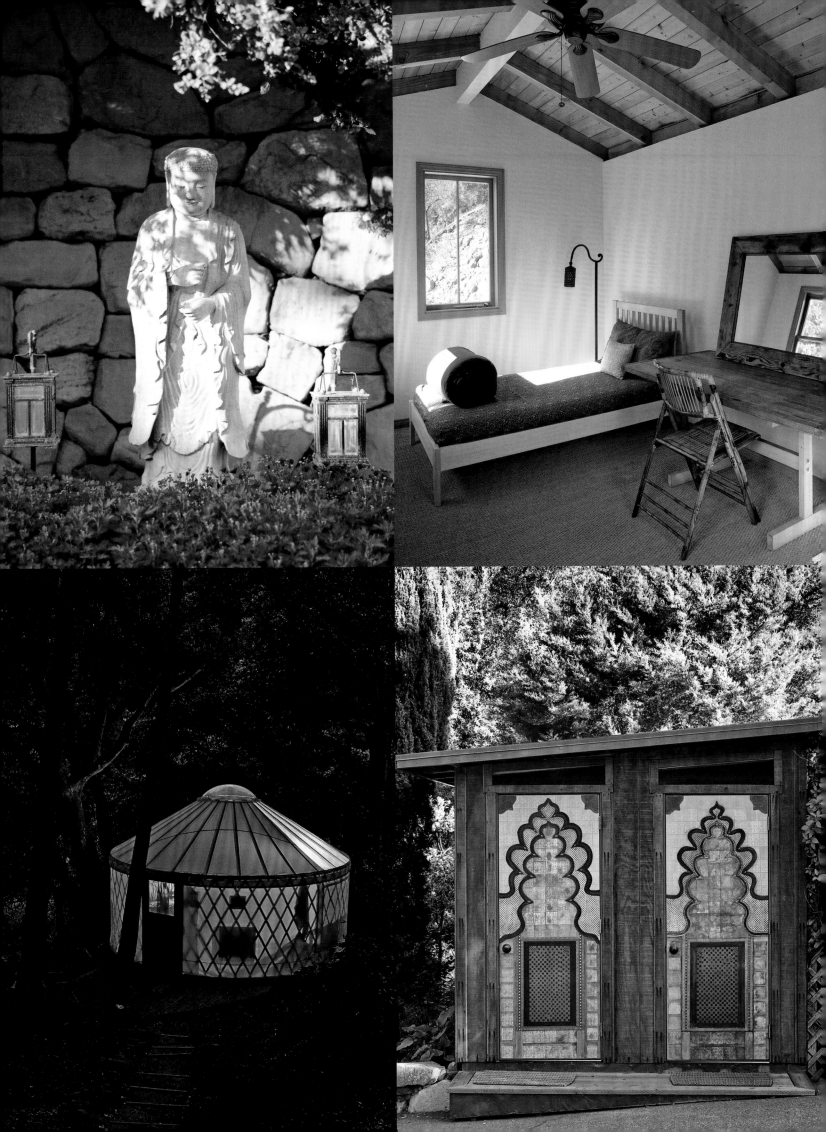

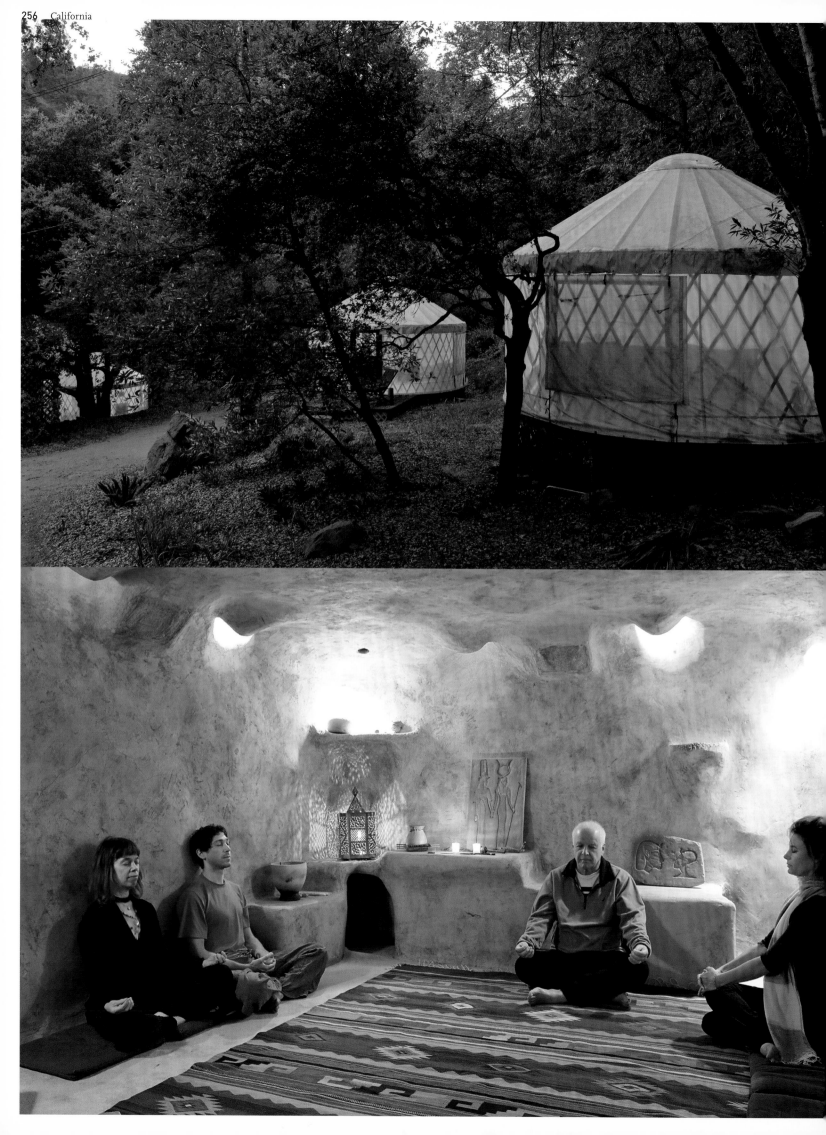

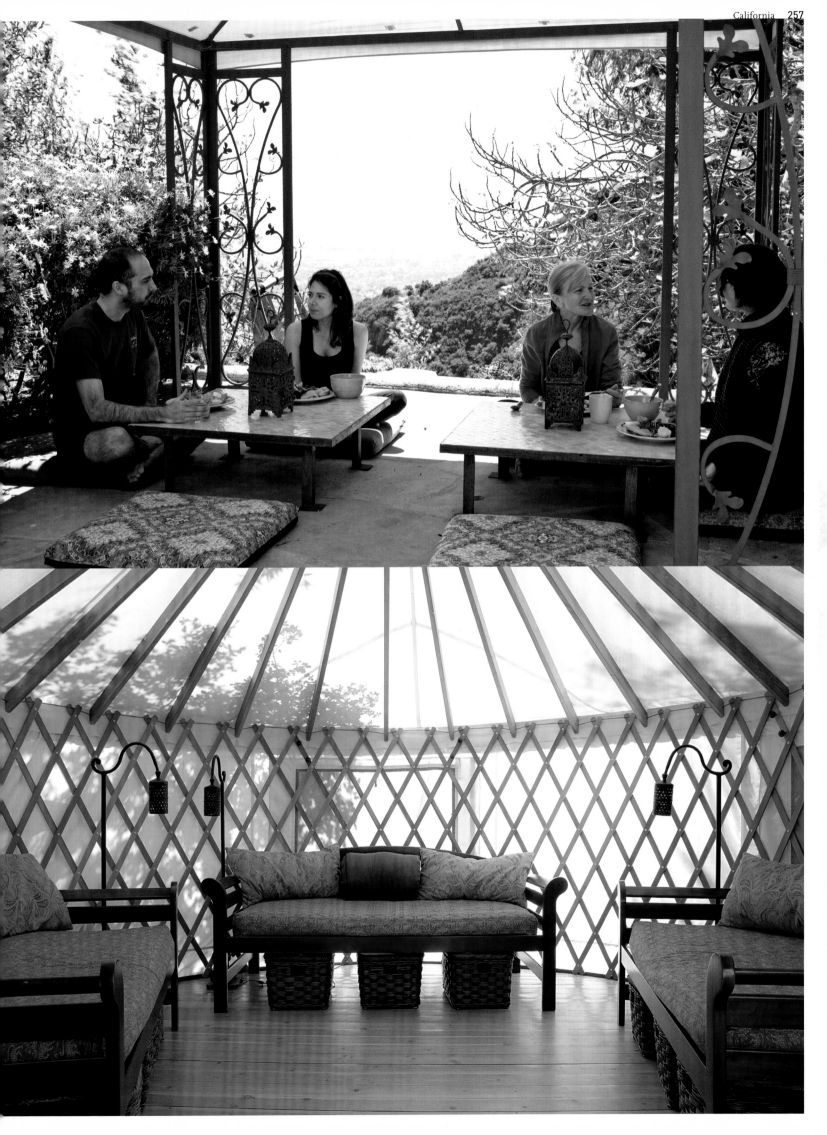

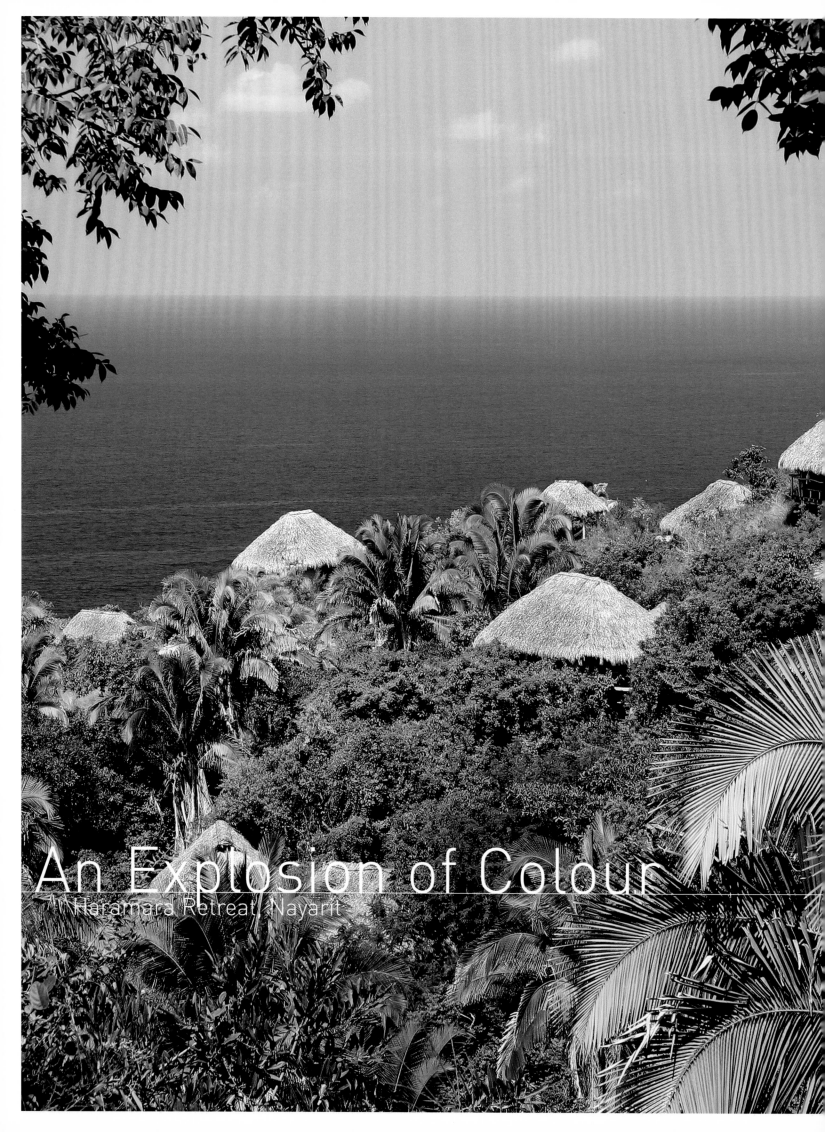

An Explosion of Colour

Haramara Retreat, Nayarit

Haramara Retreat, Nayarit

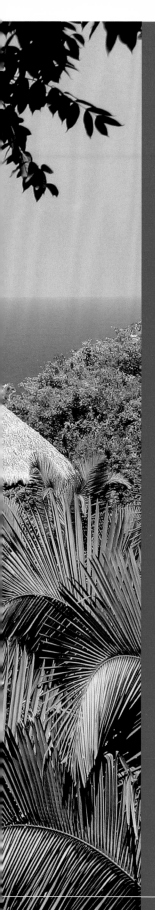

An Explosion of Colour
How many shades of green are there? When does the green of the grasses, bushes, ferns and the pine forests on the mountain crests on the horizon disappear into the white-blue of the sky, merging from there into the turquoise-blue of the sea, and transform itself from the grey-brown of the forgotten rocks on the beach into the golden yellow of the sand? Wherever you look at the Haramara Retreat, colours explode. The Yoga sessions in the Yoga pavilion that is open 360 degrees and stands high on the hill are an adventure in themselves. A fabulous view onto the entangled jungle all about you comes as the reward after intense practice. If the thicket in your own head has not been wonderfully cleared after that, Vipassana meditation is a possibility. Or simply the luxury of a good old-fashioned midday nap. When the sky hovers hot over Haramara, time stands still for a couple of hours. And the spirit finds peace. If you hadn't booked one of the world-class massages, wild horses couldn't drag you from the hand-woven linen of the romantic and charmingly furnished bungalows. Perhaps the whales – here too, by the way – might just manage it.
Books to pack: "The Maya End Times" by Patricia Mercier and "Living Yoga" by Christy Turlington.

Haramara Retreat	
Tamarindos 13	
Sayulita, Nayarit	
Mexico	
Tel. +52 29 329 291 3038	
haramara@comcast.net	
www.haramararetreat.com	

DIRECTIONS	40 min north of Puerto Vallarta Airport. Airport transfer by arrangement.
YOGA	Hatha, Ashtanga, Sivananda, Iyengar, Anusara, Kundalini, Istha.
TEACHERS	Rodney Yee, Marsha Nieland, Desiree Rumbaugh, Sherri Baptiste, Jonny Kest, Denise Kaufman, Dave Stringer.
ROOMS	15 rooms with one, two or more beds for max. 40 guests. Additional dormitory for 8 guests.
FOOD	Vegan and vegetarian, with fish and seafood.
TREATMENTS	Massages and facials.
RECREATION	Snorkelling, whale watching, surfing and jungle hikes.

Farbexplosion

Wie viele Schattierungen von Grün gibt es? Wann taucht das Grün der Gräser, Sträucher, Farne, der Kiefernwälder auf den Bergkämmen am Horizont ins weißlich Blaue des Himmels, von dort ins Türkisblau des Meers – und verwandelt sich vom Graubraun der am Strand vergessenen Felsbrocken ins Goldgelbe des Sands? Wohin auch immer man blickt im Haramara Retreat explodieren Farben. Ein Abenteuer für sich sind die Yogastunden in dem rundum offenen Yoga-Pavillon, der hoch auf dem Hügel thront. Ein sagenhafter Ausblick auf den verknoteten Dschungel ringsum ist die Belohnung nach intensivem Üben. Wenn sich danach das Dickicht im eigenen Kopf nicht auf wundersame Weise löst, gibt es die Möglichkeit zur Vipassana-Meditation. Oder einfach den Luxus einer altmodischen Mittagsruhe. Spätestens dann, wenn der Himmel heiß über Haramara schwebt, bleibt für ein paar Stunden die Zeit stehen. Und der Geist findet Ruhe. Hätte man nicht eine der Weltklasse-Massagen gebucht, würden einen keine zehn Pferde von den handgewebten Laken der romantisch-charmant eingerichteten Bungalows holen. Höchstens Wale. Die gibt es hier nämlich auch.

Buchtipps: »Der Ruf der Mayas« von Wiek Lenssen und »Living Yoga« von Christy Turlington.

Une explosion de couleurs

Combien de tons de vert existe-t-il ? Quand exactement le vert des herbes, buissons, fougères et forêts de pins sur les cimes montagneuses à l'horizon se fond-il au bleu pâle du ciel, puis dans le bleu turquoise de la mer, avant de passer du gris brun des rochers oubliés sur la plage au jaune doré du sable ? Au Hamarara Retreat, où que le regard se pose, les couleurs explosent. Les séances de yoga, qui ont lieu dans le pavillon de yoga ouvert à 360 degrés et trônant tout en haut de la colline, sont un véritable événement. Une splendide vue panoramique sur la forêt vierge enchevêtrée tout autour est la récompense après un entraînement intensif. Si, après cela, la jungle de l'esprit n'est toujours pas défrichée, une méditation Vipassana est possible. Ou tout simplement le luxe d'une sieste classique. Au plus tard à cet instant-là, tandis que le ciel brûlant plane au-dessus de Hamarara, le temps s'arrête pour quelques heures. Et l'esprit trouve la paix. Si l'on n'était pas inscrit à l'un des massages haut de gamme, dix chevaux ne pourraient pas vous tirer des toiles de lin tissées main des charmants bungalows romantiques. Tout au plus des baleines. Parce qu'il y en a ici aussi.

Livres à emporter: : « Le code Maya » de Barbara Hand Clow et « Living Yoga » de Christy Turlington.

ANREISE	40 min vom Flughafen Puerto Vallarta entfernt. Flughafentransfer nach Absprache.	
YOGA	Hatha, Astanga, Sivananda, Iyengar, Anusara, Kundalini, Istha.	
GASTLEHRER	Rodney Yee, Marsha Nieland, Desiree Rumbaugh, Sherri Baptiste, Jonny Kest, Denise Kaufman, Dave Stringer.	
ZIMMER	15 Einzel-, Doppel und Mehrbettzimmer für max. 40 Gäste. Zusätzlicher Schlafsaal für 8 Gäste.	
KÜCHE	Vegan und vegetarisch, Fisch und Meeresfrüchte.	
ANWENDUNGEN	Massagen und Facials.	
FREIZEIT	Schnorcheln, Whale Watching, Surfen und Dschungelwanderungen.	

ACCÈS	Situé à 40 min de l'aéroport de Puerto Vallarta.
YOGA	Hatha, Ashtânga, Shivananda, Iyengar, Anusara, Kundalinî, Ishta.
PROFESSEURS	Rodney Yee, Marsha Nieland, Desiree Rumbaugh, Sherri Baptiste, Jonny Kest, Denise Kaufman, Dave Stringer.
CHAMBRES	15 chambres simples, doubles et à plusieurs lits pour 40 personnes max. Dortoir supplémentaire pour 8 personnes.
RESTAURATION	Végétalienne, végétarienne, poisson et fruits de mer.
TRAITEMENTS	Massages et soins du visage.
ACTIVITÉS	Plongée, observation des baleines, randonnées.

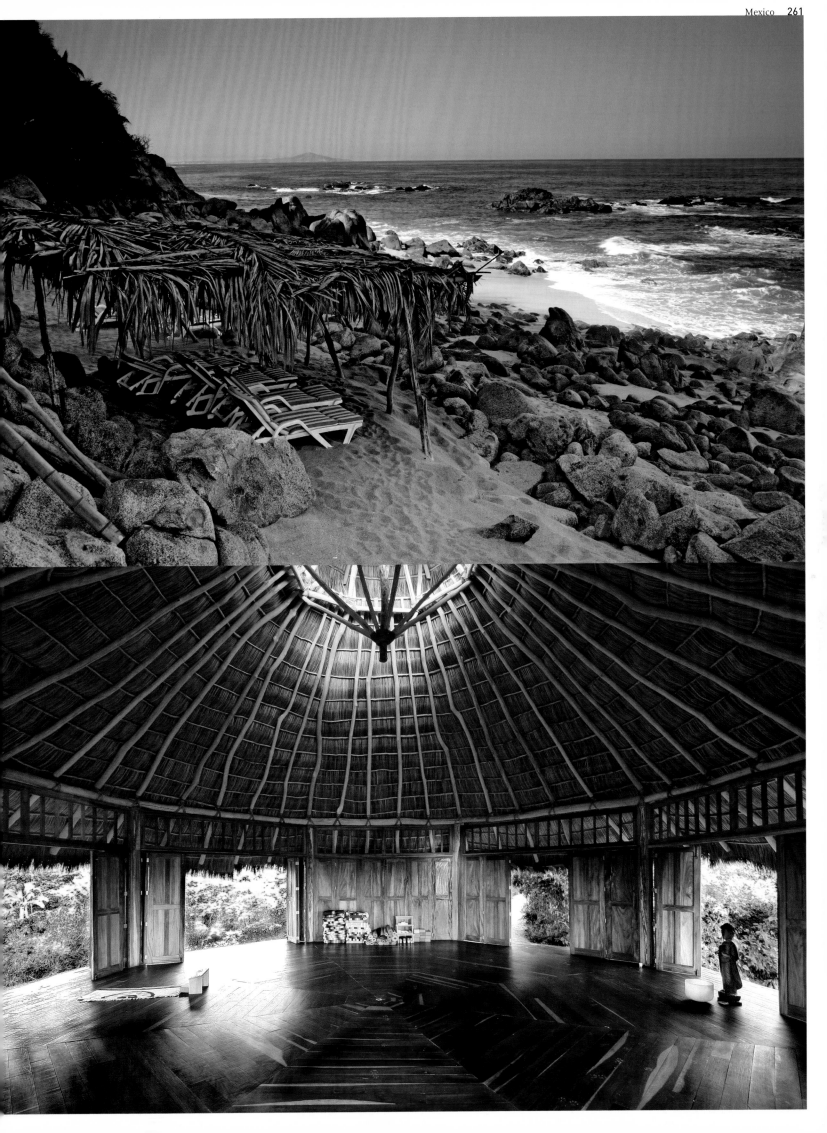

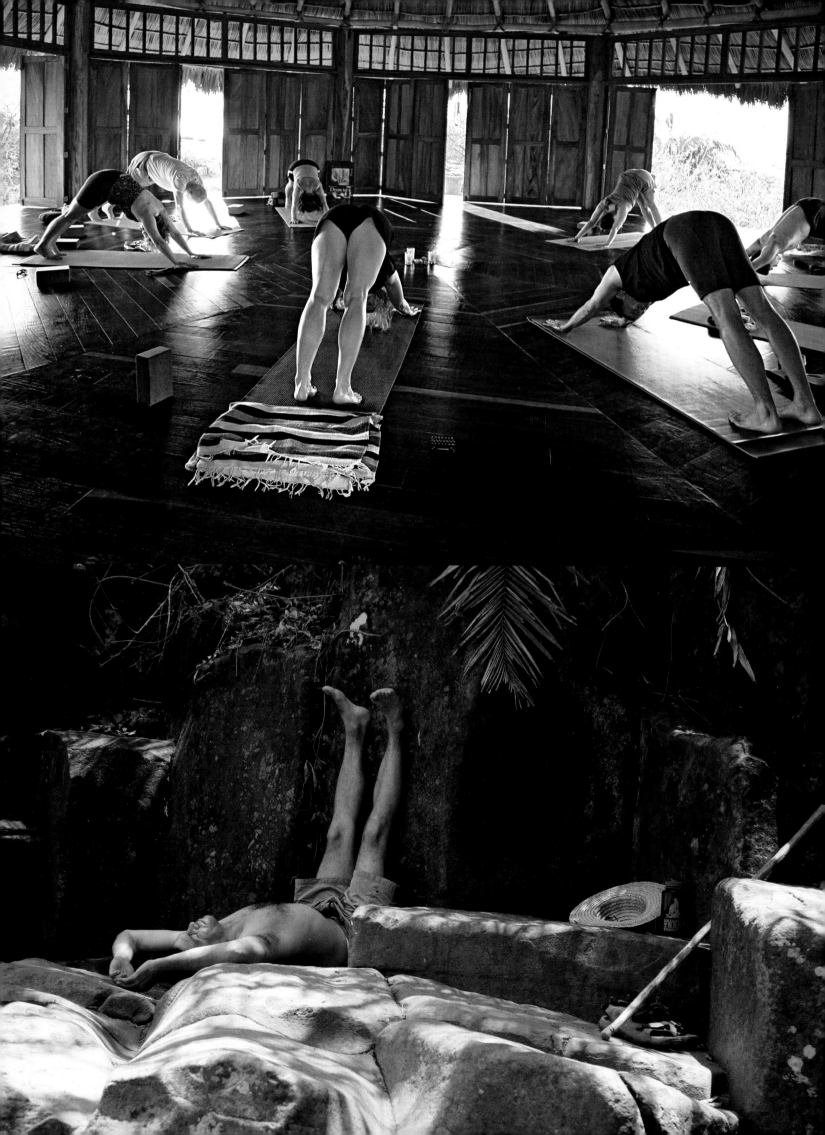

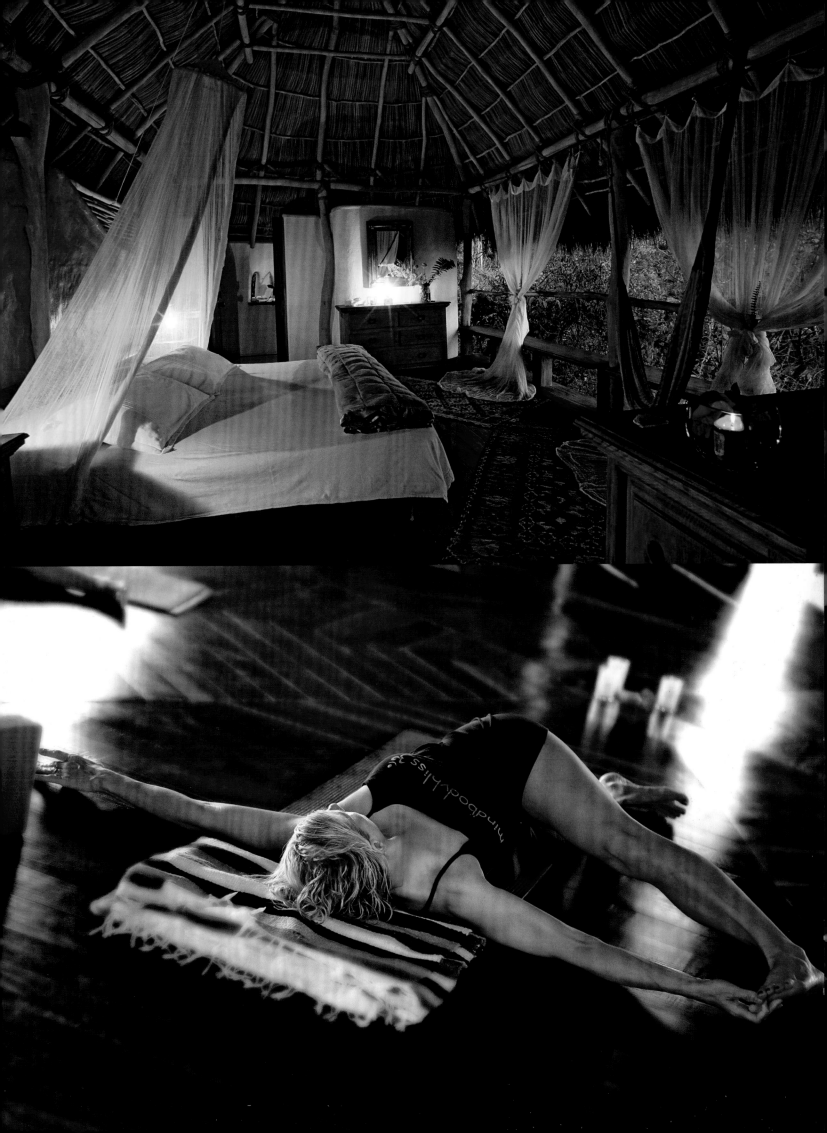

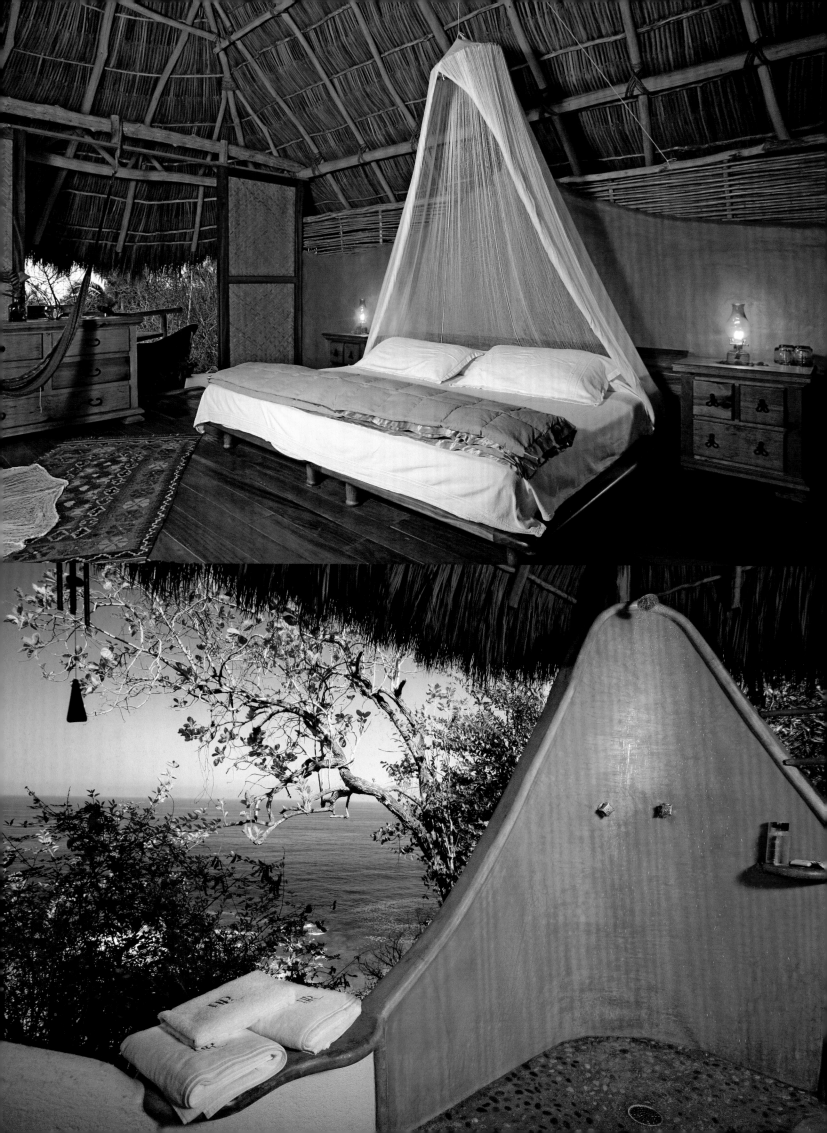

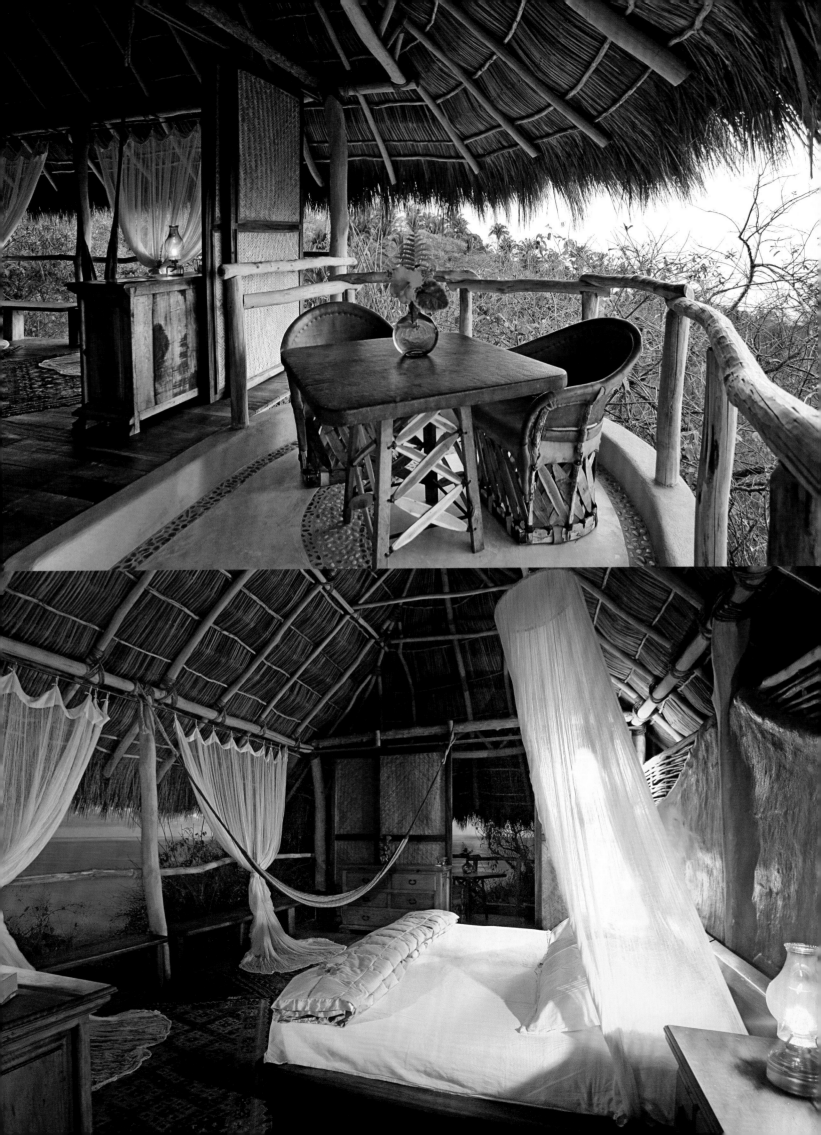

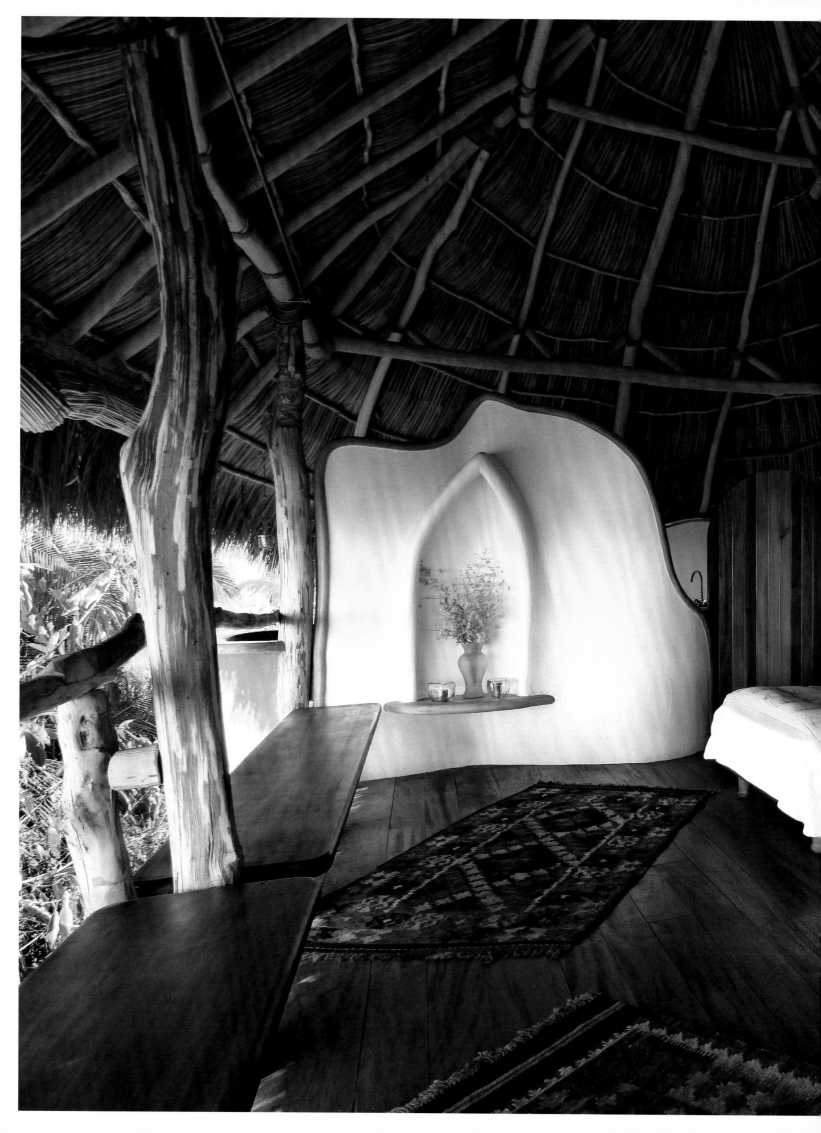

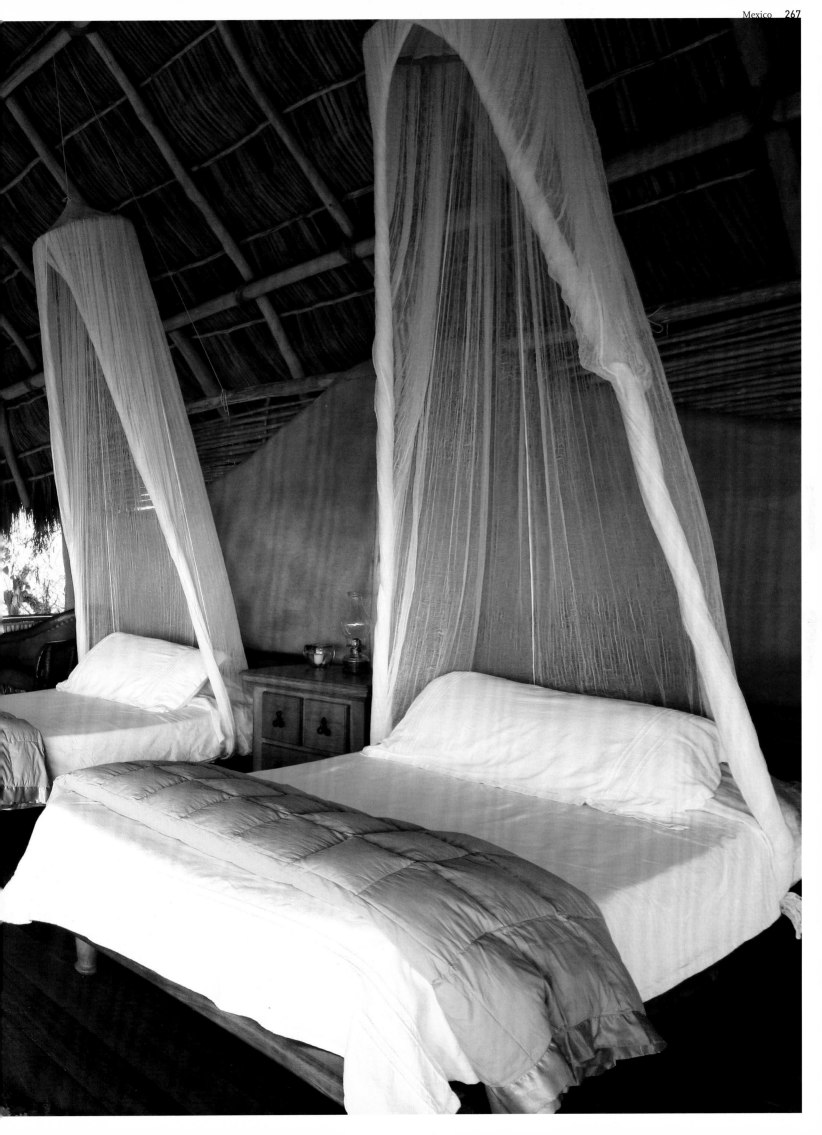

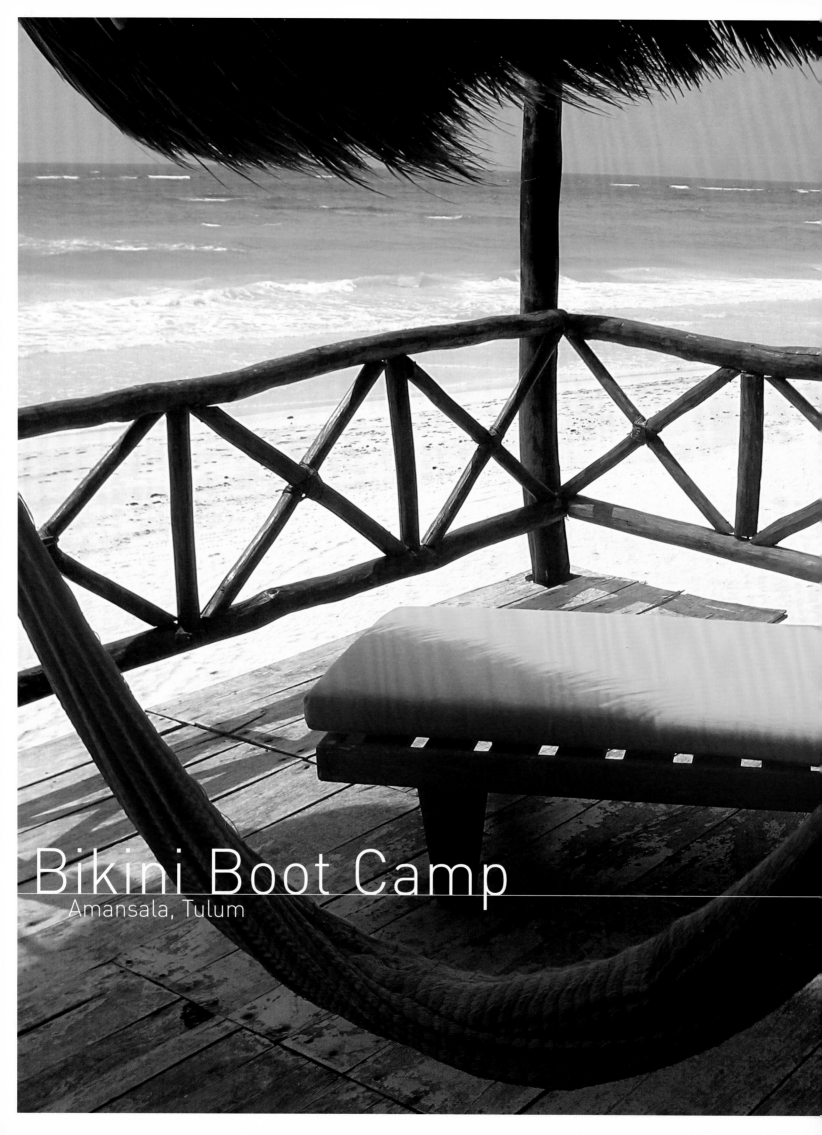

Bikini Boot Camp
Amansala, Tulum

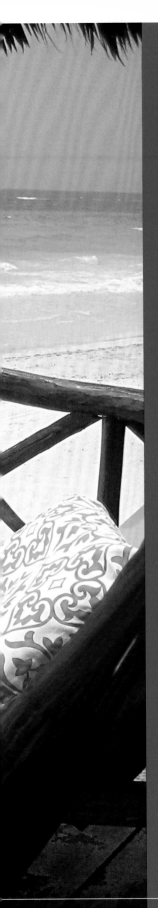

Amansala, Tulum

Bikini Boot Camp

An instructor in Wellington boots who makes a row of shivering girls do sit-ups in the wet sand before sunrise? And in bikinis? Wrong. Amansala means "peaceful water" and in this solar-powered resort right beside the sea the guest is permitted to calmly select from the numerous activities on offer. Power Yoga perhaps, or maybe you'd prefer relaxing Restorative Yoga, a day trip on a bike, a sightseeing tour of the Mayan ruins, a kayak tour or a treatment with Mayan clay. If the bikini is a little too tight, why not sign up for the boot camp? You'll begin the day with a brisk power walk, and then after Yoga, swimming, massages and another march, after tasty grilled fish and a fresh pineapple juice, sink into the distinctly non-rustic Frette linen under the mosquito net in your little hut. If need be you can still drink one of the best margaritas in the world on the veranda of the hippy-chic little wooden houses. In the candlelight, no one will see you.

Books to pack: "The Girls' Guide to Hunting and Fishing" by Melissa Bank and "The Tortilla Curtain" by T. C. Boyle.

Amansala & Casa de Miel Eco Chic Resort
Km 5.5 Boca Paila
Tulum
Mexico
Tel. +52 998 185 7428
casademiel.tulum@yahoo.com
www.amansala.com or www.casademiel.com

DIRECTIONS	2 hrs south of Cancun Airport.
YOGA	Hatha, Ashtanga, Sivananda, Iyengar, Anusara, Vinyasa Flow.
TEACHERS	Jessica Belafonte, Cole Williston, Ian Lopatin.
ROOMS	12 huts and 4 small rooms for max. 40 guests.
FOOD	According to the needs of the group vegetarian-vegan with fish, Mexican specialities like ceviche, tacos, mango, papaya, jicama, jalapeño.
TREATMENTS	Massage, treatments with Mayan clay.
RECREATION	Swimming, hiking, snorkelling, kayaking, day trips to Mayan ruins.

Bikini Boot Camp

Ein Ausbilder in Gummistiefeln, der eine Reihe zitternder Mädchen im nassen Sand vor Sonnenaufgang Sit-ups machen lässt? Im Bikini? Falsch. Amansala bedeutet »friedliches Wasser«, und in diesem solarbetriebenen Resort direkt am Meer darf der Gast in aller Ruhe entscheiden, welches der vielen Angebote er wahrnehmen möchte. Power-Yoga oder lieber Yoga zur Entspannung (Restorative), Ausflüge mit dem Fahrrad, eine Besichtigung der Maya-Ruinen, eine Kajaktour oder eine Behandlung mit Maya-Tonerde? Sollte der Bikini zu sehr zwicken, warum sich nicht doch dem Boot Camp anschließen? Und den Tag mit einem strammen Power-Walk beginnen, um nach Yoga, Schwimmen, Massagen, erneutem Marsch, nach würzig gegrilltem Fisch und einem frischen Ananassaft in seiner kleinen Hütte unter das Moskitonetz in die völlig unbäuerlichen Frette-Laken zu sinken. Zur Not kann man immer noch auf der Veranda der hippieschicken Holzhäuschen einen der besten Margaritas der Welt trinken. Bei Kerzenlicht sieht das keiner so genau.
Buchtipps: »Wie Frauen fischen und jagen« von Melissa Bank und »América« von T. C. Boyle.

Bikini Boot Camp

Un instructeur en bottes de caoutchouc qui, avant l'aube, fait faire dans le sable mouillé des abdominaux à une rangée de filles grelottantes ? En bikini ? Erreur. Amansala signifie « eau paisible », et dans ce site en bordure de mer, alimenté à l'énergie solaire, le client peut choisir en toute quiétude ce qu'il aimerait faire parmi les nombreux programmes qui lui sont proposés. Yoga dynamique ou plutôt yoga de relaxation (restoratif), des randonnées à vélo, une visite des sites mayas, un tour en kayak ou un traitement à base d'argile maya ? Si le bikini vous serre un peu trop, pourquoi ne pas aller rejoindre le camp d'entraînement ? Et commencer la journée par une marche soutenue, et après le yoga, la nage, les massages, une nouvelle marche, après avoir dégusté un poisson grillé aux épices et un jus d'ananas frais, se laisser tomber dans des draps de lin griffé Frette sous la moustiquaire de sa petite hutte. Au besoin, on peut toujours boire une des meilleures Margaritas du monde sur la véranda des jolies maisonnettes de bois de style hippie. A la lueur des bougies personne n'y regarde de si près.
Livres à emporter : « Manuel de chasse et de pêche à l'usage des filles » de Melissa Bank et « América » de T. C. Boyle.

ANREISE	2 Std. südlich vom Flughafen Cancun.
YOGA	Hatha, Astanga, Sivananda, Iyengar, Anusara, Vinyasa Flow.
GASTLEHRER	Jessica Belafonte, Cole Williston, Ian Lopatin.
ZIMMER	12 Hütten und 4 kleine Zimmer.
KÜCHE	Je nach Gruppe vegetarisch-vegan, mit Fisch, mexikanische Spezialitäten wie Ceviche, Tacos, Mango, Papaya, Jicama, Jalapeño.
ANWENDUNGEN	Massage, Behandlung mit Maya-Tonerde.
FREIZEIT	Schwimmen, Wandern, Schnorcheln, Kajak, Ausflüge zu Maya-Ruinen.

ACCÈS	Situé à 2 h au sud de l'aéroport de Cancun.
YOGA	Hatha, Ashtânga, Shivananda, Iyengar, Anusara, Vinyasa Flow.
PROFESSEURS	Jessica Belafonte, Cole Williston, Ian Lopatin.
CHAMBRES	12 huttes et 4 petites chambres pour 40 personnes max.
RESTAURATION	Selon le groupe, cuisine végétarienne-végétalienne avec poisson, spécialités mexicaines comme le ceviche, les tacos, la mangue, la papaye, le jicama, le piment japaleño.
TRAITEMENTS	Massage, traitement à base d'argile maya.
ACTIVITÉS	Natation, randonnées, plongée libre, kayak, visites des sites mayas.

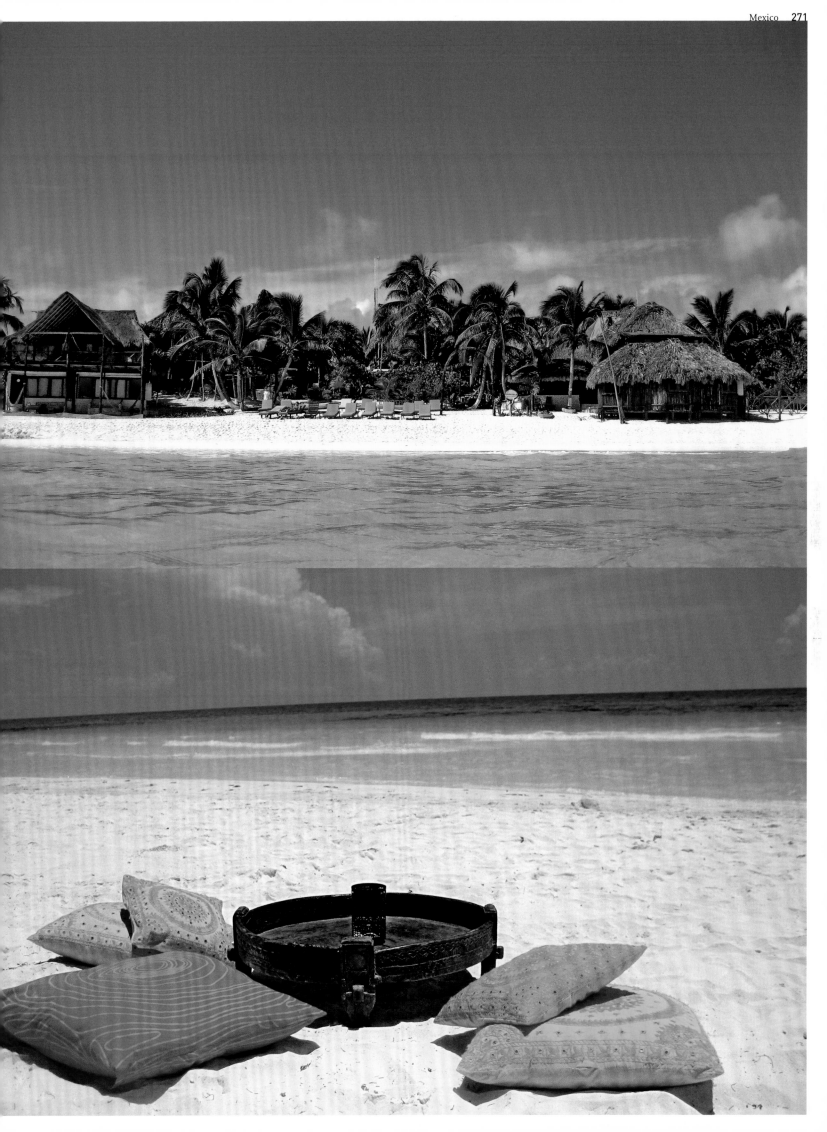

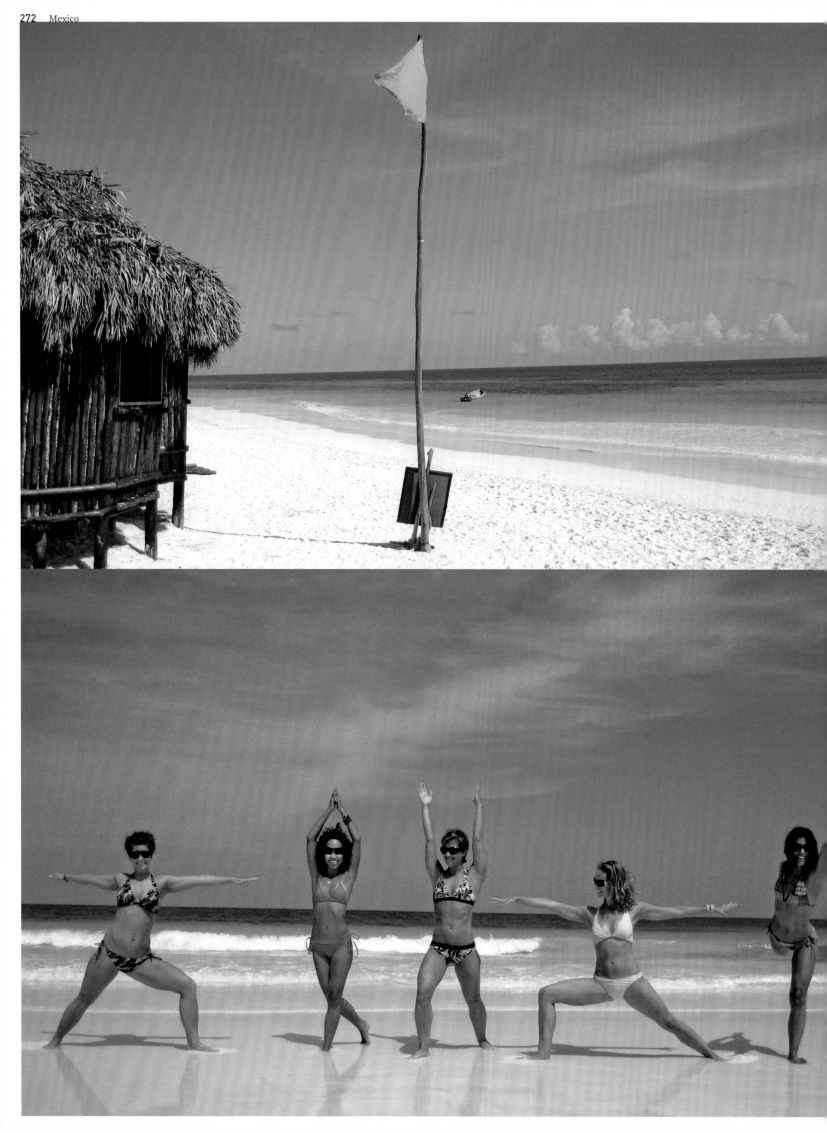

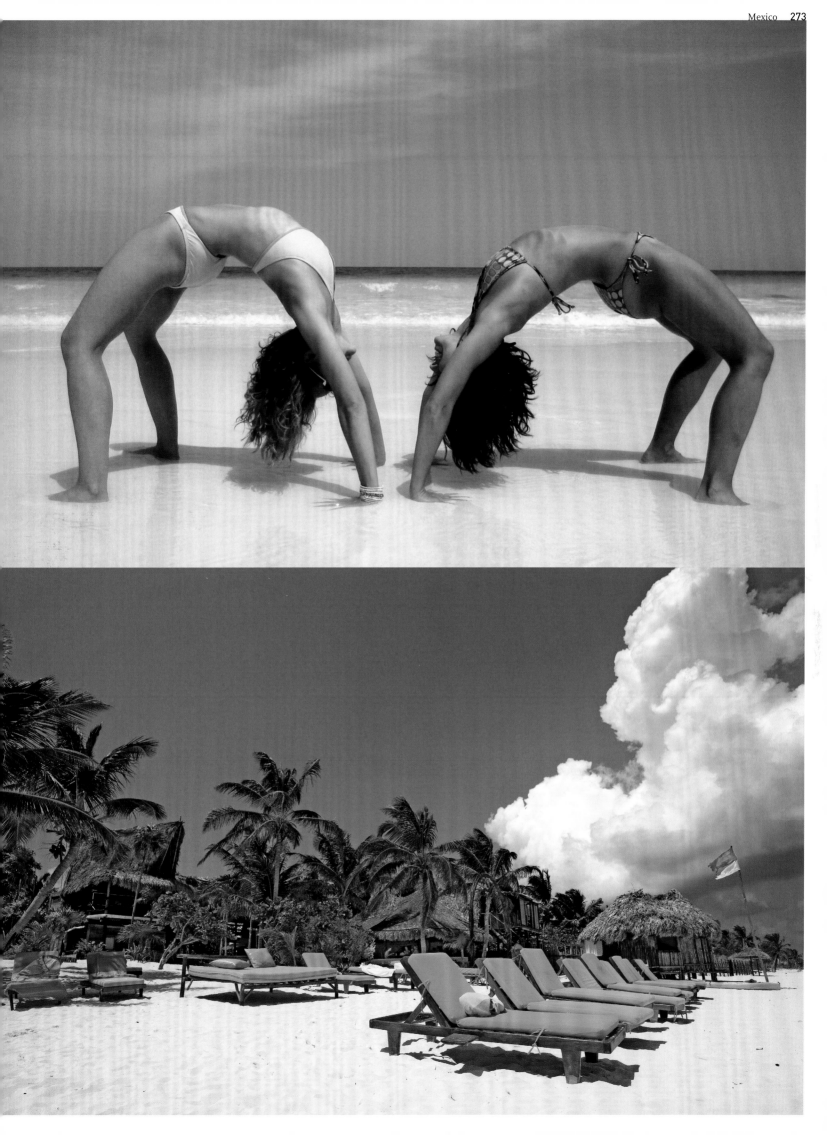

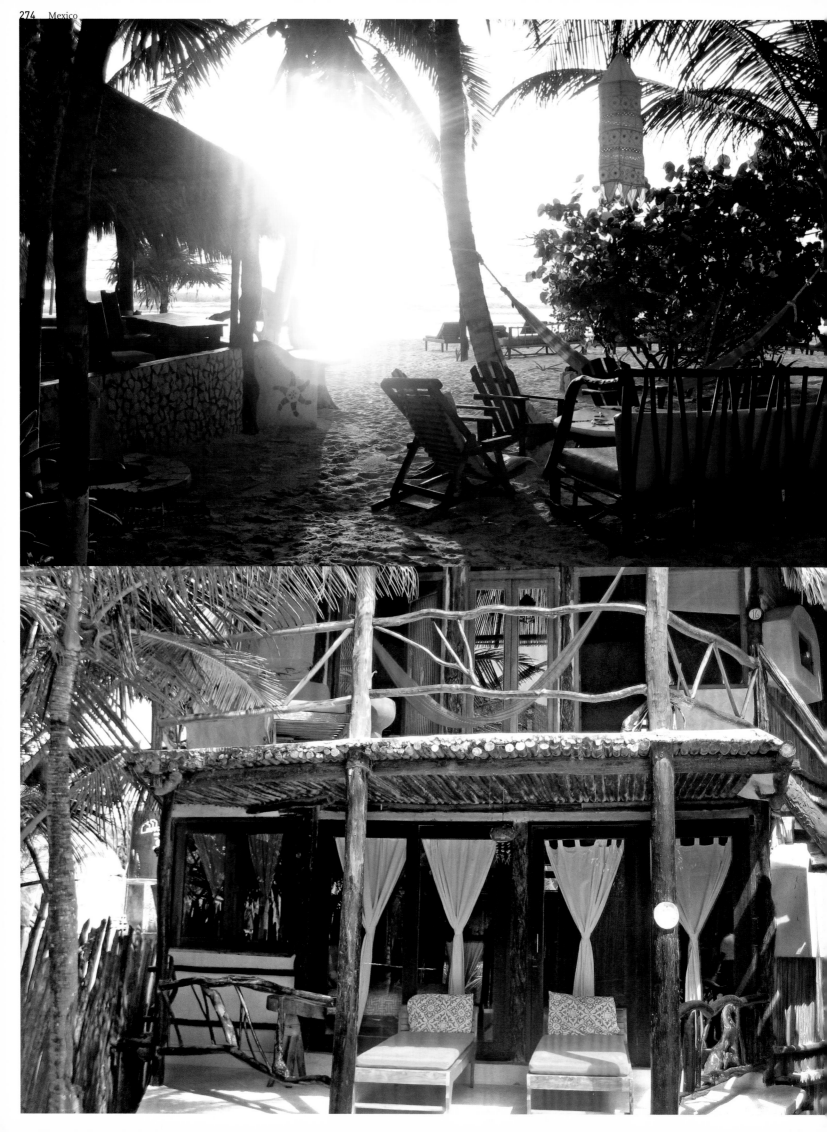

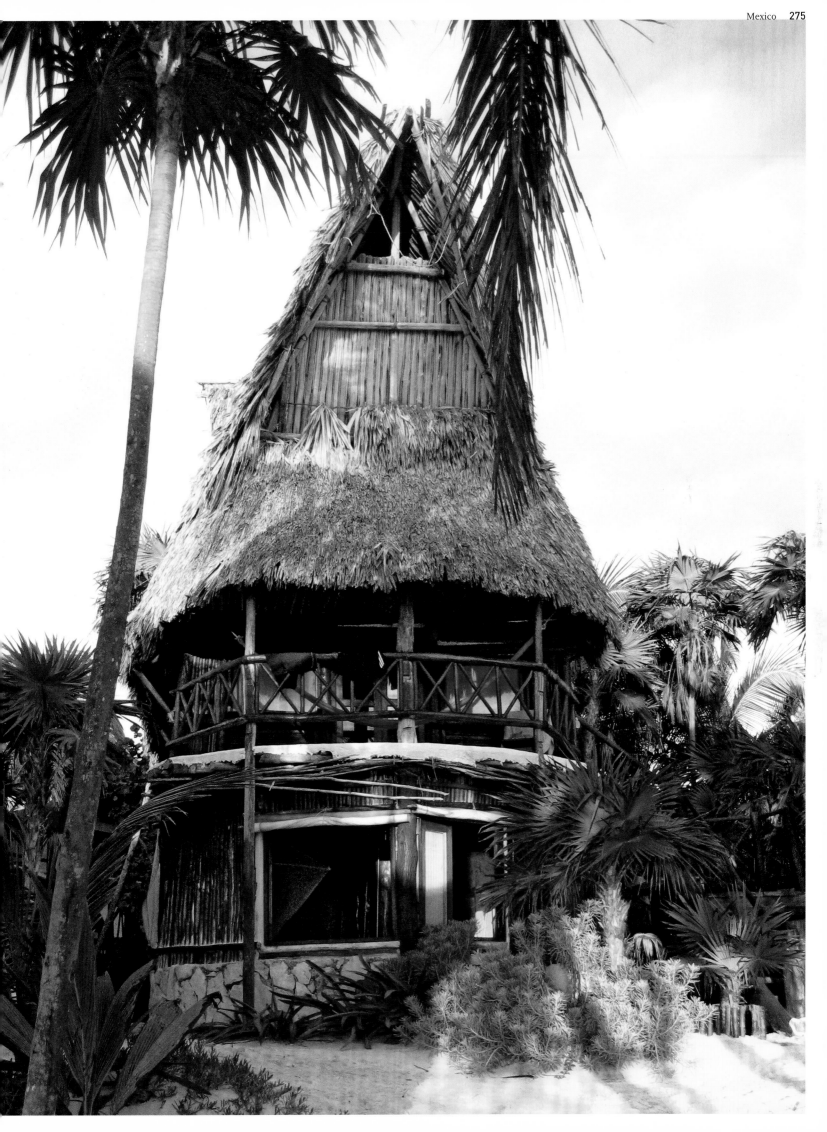

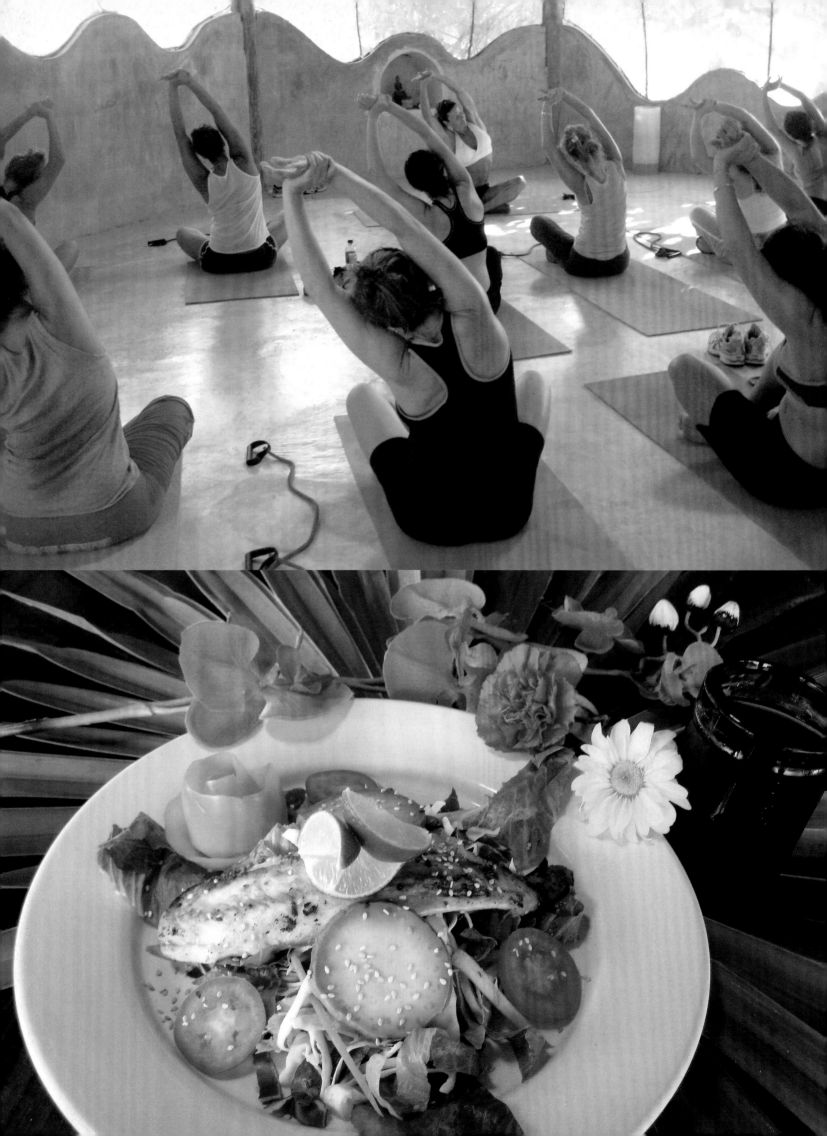

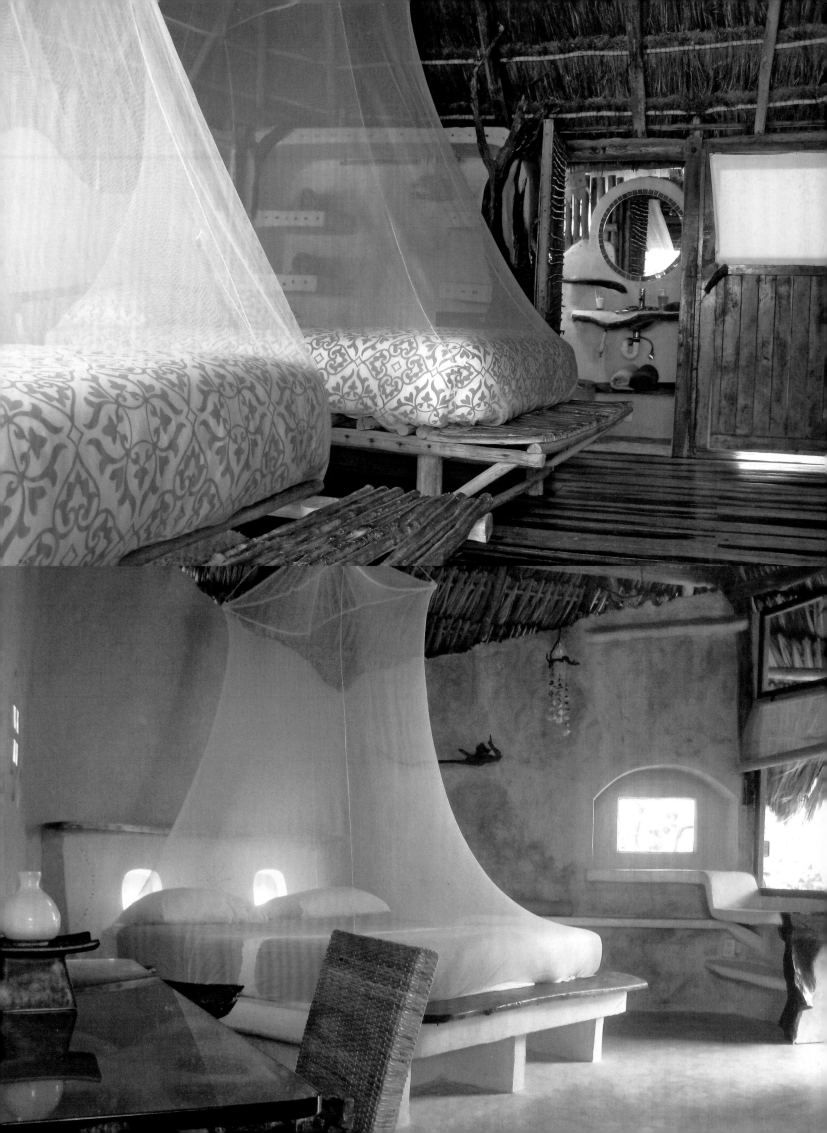

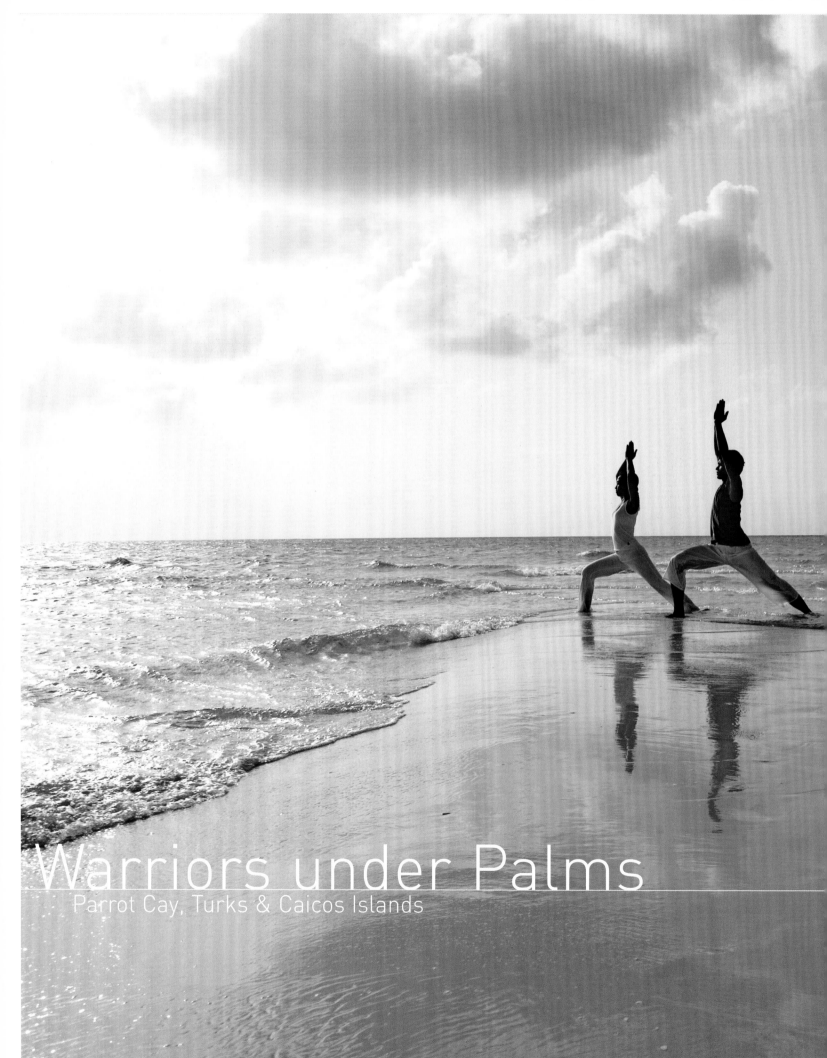

Warriors under Palms
Parrot Cay, Turks & Caicos Islands

Parrot Cay, Turks & Caicos Islands

Warriors under Palms

Outside it is well over 86 degrees Fahrenheit; inside the ventilator whirrs, and the sweating guests hold Downward Facing Dog. Was that more than five breaths? The cheek of it. Why not pack up and amble over to Keith Richards' place for a drink? Or to Donna Karan's – she does Yoga too. But the almost unnatural blue of the Caribbean, which reminds one of a drink for the ladies, or a visit to the world's most elegant spa, quickly calms the temper. What's the use anyway? There is no escape from this small private island, which lies in the Caribbean as though James Bond had taken up residence there as a pensioner. And why would you want to leave? Private butlers fulfil every wish, and the scent of hibiscus flowers hangs heavy in the air above the floodlit tennis courts and the infinity pool. Supermodels, world-famous Yogis and their followers escape here to enjoy, to a soundtrack of silver herons and the quietly hissing spray of the sea, what Shambala means in Sanskrit: peace and harmony. Maybe a facial, too, from the specialist Dr. Nicholas Perricone, and the best "organic" piña colada in the world.

Book to pack: "The Power of Now" by Eckhart Tolle.

Parrot Cay	
P.O. Box 164	
Providenciales, Turks & Caicos Islands	
British West Indies	
Tel. +1 649 946 7788	
Fax +1 649 946 7789	
info@parrotcay.como.bz	
www.parrotcay.como.bz	

DIRECTIONS	One of the 40 small Turks & Caicos Islands. About 70 min flying time southwest of Miami. Airport transfer from the main island of Providenciales by boat included in the price.
YOGA	Iyengar, Vinyasa, Hatha, Anusara.
TEACHERS	Erich Schiffmann, Elena Brower, Rodney Yee, Colleen Saidman.
ROOMS	A total of 60 rooms, including beach houses and villas.
FOOD	Caribbean, Southeast Asian, Continental, Italian.
TREATMENTS	Holistic therapies, reflex zone massage, Ayurveda, massage, facial treatments, Abhyanga package.
RECREATION	Pilates, catamaran sailing, water-skiing, diving, tennis, swimming.

Krieger unter Palmen

Draußen sind es weit über 30 Grad, drinnen surrt der Ventilator, schwitzend harren die Gäste im herabschauenden Hund aus. Das waren doch mehr als fünf Atemzüge? Frechheit. Warum nicht zusammenpacken und hinüber zu Keith Richards schlendern auf einen Drink? Oder zu Donna Karan, die macht doch auch Yoga. Doch das fast schon unnatürliche Blau der Karibik, das an einen Drink für Ladys erinnert, oder ein Besuch im elegantesten Spa der Welt besänftigt schnell die Gemüter. Was würde es auch nützen? Es gibt kein Entkommen von dieser kleinen Privatinsel, die in der Karibik liegt, als warte sie darauf, dass sich James Bond dort als Rentner niederlässt. Und warum auch? Private Butler erfüllen einem jeden Wunsch, schwer hängt der Duft nach Hibiskusblüten über den von Flutlicht erhellten Tennisplätzen und dem Infinity-Pool. Supermodels, weltberühmte Yogis und ihre Anhänger flüchten hierher, um beim Soundtrack von Silberreihern und leise zischender Gischt des Meeres zu genießen, was Shambala auf Sanskrit bedeutet: Frieden und Harmonie. Vielleicht noch ein Facial des Spezialisten Dr. Nicholas Perricone und den besten »organic« Piña Colada der Welt.

Buchtipp: »Jetzt! Die Kraft der Gegenwart« von Eckhart Tolle.

Guerriers sous les palmiers

A l'extérieur, le thermomètre grimpe bien au-dessus de 30 degrés, à l'intérieur le ventilateur bourdonne, les hôtes en sueur gardent stoïquement la posture du « chien tête en bas ». Mais c'était plus que cinq inspirations, non ? Quel toupet. Pourquoi ne pas plier bagage et aller tranquillement prendre un pot chez Keith Richards ? Ou chez Donna Karan, car elle aussi fait du yoga. Cependant, le bleu presque irréel des Caraïbes, couleur d'un drink pour dames, ou un passage dans le spa le plus élégant du monde, calme vite les esprits. D'ailleurs, à quoi bon ? On ne s'évade pas de cette petite île privée, posée là dans la mer des Caraïbes, comme si James Bond s'y était installé à l'âge de la retraite. Et puis, pourquoi s'enfuir ? Un maître d'hôtel à votre service satisfait tous vos désirs, le parfum lourd des fleurs d'hibiscus plane au-dessus des courts de tennis baignés par la lumière des projecteurs et de la piscine à débordement. Top modèles, yogis mondialement connus et leurs adeptes viennent se réfugier ici et, avec en fond sonore les cris des grandes aigrettes et le bruit de l'écume frémissante, goûtent le shambala, qui signifie en sanskrit : paix et harmonie. Peut-être encore un traitement facial du Dr Nicholas Perricone, expert en la matière, et le meilleur drink bio au monde, une Piña Colada.

Livre à emporter : « Le Pouvoir du moment présent » d'Eckhart Tolle.

ANREISE	Eine der 40 kleinen Turks- und Caicosinseln. Etwa 70 min Flugzeit südöstlich von Miami gelegen. Flughafentransfer von der Hauptinsel Providenciales per Boot.
YOGA	Iyengar, Vinyasa, Hatha, Anusara.
GASTLEHRER	Erich Schiffmann, Elena Brower, Rodney Yee, Colleen Saidman.
ZIMMER	60 Zimmer inklusive Beach-Häuser und Villen.
KÜCHE	Karibisch, südostasiatisch, kontinental, italienisch.
ANWENDUNGEN	Reflexzonenmassage, Ayurveda, Massage, Gesichtsbehandlungen, Abhyanga-Package.
FREIZEIT	Pilates, Katamaransegeln, Wasserski, Tauchen, Tennis, Schwimmen.

ACCÈS	Une des 40 petites îles Turques-et-Caïques. Située à environ 70 min de vol au sud-est de Miami. Transfert par bateau inclus, de l'aéroport de l'île principale.
YOGA	Iyengar, Vinyasa, Hatha, Anusara.
PROFESSEURS	Erich Schiffmann, Elena Brower, Rodney Yee, Colleen Saidman.
CHAMBRES	60 chambres, y compris maisons de plage et villas.
RESTAURATION	Cuisine des Caraïbes, du Sud-Est asiatique, italienne.
TRAITEMENTS	Thérapies intégrales, massages des zones de réflexe, Ayurveda, massage, soins du visage, Abhyanga-Package.
ACTIVITÉS	Pilates, nautisme (catamaran), ski nautique, plongée, tennis, natation.

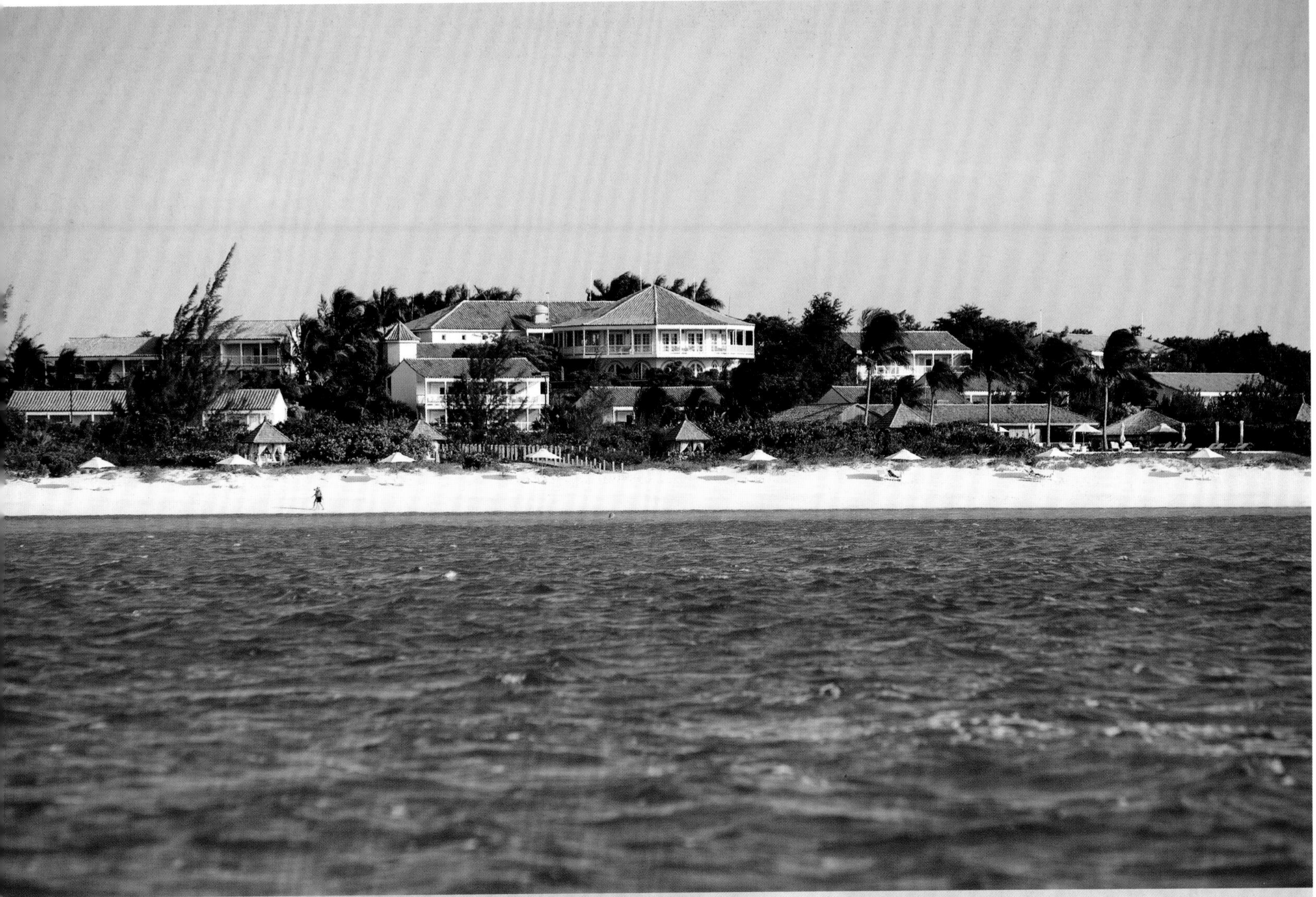

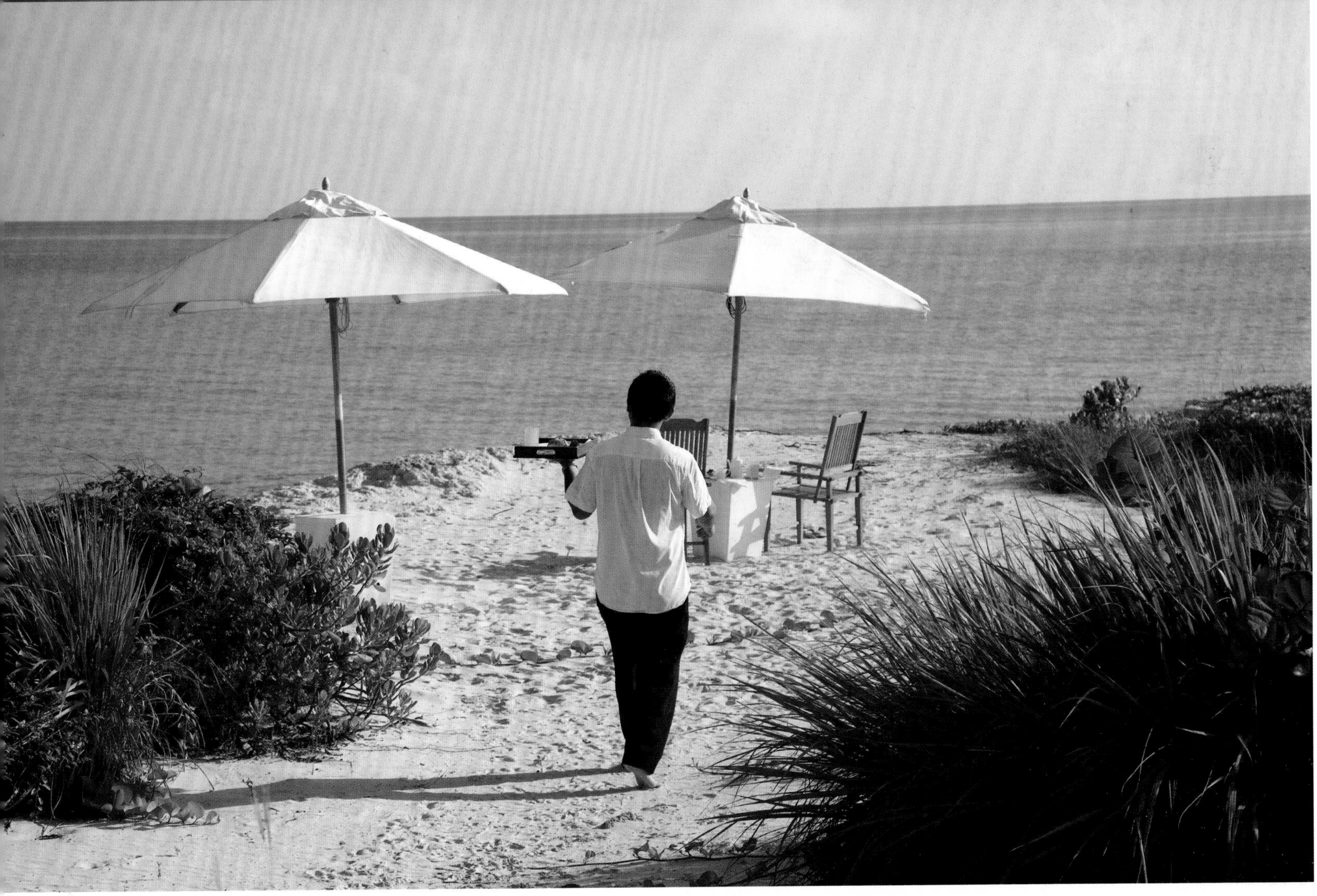

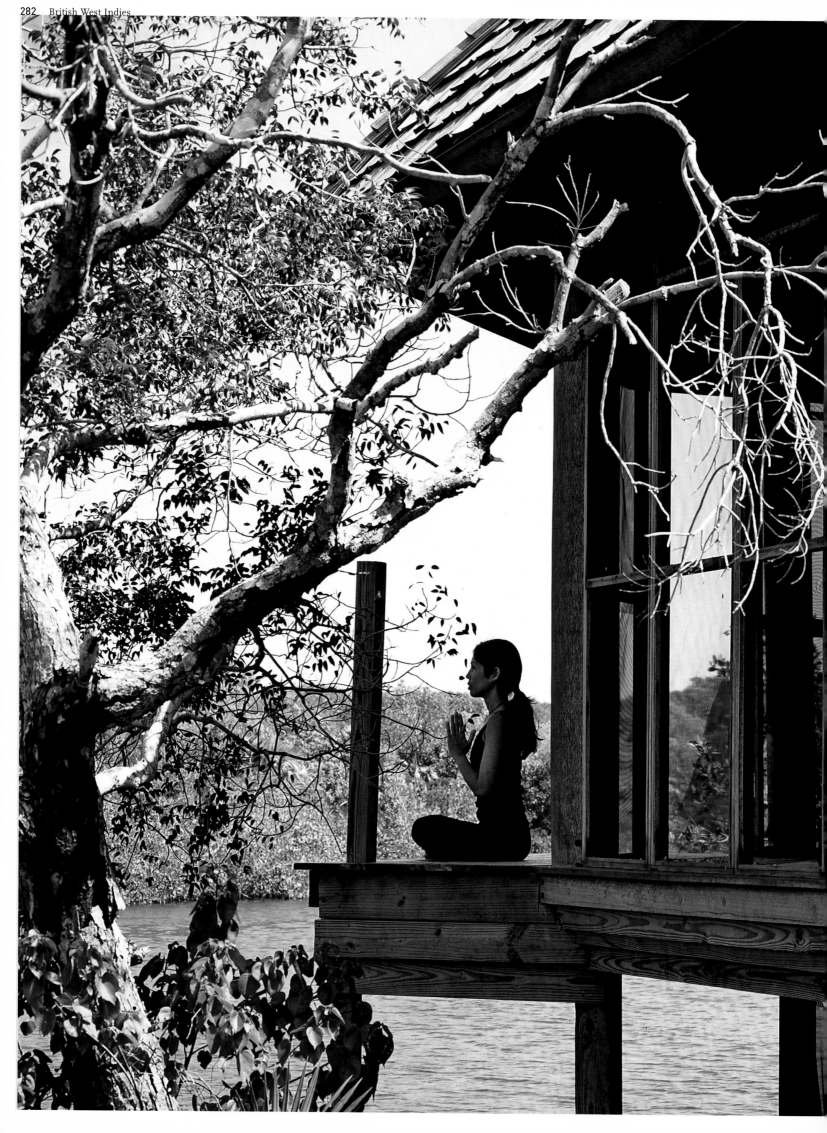

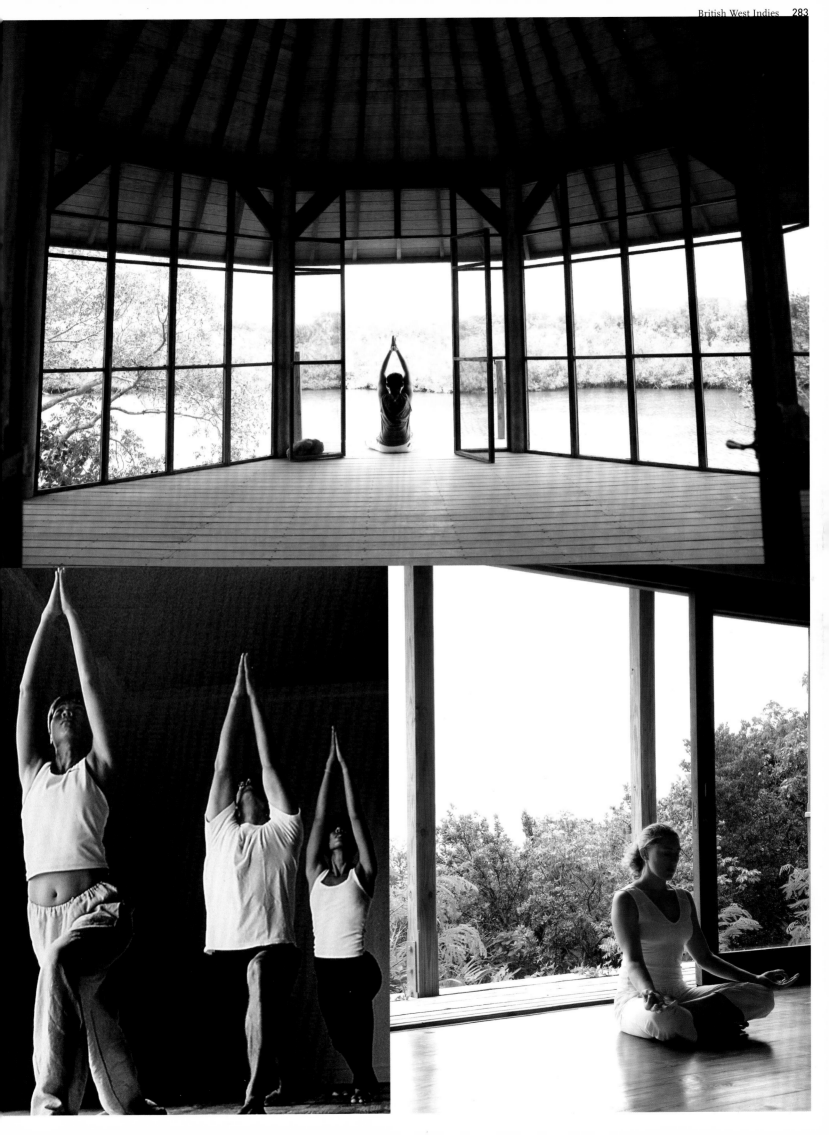

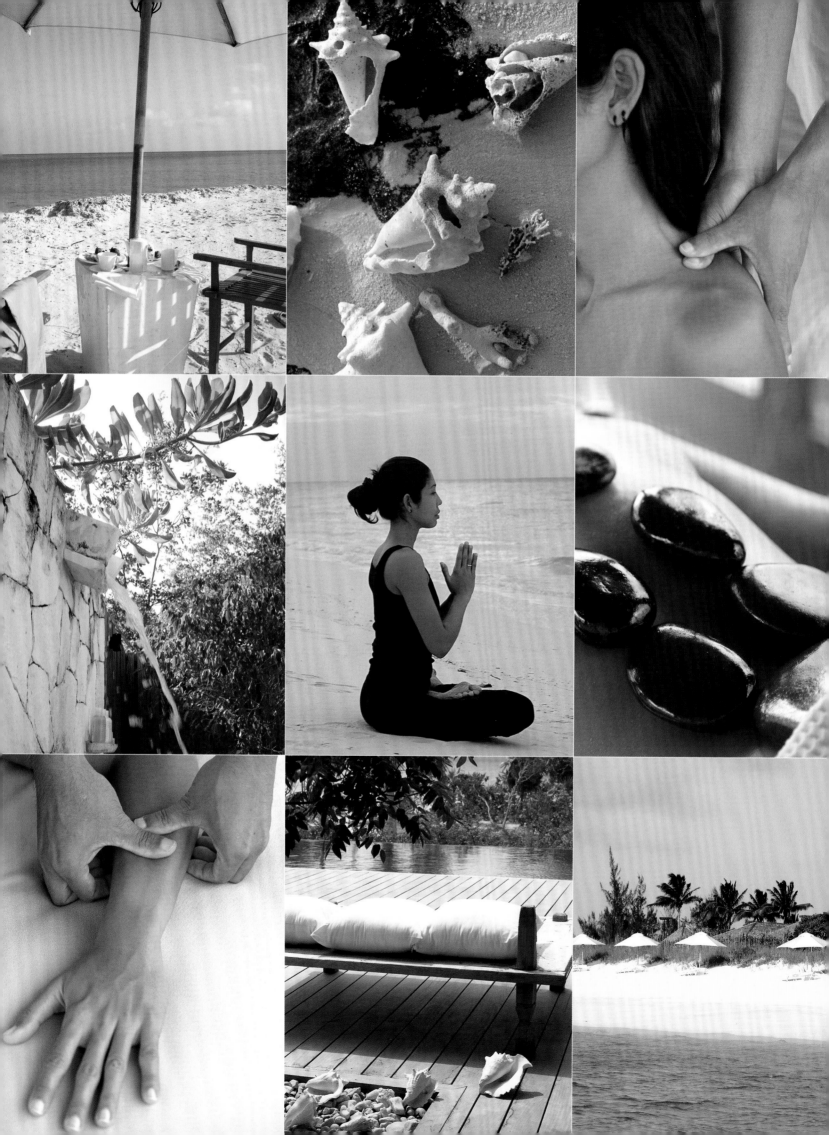

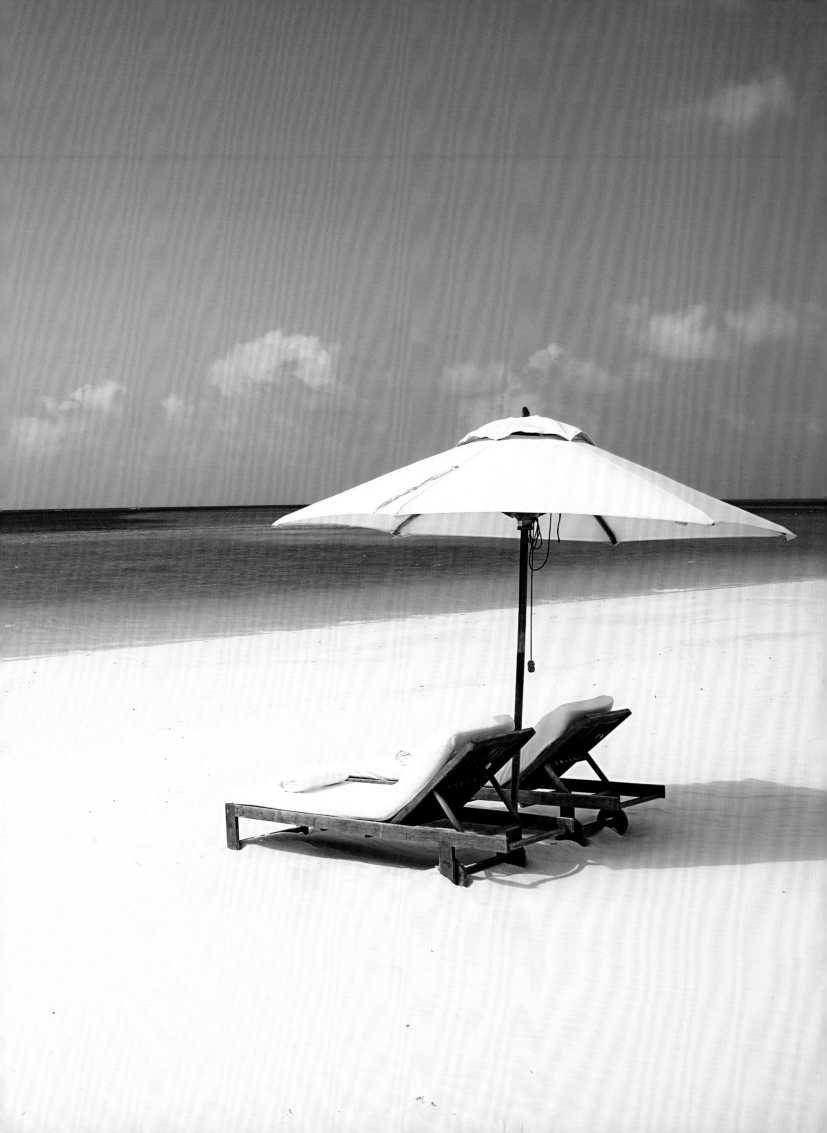

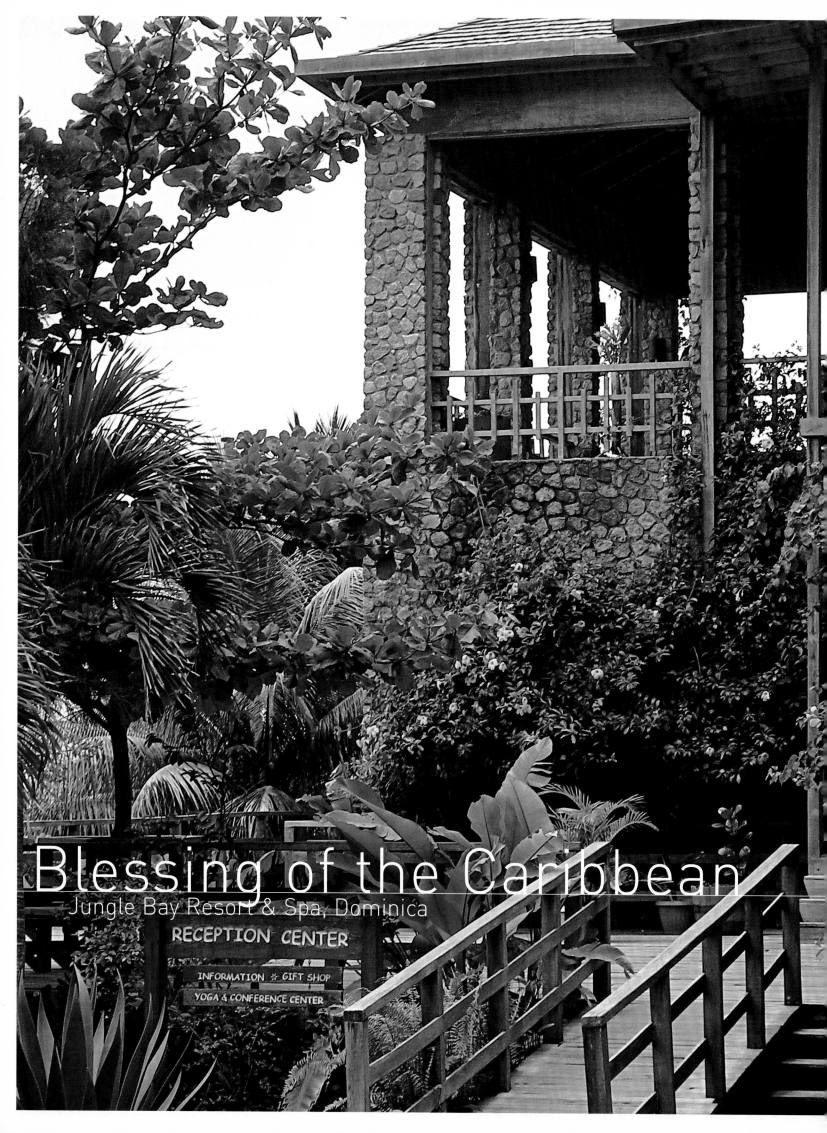

Blessing of the Caribbean
Jungle Bay Resort & Spa, Dominica

RECEPTION CENTER

INFORMATION ❀ GIFT SHOP
YOGA & CONFERENCE CENTER

Jungle Bay Resort & Spa, Dominica

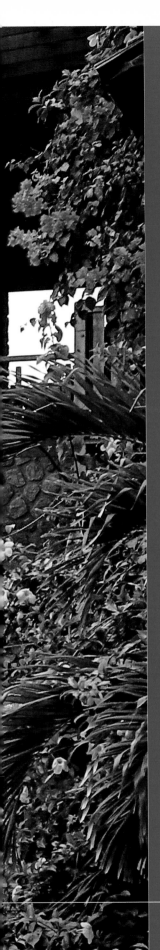

Blessing of the Caribbean
If the Dominican Republic is the Pamela Anderson of the Caribbean – shining surface, instant fun, occasionally chaotic – then Dominica is the Julia Roberts of the Lesser Antilles: intense, idiosyncratic, unpolished, but really quite sexy. With its black sandy beaches, primeval rain forest, huge ferns, orchids, banana trees and red-throated parrots, the Morne Trois Pitons National Park is on Unesco's World Heritage list. At daybreak in the Jungle Bay eco lodge, opened in 2005, you can face east for a sun salutation on the veranda; but if you oversleep you can also have a good stretch later in the large hall of volcanic stone. Sometimes the view over the Atlantic is enough to make you feel somewhat closer to heaven. Those who survive the ten-hour trek through mud and over steep cliffs to the 4747-foot-high Mount Diablotin will need a deep-tissue massage in the spa pavilion, built on the slope as if hovering above the surf. Curse of the Caribbean? On the contrary. The place is a blessing.
Book to pack: "The Green Pope" by Miguel Angel Asturias.

Jungle Bay Resort & Spa	
Point Mulatre, Roseau	
Commonwealth of Dominica	
British West Indies	
Tel. +1 767 446 1789	
Fax +1 767 446 1090	
info@junglebaydominica.com	
www.junglebaydominica.com	

DIRECTIONS	Dominica lies in the eastern Caribbean between Guadeloupe and Martinique and has two small airports: Melville Hall Airport and Canefield Airport.
YOGA	Hatha, Anusara, Vinyasa Flow.
TEACHERS	Sheree Mullen, Chrissy Carter, Nikki Vilella.
ROOMS	35 huts with a king-size bed or 2 double beds.
FOOD	Caribbean, freshly caught fish, breadfruit salad, beetroot salad, baked bananas, fresh tamarind juice.
TREATMENTS	Massage, facial, pedicure, manicure, aromatherapy, detoxifying body rub, honeymoon massage.
RECREATION	Tai Chi, hiking, day trips, mountain biking, snorkelling, kayaking, diving.

Segen der Karibik

Wenn die Dominikanische Republik die Pamela Anderson der Karibik ist – glänzende Oberfläche, schneller Spaß, gelegentlich chaotisch – ist Dominica die Julia Roberts der Kleinen Antillen: intensiv, eigen, unpoliert, dabei durchaus sexy. Mit seinen schwarzen Sandstränden, urzeitlichem Regenwald, dicken Farnen, Orchideen, Bananenbäumen und rothalsigen Papageien gehört der Morne Trois Pitons National Park zum UNESCO-Welterbe. In der 2005 eröffneten Jungle-Bay-Öko-Lodge kann man bereits in der Morgendämmerung auf der Veranda seine Sonnengrüße Richtung Osten richten, oder aber, sollte man verschlafen, sich später in der großen Halle aus Vulkanstein dehnen. Manchmal genügt schon der Blick über den Atlantik, um sich dem Himmel etwas näher zu fühlen. Wer die zehnstündige Wanderung durch Matsch und über steile Felsen zum 1.447 Meter hohen Mount Diablotin übersteht, wird eine Deep-Tissue-Massage im Spa-Pavillon brauchen, der oberhalb der Brandung gleichsam schwebend in den Hang gebaut ist. Fluch der Karibik? Im Gegenteil. Der Platz ist ein Segen.

Buchtipp: »Der grüne Papst« von Miguel Angel Asturias.

Le paradis est aux Caraïbes

Si la République dominicaine est la Pamela Anderson des Caraïbes – look éblouissant, plaisir facile, quelquefois chaotique –, la Dominique est la Julia Roberts des Petites Antilles : intense, capricieuse, naturelle mais ô combien sexy. Avec ses plages de sable noir, sa forêt pluviale, ses fougères touffues, ses orchidées, ses bananiers et ses perroquets à cou rouge, le Parc national de Morne Trois Pitons est classé au patrimoine mondial de l'UNESCO. Dans les pavillons écologiques de Jungle Bay, inaugurés en 2005, on peut adresser sur la véranda, dès l'aurore, un salut au soleil en se tournant vers l'est, ou plus tard, si l'on a dormi trop longtemps, faire des exercices d'assouplissement dans la grande salle en pierre volcanique. Parfois, un regard posé sur l'Atlantique suffit pour se sentir plus près du ciel. Pour qui vient de marcher dix heures dans la boue au-dessus des roches escarpées du Mont Diablotin (1 447 mètres), un massage en profondeur dans le pavillon Spa, suspendu à même le coteau au-dessus du ressac, s'impose. Pas de pirates ni de malédiction ici, au contraire, cet endroit est béni des dieux.

Livre à emporter : « Le Pape Vert » de Miguel Angel Asturias.

ANREISE	Dominica liegt in der Ostkaribik zwischen Guadeloupe und Martinique und hat zwei kleine Flughäfen: Melvill Hall Airport oder Canefield Airport.	ACCÈS	La Dominique se trouve entre la Guadeloupe et la Martinique et dispose de deux petits aéroports: Melvill Hall Airport et Canefield Airport.
YOGA	Hatha, Anusara, Vinyasa Flow.	YOGA	Hatha, Anusara, Vinyasa Flow.
GASTLEHRER	Sheree Mullen, Chrissy Carter, Nikki Vilella.	PROFESSEURS	Sheree Mullen, Chrissy Carter, Nikki Vilella.
ZIMMER	35 Hütten mit einem Kingsize-Bett oder 2 Doppelbetten.	CHAMBRES	35 bungalows avec un lit extra-large ou deux lits.
KÜCHE	Karibisch, frischer Fisch, Brotfruchtsalat, Rote-Bete-Salat, geröstete Bananen, frischer Tamarindensaft.	RESTAURATION	Caraïbe, poisson pêché sur place, salade d'uru, salade de betterave rouge, bananes grillées, jus de tamarin.
ANWENDUNGEN	Massage, Facial, Pediküre, Maniküre, Aromatherapie, Detox-Body-Rub, Honeymoon-Massage.	TRAITEMENTS	Massage, facial, pédicurie, manucurie, aromathérapie, massage de détoxication, massage « lune de miel ».
FREIZEIT	Tai Chi, Wandern, Ausflüge, Mountainbike, Schnorcheln, Kajak, Tauchen.	ACTIVITÉS	Tai Chi, randonnées, excursions, VTT, plongée libre, kayak, plongée sous-marine.

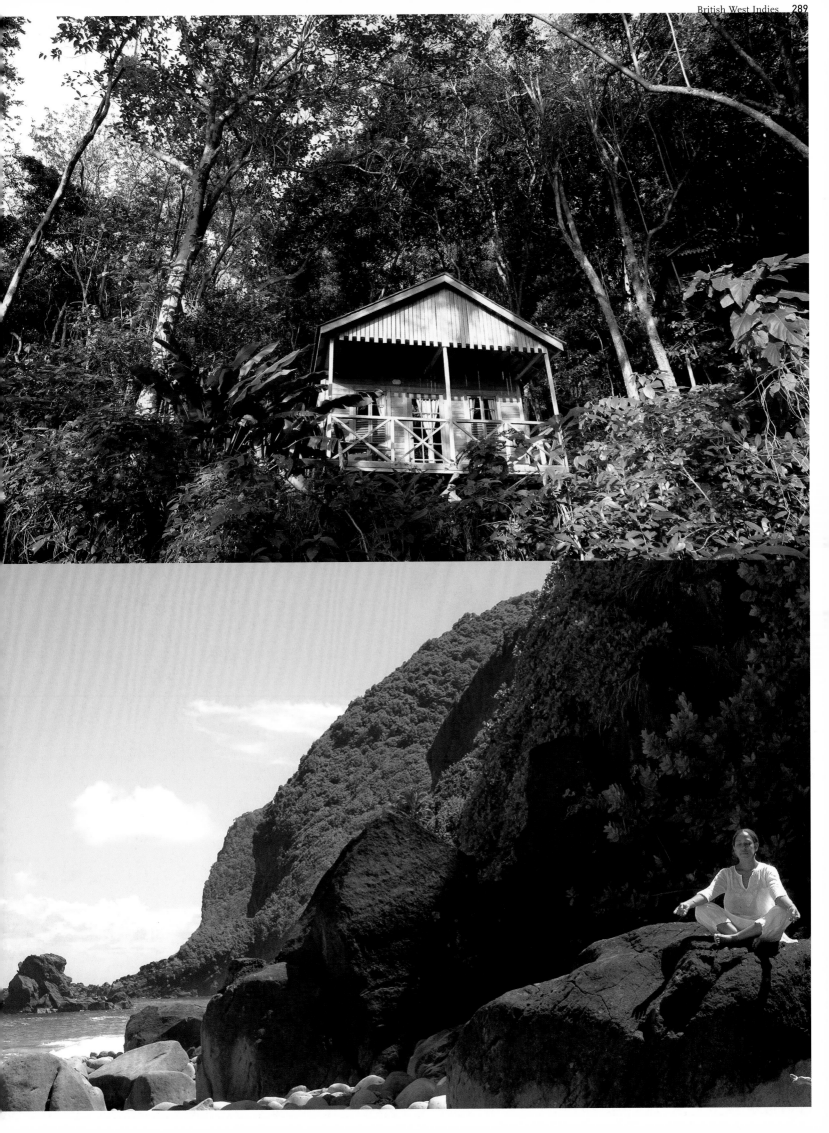

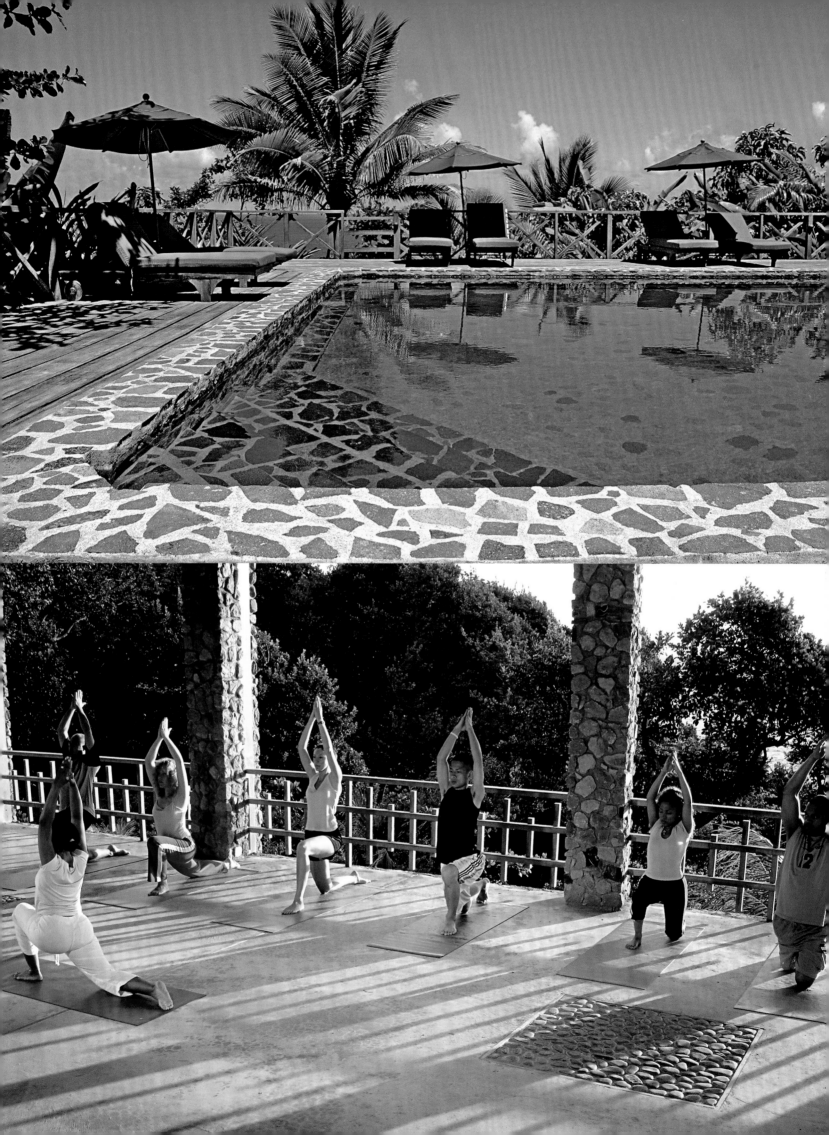

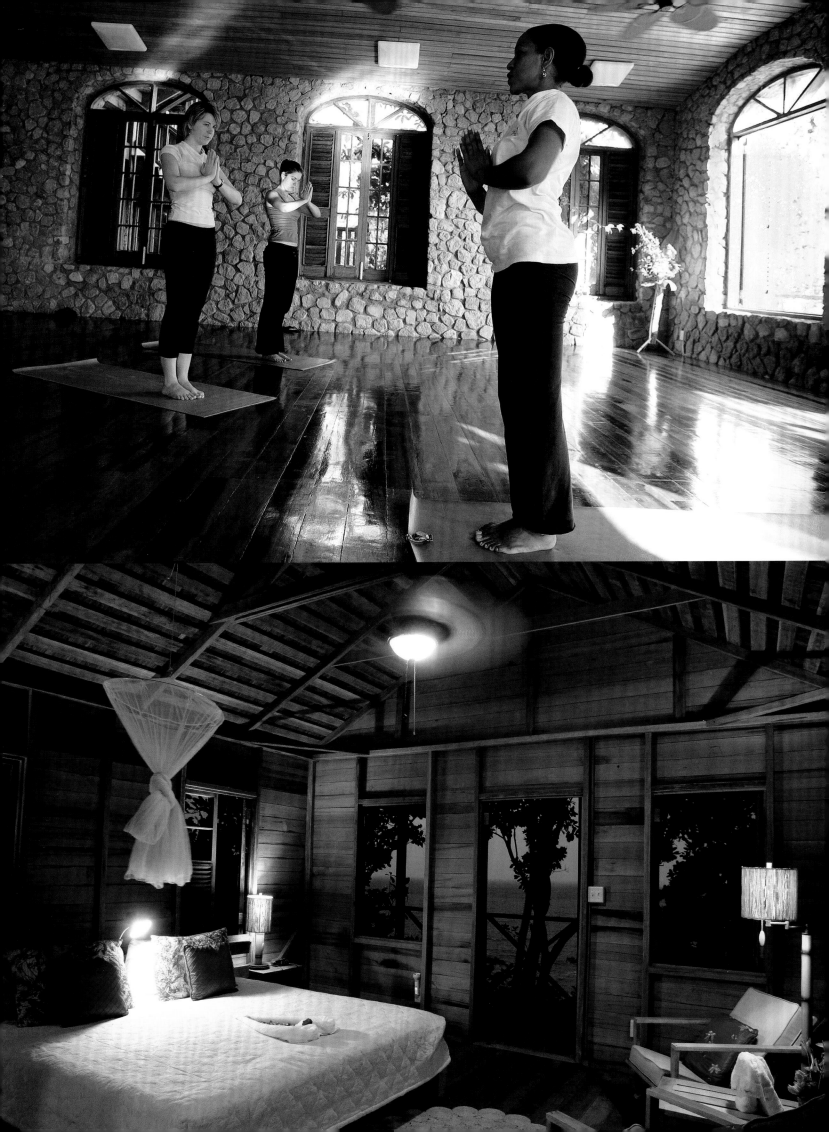

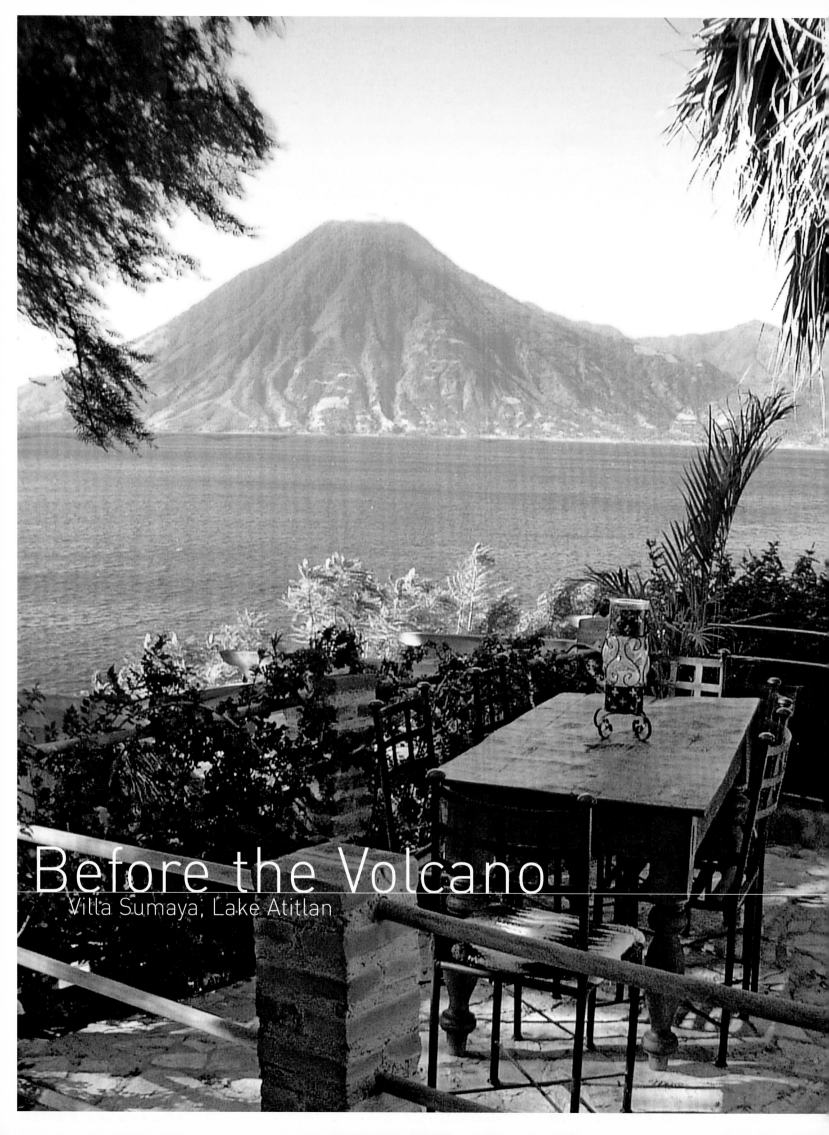

Before the Volcano
Villa Sumaya, Lake Atitlan

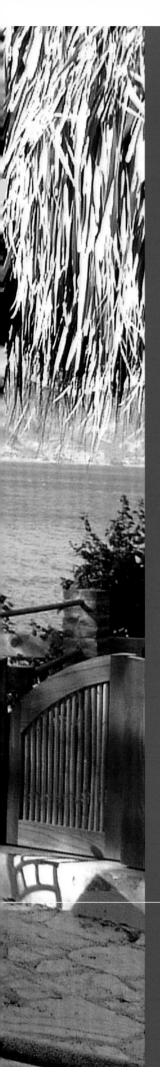

Villa Sumaya, Lake Atitlan

Before the Volcano

The morning fog banks rise, clearing the view onto the mighty volcano on the opposite shore of the unique deep blue lake, and from the kitchen comes the aroma of freshly baked bread and coffee. Even if the advanced civilisation of the Mayas met its mysterious end more than a thousand years ago, the fertile soil of the mountain ridge, the lakes and the avocado and coffee forests became home to the Cack'chiquel, Quek'chi, Mam and Tzutujil – ethnic Mayan groups whose traditional culture still exists today. How did they pass the time back then? In Villa Sumaya, at any rate, there is no reason for cultural pessimism. Under the huge dome of the straw roof, not only is Yoga practised on the parquet floor, but also, mindful of the ruins of a unique civilisation, an insight is gained into the transitoriness of one's own culture. But as long as there is the solar-heated pool and fresh enchiladas, home-made sauces with chilli peppers and organic fruit, no problem. The rest is taken care of by the sweet Guatemalan worry dolls, which are on sale in the hotel's delightful shop, Spirit Dog.

Book to pack: "Under the Volcano" by Malcolm Lowry.

Villa Sumaya	
Santa Cruz La Laguna,	
Lake Atitlan	
Guatemala	
Tel. +502 402 61390 and +502 402 61455	
info@villasumaya.com	
www.villasumaya.com	

DIRECTIONS	Located on the shores of Lake Atitlan at an elevation of 5,000 feet, about 3 hrs drive from the airport in Guatemala City.
YOGA	Hatha, Iyengar.
TEACHERS	Paula Tursi, Will Duprey, Laurie Ellis Young.
CLASSES	Maya seminar, Spanish course, creative writing.
ROOMS	15 rooms, max. 33 guests.
FOOD	Slow Food, fish, local specialities.
TREATMENTS	Massage.
RECREATION	Pool, hot tub, sauna, kayaking, diving, water-skiing, hiking, horseback riding, birdwatching, boat trips.

Vor dem Vulkan

Die morgendlichen Nebelbänke heben sich, der Blick wird frei auf die mächtigen Vulkane am anderen Ufer des einzigartigen tiefblauen Sees, und aus der Küche dringt der Geruch nach frisch gebackenem Brot und Kaffee. Auch wenn die Hochkultur der Mayas vor mehr als 1000 Jahren ihr mysteriöses Ende fand, wurden die fruchtbare Erde der Bergzüge, die Seen, Avocado- und Kaffeewälder zur Heimat der Cack'chiquel, Quek'chi, Mam und Tzutujil – ethnische Maya-Gruppen, deren traditionelle Kultur noch heute besteht. Wie sie sich damals wohl die Zeit vertrieben haben? In der Villa Sumaya besteht jedenfalls kein Grund zum Kulturpessimismus. Unter der riesigen Kuppel des Strohdachs wird auf Holzparkett nicht nur Yoga geübt, sondern eingedenk der Ruinen einer einzigartigen Zivilisation auch die Einsicht in die Vergänglichkeit der eigenen Kultur. Solange es den solargeheizten Pool und frische Enchiladas, selbst gemachte Soßen aus Chillies und naturbelassenes Obst gibt, ist das kein Problem. Den Rest erledigen die niedlichen guatemaltekischen Sorgenpüppchen, die es in dem entzückenden Laden, Spirit Dog, im Hotel zu kaufen gibt.
Buchtipp: »Unter dem Vulkan« von Malcolm Lowry.

Face au volcan

Les nappes de brumes matinales s'évaporent, libérant la vue sur les puissants volcans dressés sur l'autre rive du fantastique lac d'un bleu profond, tandis que de la cuisine monte l'odeur de pain frais et de café. Si la civilisation maya s'éteignit mystérieusement il y a plus de mille ans, la terre fertile des flancs de montagne, les lacs, les forêts d'avocatiers et de caféiers sont devenus la patrie des Cack'chiquel, Quek'chi, Mam et Tzutujil, groupes ethniques mayas dont la culture traditionnelle subsiste de nos jours. Comment ont-ils tué le temps autrefois ? Dans la Villa Sumaya, en tout cas, il n'y a aucune raison de s'adonner à une vision pessimiste de la civilisation. Sous l'immense voûte du toit de paille ont lieu des séances de yoga sur le parquet en bois mais aussi, face aux ruines d'une civilisation extraordinaire, on prend conscience de la fragilité de notre propre culture. Pas de souci, tant qu'il y aura la piscine chauffée au soleil et des enchiladas, les sauces maison à base de piment fort et les fruits bio. Les ravissantes poupées anti-soucis guatémaliennes que l'on peut acheter à l'hôtel dans le joli magasin Spirit Dog se chargent du reste.
Livre à emporter : « Au-dessous du volcan » de Malcolm Lowry.

ANREISE	Am Ufer des Lake Atitlan auf 1.500 Höhenmetern gelegen, etwa 3 Std. Autofahrt vom Flughafen in Guatemala City entfernt.
YOGA	Hatha, Iyengar.
GASTLEHRER	Paula Tursi, Will Duprey, Laurie Ellis Young.
ZIMMER	15 Zimmer, max. 33 Gäste.
KÜCHE	Slow Food, Fisch, lokale Spezialitäten.
ANWENDUNGEN	Massagen.
FREIZEIT	Maya-Seminar, Spanischkurs, kreatives Schreiben, Pool, Hot Tub, Sauna, Kajak, Tauchen, Wasserski, Wandern, Reiten, Vogelschau, Bootsfahrten.

ACCÈS	Au bord du lac Atitlán situé à 1 500 m d'altitude, env. à 3 h de voiture de l'aéroport de Guatemala ville.
YOGA	Hatha, Iyengar.
PROFESSEURS	Paula Tursi, Will Duprey, Laurie Ellis Young.
CHAMBRES	15 chambres, 33 hôtes max.
RESTAURATION	Slow Food, poisson, spécialités locales.
TRAITEMENTS	Massages.
ACTIVITÉS	Séminaire maya, cours d'espagnol, écriture créative, piscine, bain tourbillon, sauna, kayak, plongée sous-marine, ski nautique, randonnées, équitation, observation d'oiseaux, promenades en bateau.

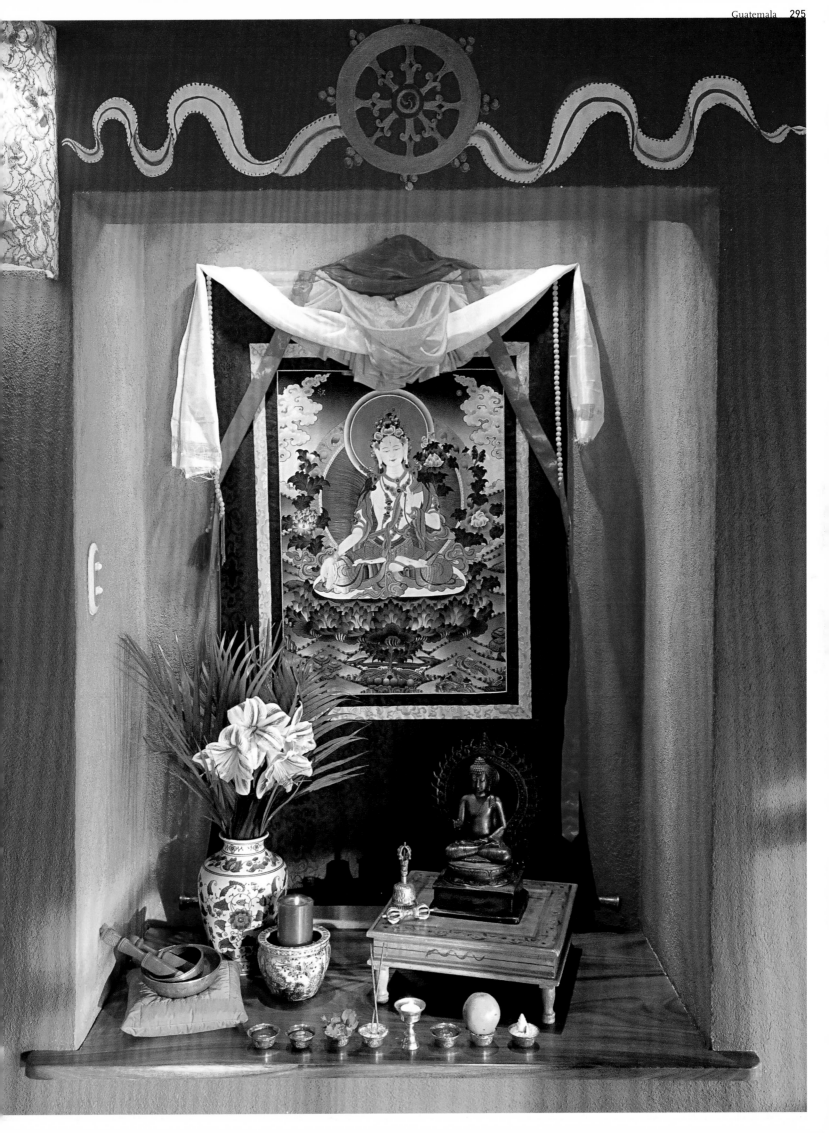

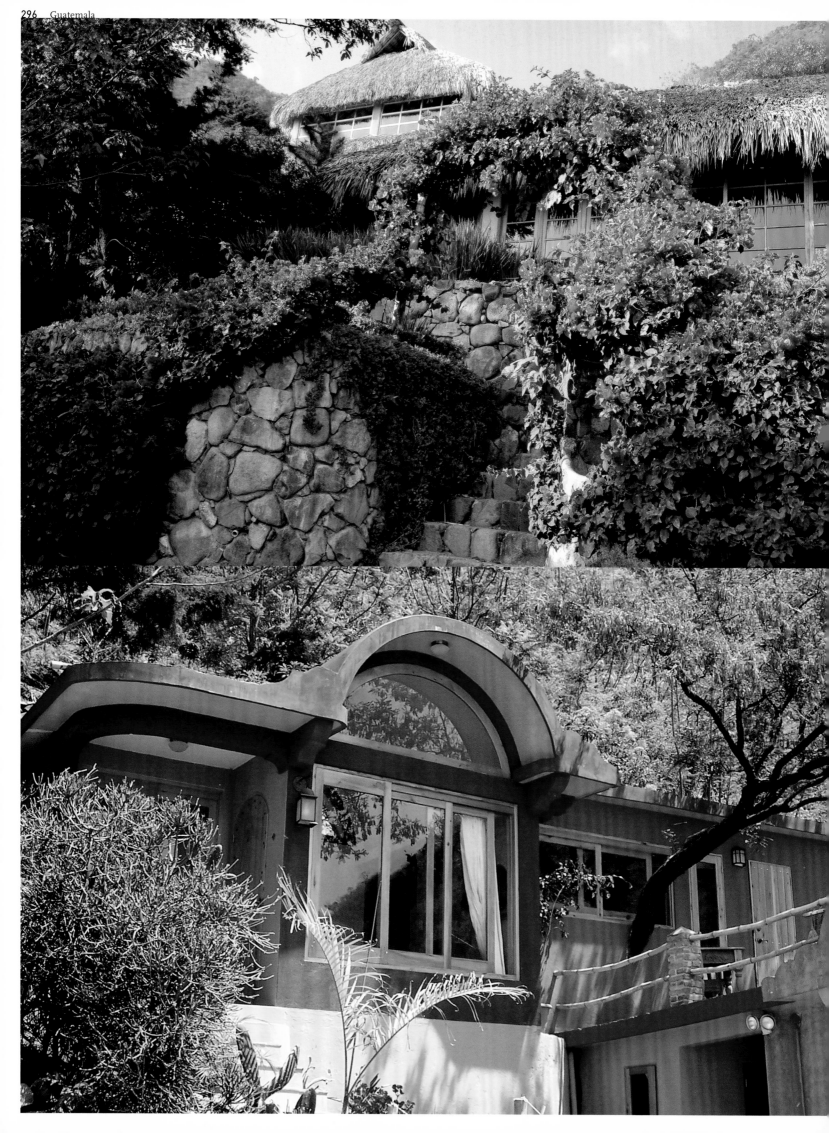

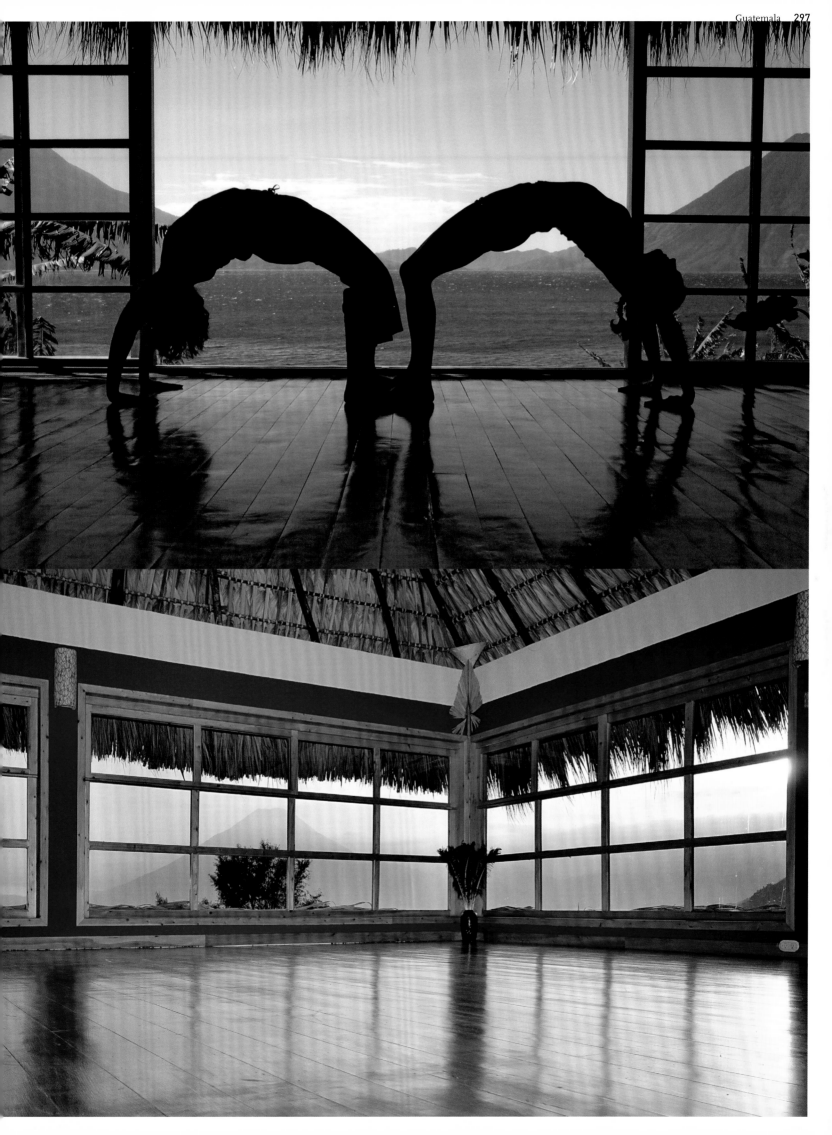

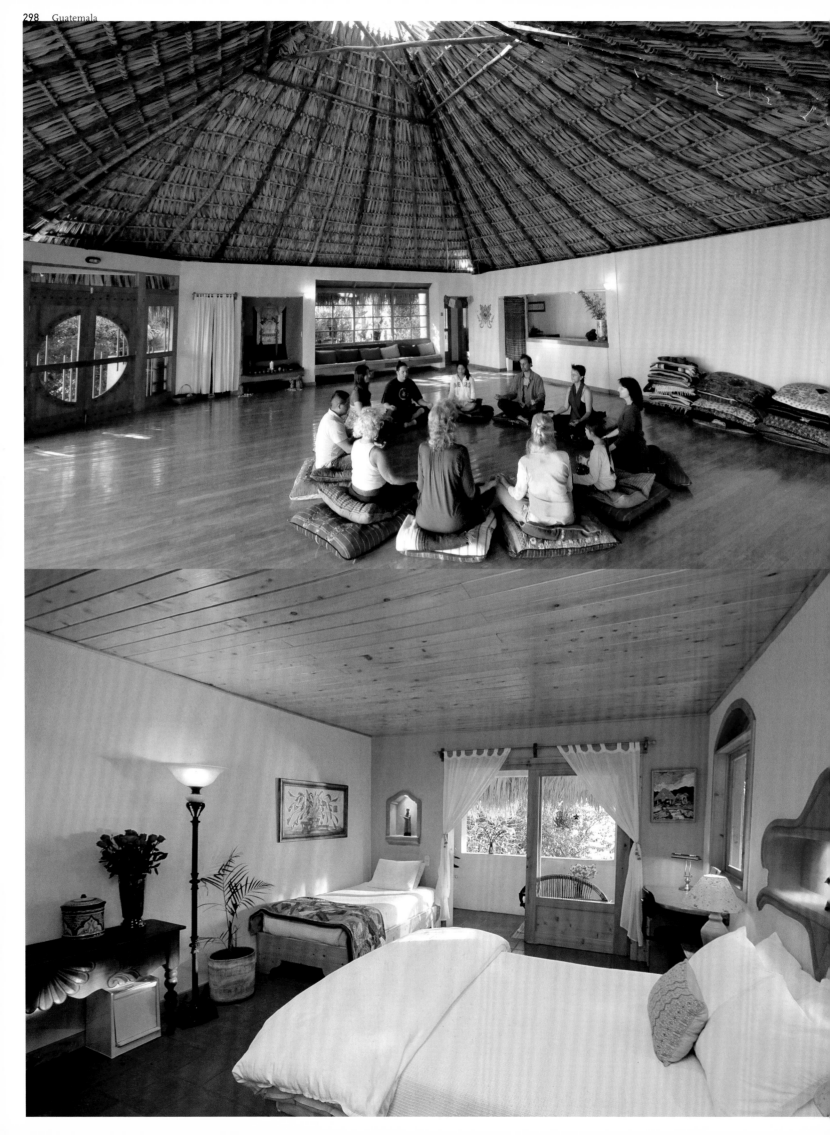

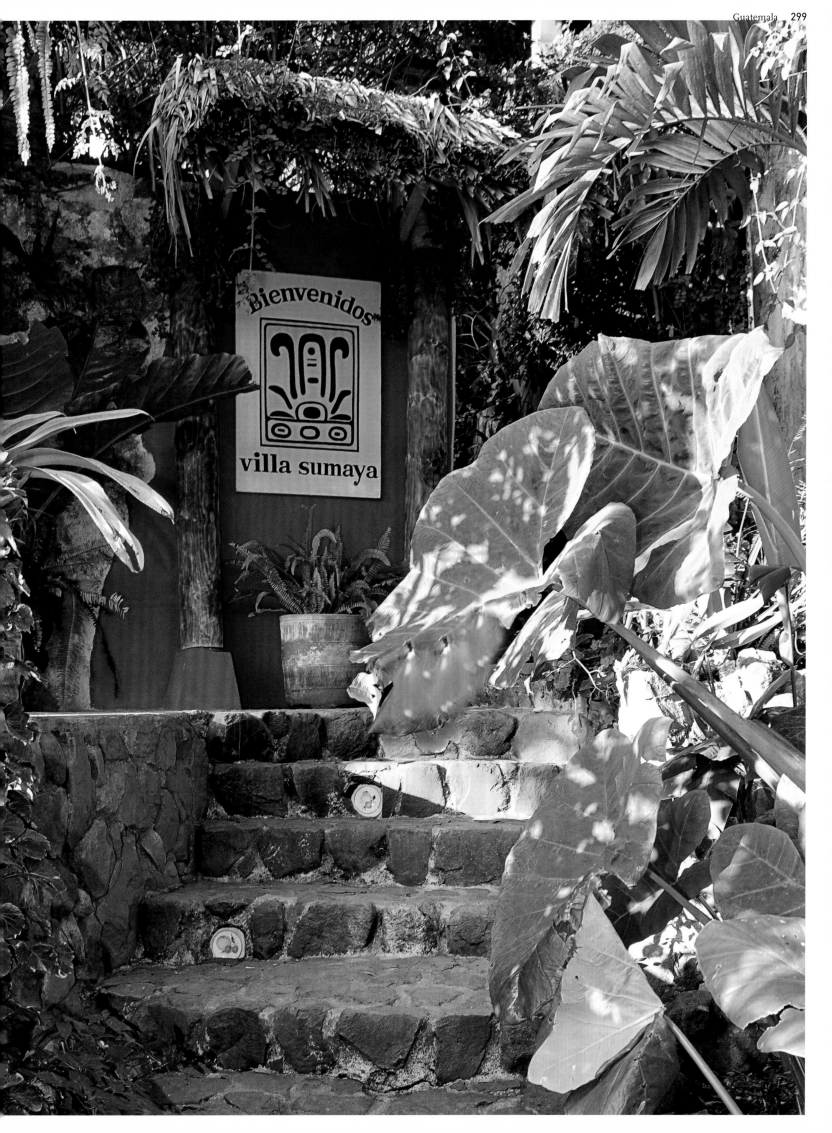

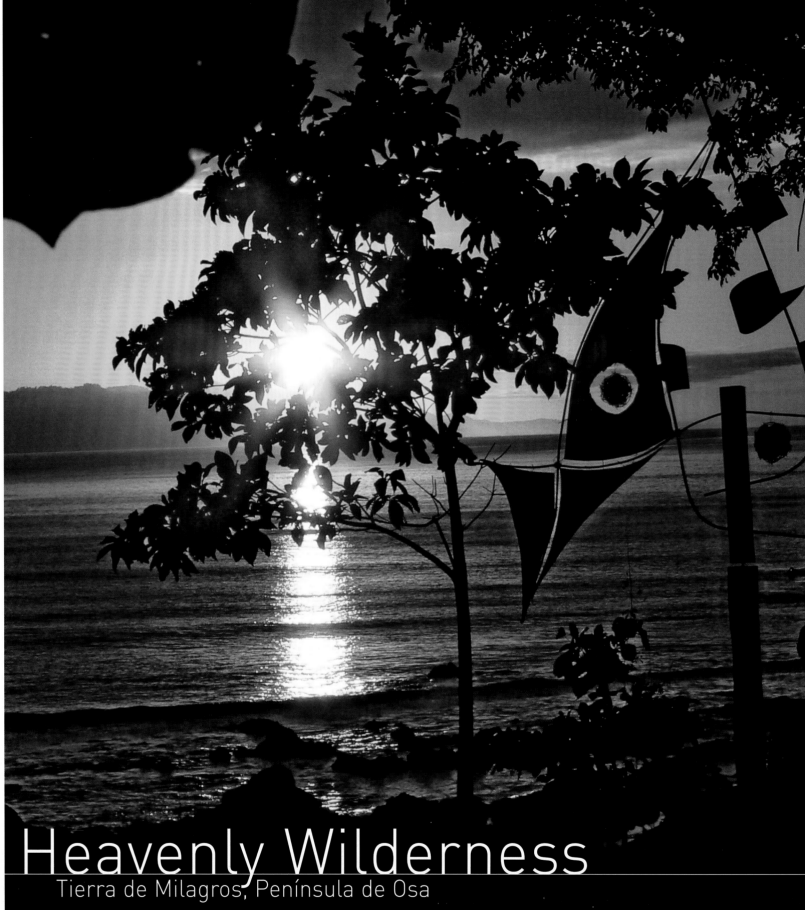

Heavenly Wilderness
Tierra de Milagros, Península de Osa

Tierra de Milagros, Península de Osa

Heavenly Wilderness

Let's not talk of paradise from the off; let's talk for the time being of a tiny country located between the Pacific and the Caribbean, of a couple of straw-covered huts in the midst of an enchanted botanical garden, of colourful hammocks woven for eternity and of a beach to whose flotsam and jetsam you would happily belong. Naturally, only the strongest in character and most flipped-out of New York's teachers ask their followers to come here. Nowhere else can monkeys, hanging casually from the auditorium's branches, see such intensive, imaginative Asana sessions as those that are held here on the spectacular Yoga platform directly at the ocean's edge. They scrutinise their relations from the city and wonder why they are contorting themselves so. There is laughter and the chattering of a multitude of voices from the balcony. The birds in the giant trees have the answer: because they still have the urban jungle in their heads. But watch out: after the shortest time, on the most beautiful patch of this small country, the people, too, swing wildly and daringly through the day. They drink ice-cool guava juice and, as they do so, they become more and more beautiful.

Books to pack: "How to Be Wild" by Simon Barnes and "I Am That" by Sri Nisargadatta Maharaj.

Tierra de Milagros	
Rio Carbonera	
Puerto Jimenez, Península de Osa	
Costa Rica	
Tel. +506 8387 6058	
info@tierrademilagros.com	
www.tierrademilagros.com	

DIRECTIONS	Located directly on the Golfo Dulce. 50-min flight from San José, capital of Costa Rica.
YOGA	Hatha, Ashtanga, Sivananda, Iyengar, Anusara.
TEACHERS	Schuyler Grant, Alison Novie, Sianna Sherman, Douglas Brooks, Kenneth Graham.
ROOMS	15 rooms for max. 30 guests.
FOOD	Organic vegetarian.
TREATMENTS	Facials, wraps, scrubs, massage, acupuncture.
RECREATION	Surfing, kayaking, horseback riding, hiking, swimming with dolphins.

Himmlische Wildnis

Reden wir nicht gleich vom Paradies, reden wir zunächst von einem winzigen Land, eingeklemmt zwischen Pazifik und Karibik, von ein paar strohgedeckten Hütten inmitten eines verwunschenen botanischen Gartens, von bunten Hängematten, die für die Ewigkeit geknüpft wurden, und von einem Strand, zu dessen Strandgut man gerne gehört. Logisch, dass hier die charakterstärksten und ausgeflipptesten Lehrer New Yorks ihre Anhänger herbestellen. So intensive, fantasievolle Asana-Stunden, wie sie hier auf der spektakulären Yoga-Plattform direkt am Ozean abgehalten werden, bekommen die Affen, die lässig an Ästen im Zuschauerraum hängen, woanders nicht zu sehen. Nachdenklich mustern sie ihre Verwandten aus der Stadt und fragen sich, warum die sich so verrenken. Gelächter und vielstimmiges Gezwitscher vom Balkon. Die Vögel in den Baumriesen haben die Antwort: weil sie noch den Großstadtdschungel im Kopf haben. Doch aufgepasst: Nach kürzester Zeit hangeln sich hier, am schönsten Fleck dieses kleinen Landes, auch die Menschen wild und wagemutig durch den Tag. Trinken eisgekühlten Guavensaft und werden dabei immer schöner.
Buchtipps: »How to be wild« von Simon Barnes und »Ich bin« (Teil 1, 2 und 3) von Sri Nisargadatta Maharaj.

Céleste et sauvage contrée

N'employons pas tout de suite le terme de paradis, parlons d'abord d'un minuscule pays coincé entre l'océan Pacifique et la mer des Caraïbes, de quelques cabanes aux toits de paille au cœur d'un jardin botanique ensorcelé, de hamacs multicolores fixés comme pour l'éternité et d'une plage sur laquelle on voudrait bien échouer à tout jamais. Il est donc logique que les professeurs les plus remarquables et les plus excentriques de New York fassent venir leurs adeptes ici. Nulle part ailleurs les singes qui, désinvoltes, se suspendent aux branches dans la salle, ne peuvent assister à des séances d'Âsana si intensives, si créatives qu'à celles qui se tiennent sur la spectaculaire plate-forme de yoga au bord de l'océan. D'un air pensif ils dévisagent leurs cousins de la ville en se demandant bien pourquoi ceux-ci se contorsionnent ainsi. Eclats de rire et babillages de mille et une voix résonnent du balcon. Les oiseaux nichés dans les arbres géants ont, eux, la réponse : c'est parce qu'ils ont encore dans la tête la jungle des métropoles. Mais attention : à peine installés ici dans le plus bel endroit de ce petit pays, les hommes aussi, farouches et intrépides, se déplacent du matin au soir à la force de leurs bras. Ils boivent du jus de goyave et n'en deviennent que plus beaux.
Livres à emporter : « How to be wild » de Simon Barnes et « Je suis » (tomes 1, 2 et 3) de Sri Nisargadatta Maharaj.

ANREISE	Direkt am Golfo Dulce gelegen. 50 min Flug von San José, Hauptstadt von Costa Rica.
YOGA	Hatha, Astanga, Sivananda, Iyengar, Anusara.
GASTLEHRER	Schuyler Grant, Alison Novie, Sianna Sherman, Douglas Brooks, Kenneth Graham.
ZIMMER	15 Zimmer für max. 30 Gäste.
KÜCHE	Biologisch-vegetarisch.
ANWENDUNGEN	Facials, Wraps, Scrubs, Massagen, Akupunktur.
FREIZEIT	Surfen, Kajak, Reiten, Wandern, Schwimmen mit Delfinen.

ACCÈS	Situé directement sur le Golfo Dulce. A 50 min de vol de San José, capitale de Costa Rica.
YOGA	Hatha, Ashtânga, Shivananda, Iyengar, Anusara.
PROFESSEURS	Schuyler Grant, Alison Novie, Sianna Sherman, Douglas Brooks, Kenneth Graham.
CHAMBRES	15 chambres pour 30 personnes max.
RESTAURATION	Cuisine bio et végétarienne.
TRAITEMENTS	Soins du visage, wraps, gommages, massages, acuponcture.
ACTIVITÉS	Surf, kayak, équitation, randonnées, nage avec les dauphins.

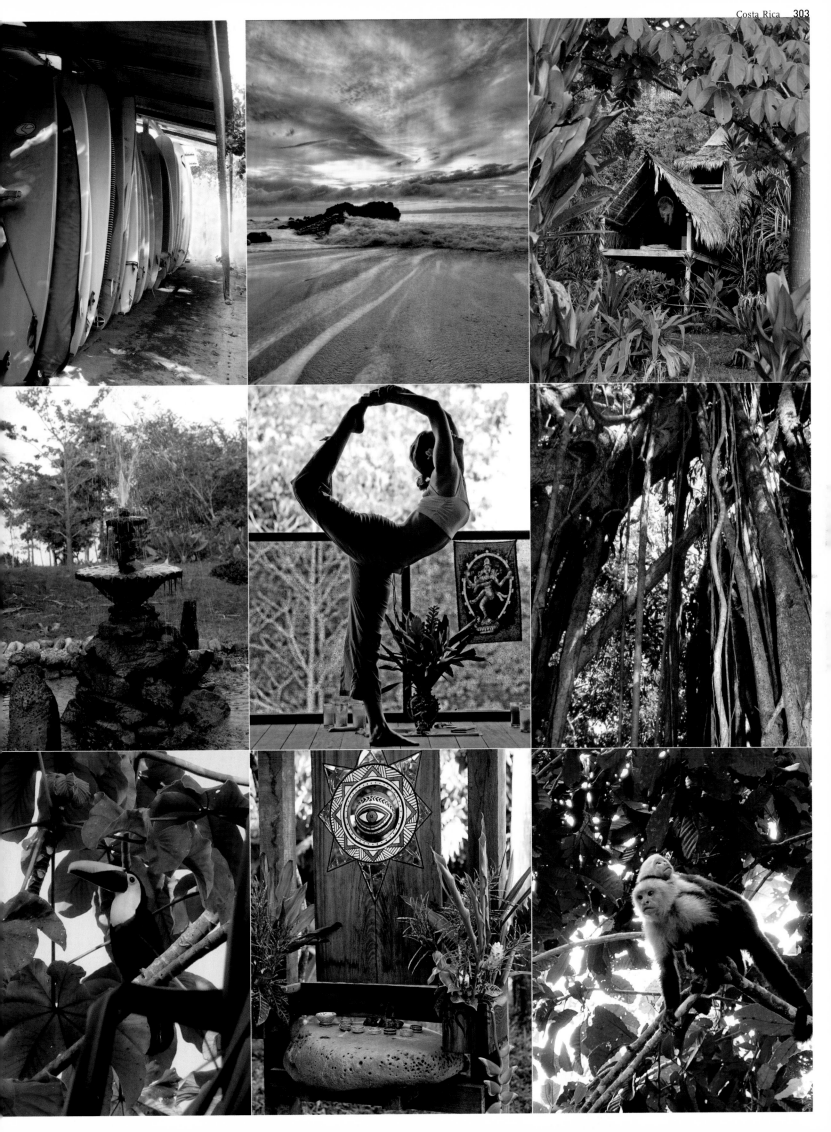

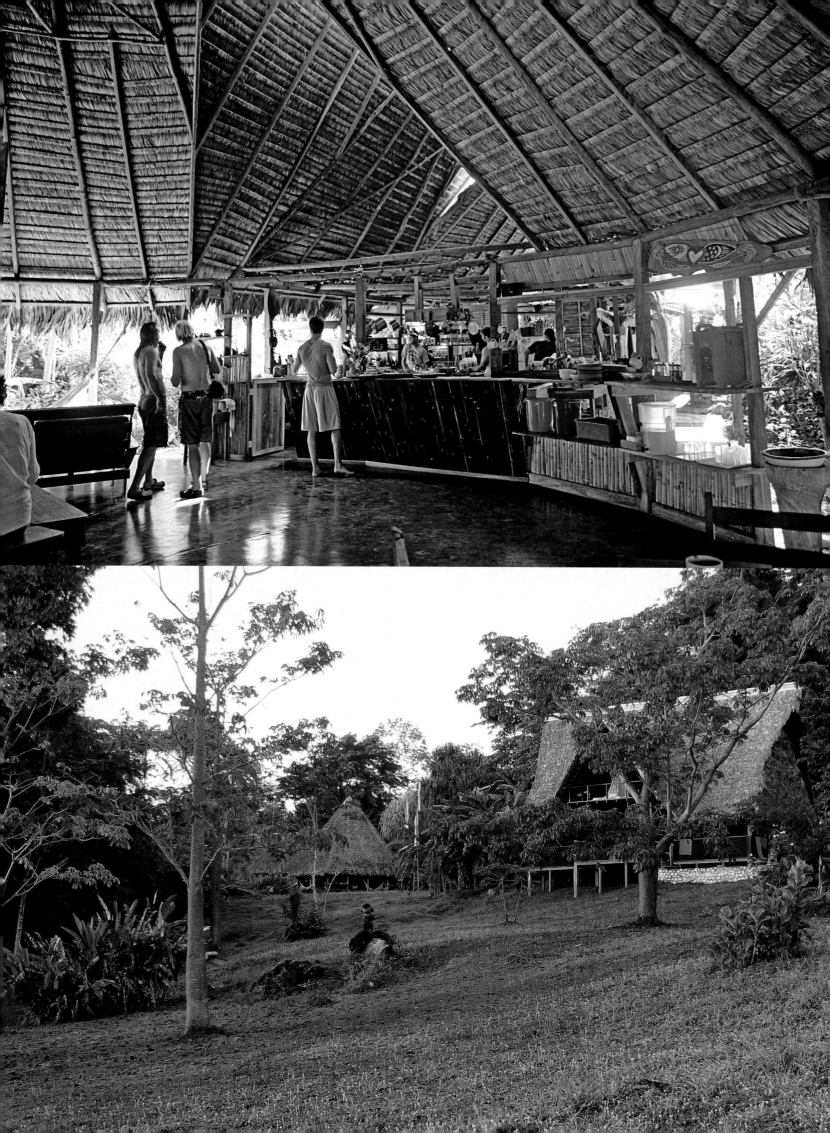

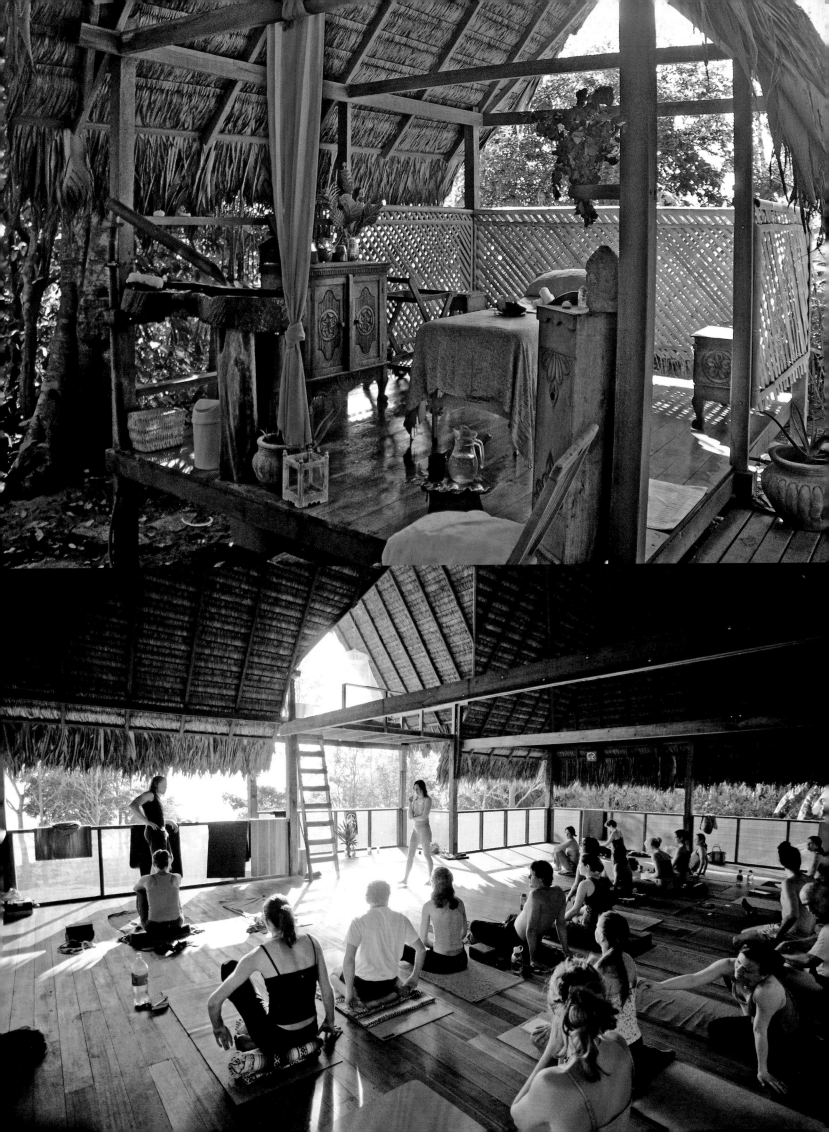

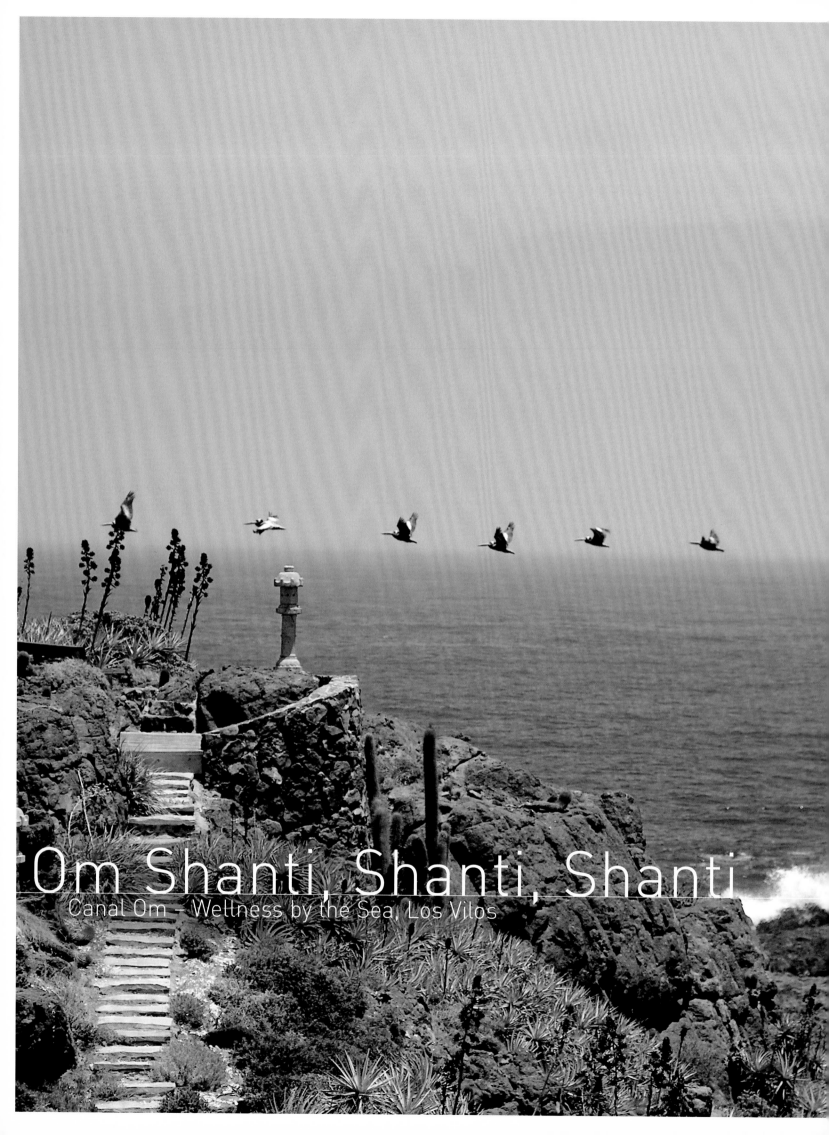

Om Shanti, Shanti, Shanti
Canal Om – Wellness by the Sea, Los Vilos

Canal Om – Wellness by the Sea, Los Vilos

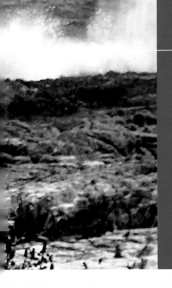

Om Shanti, Shanti, Shanti

Practise the Primary Series with the Italian Ashtanga Yoga master Lino Miele here, and the breath still flows freely in the hundredth Chaturanga. Or do backbends with the exuberantly charming Anusara teacher Amy Ippoliti until the heart is as open as the ocean. It is as if a mountain had sunk in the sea, and only the summit still juts out – that is how surreal this place at the end of the world seems. Behind are the thousand-year-old glaciers, the Chilean highlands with their desert, the canyons and cacti; in front is the Pacific. No wonder that Gustavo Ponce, founder of Canal Om, himself developed a method for Dynamic Yoga, Sattva Yoga, which he also teaches here. At the end of a quiet day, after Yoga, meditation, a long ride along the beach or a soothing bath in the saltwater pool heated to 100 degrees Fahrenheit, it is so peaceful that you can hear the stones talking. Come on, they whisper, they've lit the fire in the restaurant and a bottle of red is standing on the big table – called the monk's table here. Whoever has bagged the centrally heated, comfortable single room with a view of the barren but beautiful garden should know that though Brahmacharya perhaps literally means abstinence, the word can also be translated – as the legendary Yoga teacher Sharon Gannon has it – with "good sex".

Books to pack: "In Patagonia" by Bruce Chatwin and "House of the Spirits" by Isabel Allende.

Canal Om – Wellness by the Sea
Km 213, Panamerican Highway, close to Los Vilos
Chile
Tel. +56 2 233 1524, +56 2 233 0409 and
+56 9 9258 9041
contacto@canalom.com
and oficina@yogashala.cl
www.canalom.com

DIRECTIONS	132 miles north of Santiago. 10 miles away from Los Vilos. 2 hrs from Santiago Airport.
YOGA	Iyengar, Ashtanga, Dynamic, Kundalini, Satyananda, Sattva, Prana Shakti, Anusara.
TEACHERS	Amy Ippoliti, Lino Miele.
ROOMS	8 double rooms, 10 twin rooms and 8 single rooms for max. 30 guests.
FOOD	Vegetarian, Kundalini chef.
TREATMENTS	Massage, hydromassage, sauna, saltwater pool, thalassotherapy.
RECREATION	Tennis, horseback riding, day trips, swimming, archery.

Om Shanti, Shanti, Shanti

Hier mit dem italienischen Astanga-Altmeister Lino Miele
die erste Serie des Sonnengrußes zu üben, lässt den Atem
noch im 100. Chaturanga frei fließen. Oder mit der quirlig-
charmanten Anusara-Lehrerin Amy Ippoliti Rückbeugen
zu machen, bis das Herz so weit wie das Meer wird. Als
sei ein Berg in der See versunken, und nur die Spitze ragt
noch heraus, so surreal erscheint einem dieser Platz am
Ende der Welt. Im Rücken die 1000-jährigen Gletscher, das
chilenische Hochland mit seiner Wüste, den Schluchten
und Kakteen, vor sich der Pazifische Ozean. Kein Wunder,
dass Gustavo Ponce, Gründer von Canal Om, selbst eine
Methode für dynamisches Yoga entwickelt hat, Sattva-Yoga,
die er hier ebenfalls unterrichtet. Am Ende eines stillen
Tages, nach Yoga, Meditation, einem langen Ritt am Strand
oder einem tröstlichen Bad im auf 38 Grad erhitzten Salzwasserpool, ist es so ruhig, dass man die Steine sprechen
hört. »Los komm«, flüstern sie, »im Restaurant haben sie
Feuer im Kamin gemacht, und eine Flasche Rotwein steht
auch auf dem großen Tisch, den sie hier Mönchstisch
nennen.« Wer das zentral geheizte, gemütliche Einzelzim-
mer mit Blick in den kargschönen Garten erwischt hat,
sollte wissen, dass Brahmacharya vielleicht wortwörtlich
Enthaltsamkeit heißt, dass es aber ebenso wie von der
legendären Yogalehrerin Sharon Gannon mit »guter Sex«
übersetzt werden kann.
Buchtipps: »In Patagonien« von Bruce Chatwin und »Das
Geisterhaus« von Isabel Allende.

Om Shanti, Shanti, Shanti

Ici, effectuer la première série avec Lino Miele, le maître
italien incontesté d'Ashtânga, laisse la respiration circuler
librement même après le centième Chaturanga. Ou bien avec
Amy Ippoliti, charmante et pétulante professeur Anusara,
faire des exercices de flexion du dos jusqu'à ce que le cœur
soit aussi vaste que la mer. Comme une montagne engloutie
dans les flots et dont seulement la pointe dépasse encore,
ainsi apparaît ce site du bout du monde, tel un cliché surréa-
liste. Derrière soi, les glaciers millénaires, le haut plateau
chilien avec son désert, les gorges et les cactus et, devant soi,
l'océan Pacifique. Il n'est guère étonnant que Gustavo Ponce,
fondateur de Canal Om, ait conçu lui-même une méthode de
yoga dynamique, le Sattva Yoga, qui est également enseignée
ici. A la fin d'une journée tranquille, après le yoga, la méditation, une longue chevauchée sur la plage ou un bain récon-
fortant de 38 degrés dans la piscine à l'eau salée, tout est si
calme que l'on entend parler les pierres. Viens donc, mur-
murent-elles, au restaurant un bon feu flambe dans la cheminée et une bouteille de vin rouge t'attend aussi sur la
grande table qu'ils ont surnommée ici la table du moine.
Celui à qui échoit la confortable chambre simple, raccordée
au chauffage central, avec vue sur le jardin à la sobre beauté
devrait savoir que si Brahmacharya signifie littéralement
abstinence, il peut aussi bien être traduit par « good sex »
comme le faisait Sharon Gannon, la légendaire professeur
de yoga.
**Livres à emporter : « En Patagonie » de Bruce Chatwin et
« La Maison aux esprits » d'Isabel Allende.**

ANREISE	213 km nördlich von Santiago, 16 km von Los Vilos. 2 Std. vom Flughafen Santiago entfernt.
YOGA	Iyengar, Astanga, Dynamic, Kundalini, Satyananda, Sattva, Prana Shakti, Anusara.
GASTLEHRER	Amy Ippoliti, Lino Miele.
ZIMMER	8 Doppelbettzimmer, 10 Zweibettzimmer und 8 Einzelzimmer für max. 30 Gäste.
KÜCHE	Vegetarisch, Kundalini-Koch.
ANWENDUNGEN	Massagen, Hydromassagen, Sauna, Meerwasserpool, Thalasso-Therapie.
FREIZEIT	Tennis, Reiten, Ausflüge, Schwimmen, Bogenschießen.

ACCÈS	Situé à 213 km au nord de Santiago. A 16 km de Los Vilos. A 2 h de l'aéroport de Santiago.
YOGA	Iyengar, Ashtânga, Dynamic, Kundalini, Satyananda, Sattva, Prana Shakti, Anusara.
PROFESSEURS	Amy Ippoliti, Lino Miele.
CHAMBRES	8 chambres à lits doubles, 10 chambres à deux lits et 8 chambres simples pour 30 personnes max.
RESTAURATION	Cuisine végétarienne, cuisinier Kundalini.
TRAITEMENTS	Massages, hydromassages, sauna, piscine à l'eau de mer, thalassothérapie.
ACTIVITÉS	Tennis, équitation, excursions, natation, tir à l'arc.

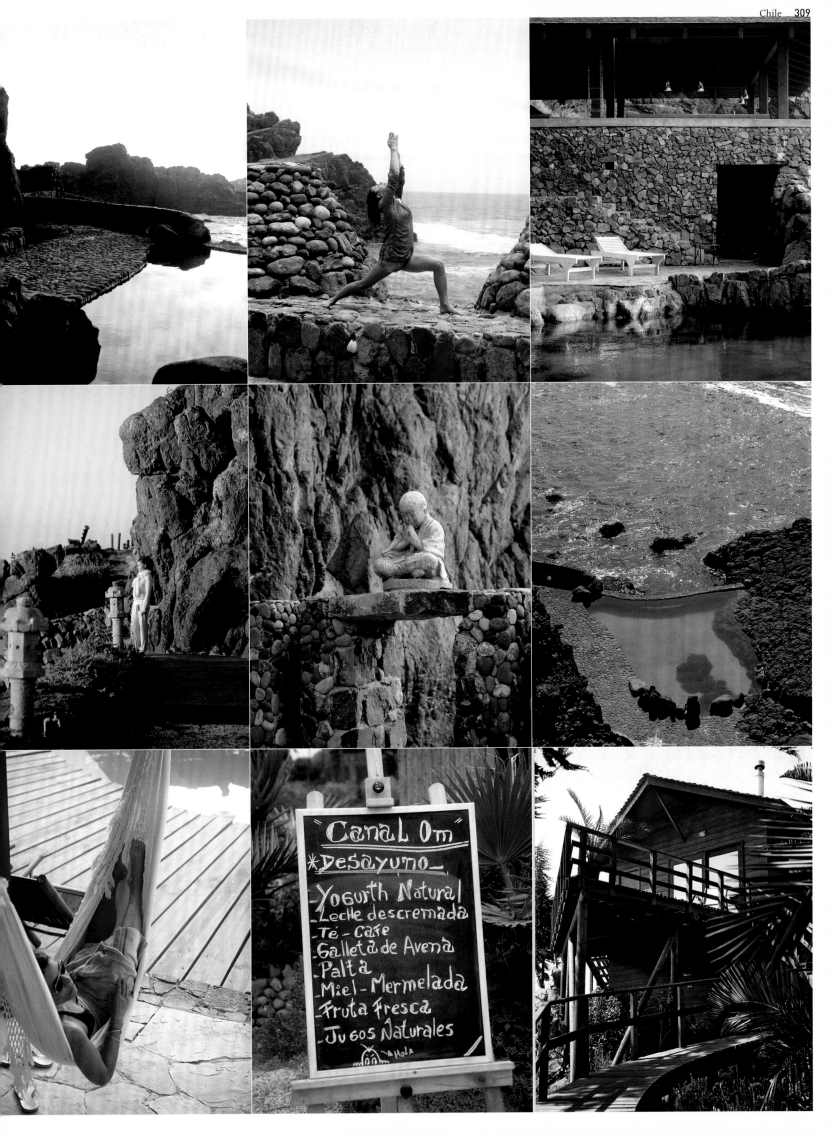

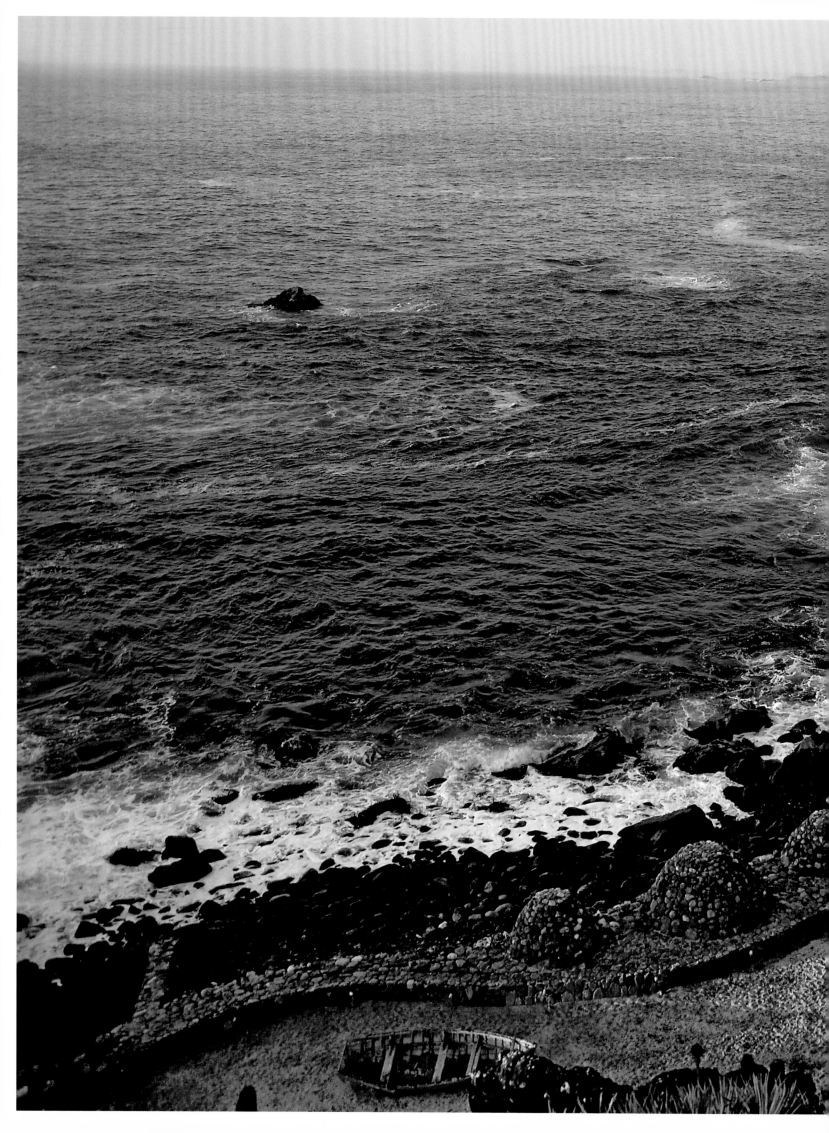

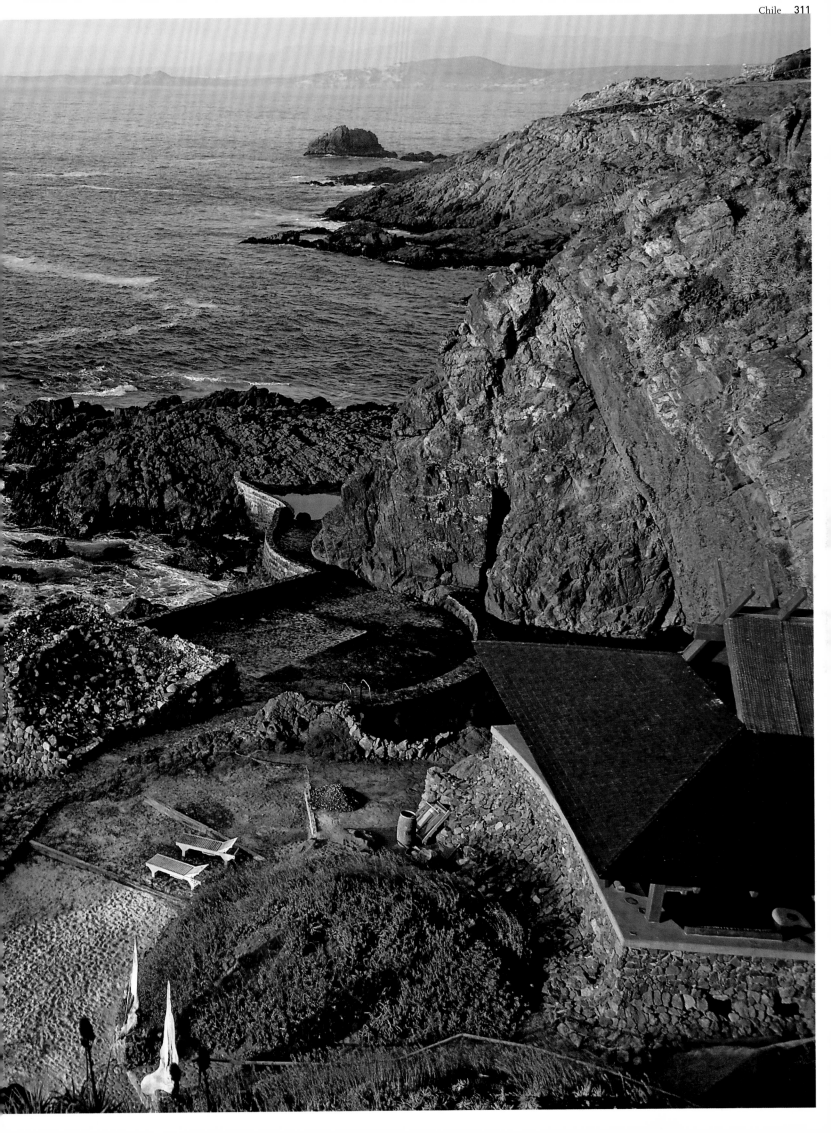

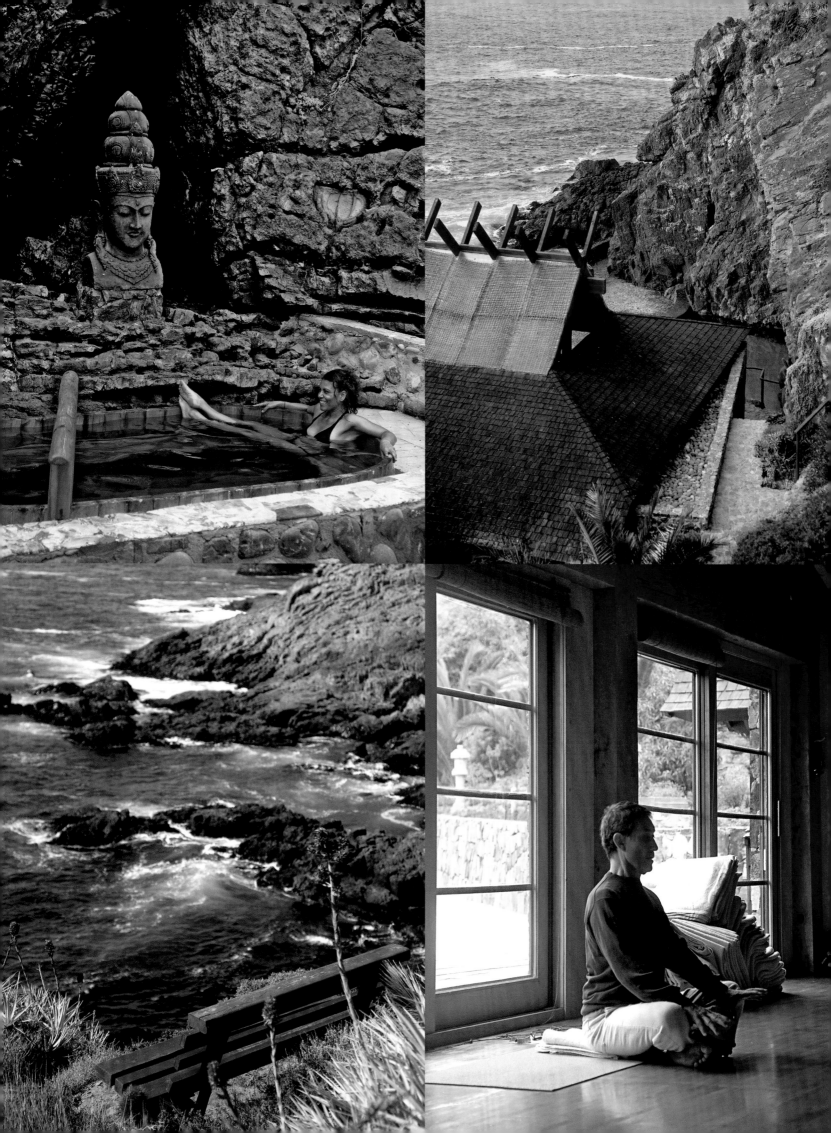

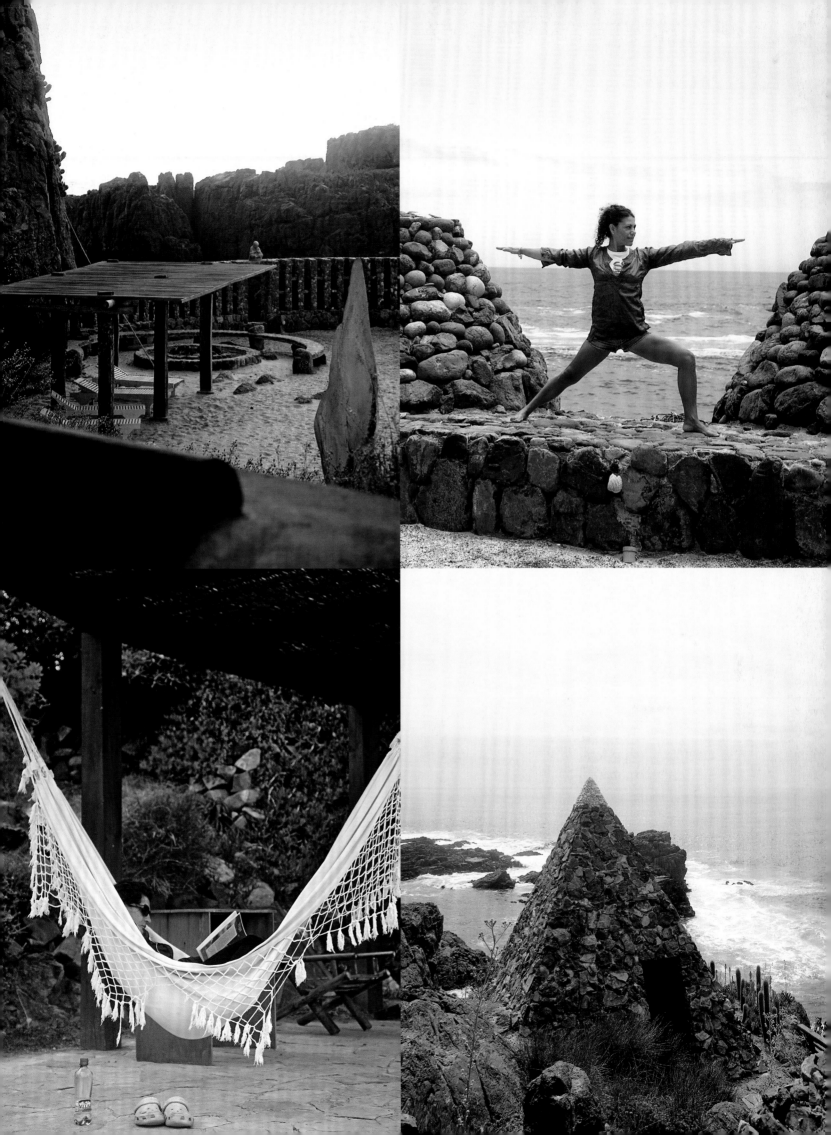

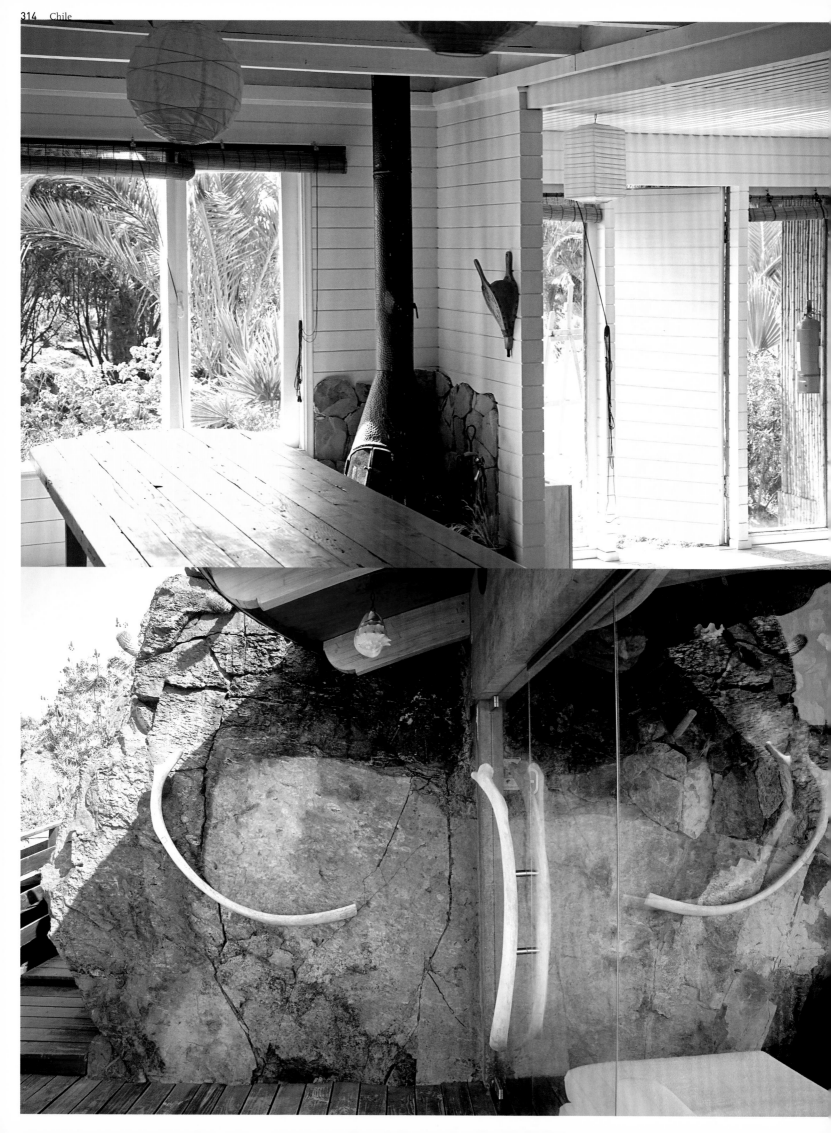

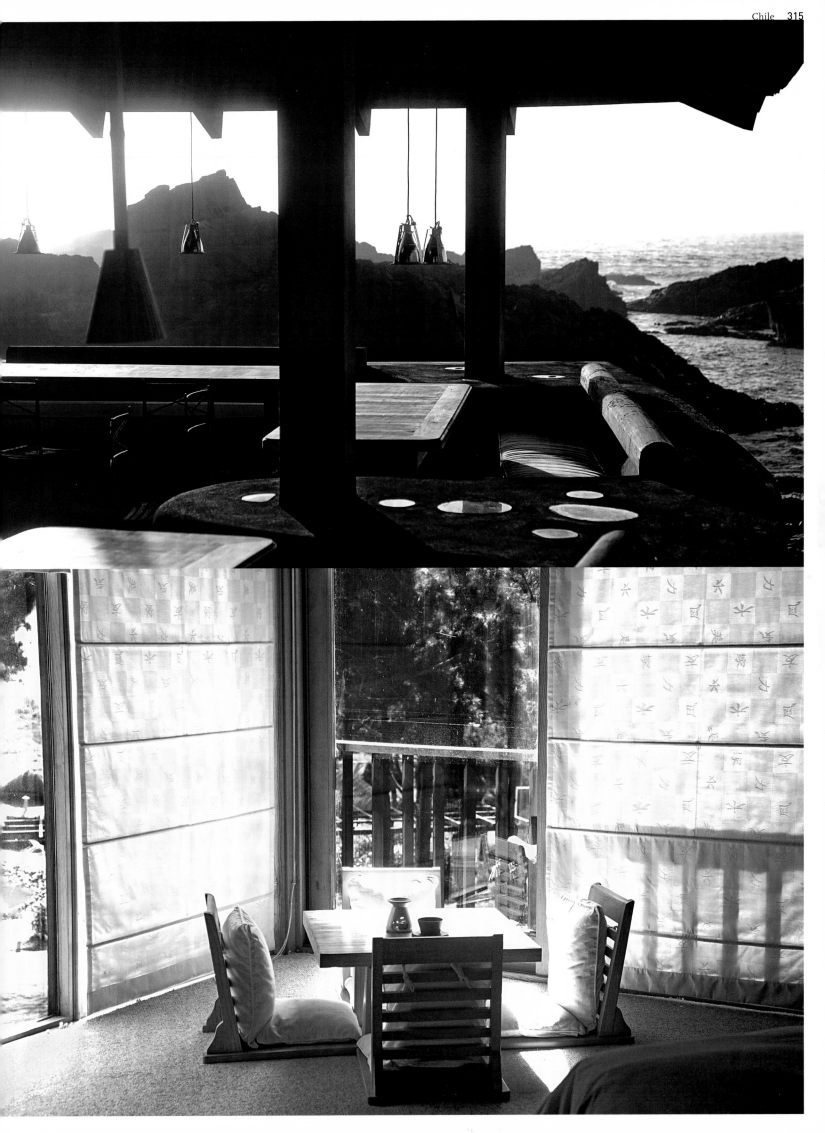

Asia

Asien

Asie

HOW TO BOOK A YOGA RETREAT: Here you can find out through which websites and links you can best make bookings for a Yoga holiday at the locations featured in this book. Otherwise, dates and offers for Yoga retreats can be found on the websites of

Europe

092–189

092 **Höllbachhof, Bavaria, Germany**
Höllbachhof: www.hoellbachhof.net
› Calendar or www.jivamuktiyoga.de
› Retreats
Yoga sessions at the Höllbachhof are
often hosted by the Jivamukti Yoga Center
in Munich.

102 **Borgo Iesolana, Tuscany, Italy**
www.yogahikes.com › dates & prices
Yoga and hiking trips at Borgo Iesolana
can be booked through yogahikes.

110 **Il Convento, Tuscany, Italy**
www.il-convento.net › Seminars &
Vacation › Seminar Calendar
A list of all current and upcoming
courses with prices and contact details.

122 **In Sabina, Latium, Italy**
www.insabina.com › Retreats
Find all Yoga course dates and contact
details here.

132 **Santa Maria del Sole, Puglia, Italy**
www.santamariadelsole.it › Retreats
A list of upcoming Yoga classes with
hyperlinks.

142 **Formentera Yoga, Formentera, Spain**
www.formenterayoga.com › Recharge
Retreats › See Schedule
The schedule of Yoga retreats with links
to register directly.

150 **Ibiza Moving Arts, Ibiza, Spain**
www.ibizamovingarts.com › Activities
Book a wellness course, a Yoga retreat or
an individual healing session.

160 **Molino del Rey, Andalusia, Spain**
www.molinodelrey.com › Bookings and
Courses
Find the dates, availability and contact
information for Yoga or wellness workshops here.

168 **Kretashala, Crete, Greece**
www.kretashala.de › Dates
An extensive schedule of Yoga courses,
many of which are in German.

174 **Atami Hotel, near Bodrum, Turkey**
www.atamihotel.com › Activities at Atami
Hotel › Yoga Holidays & Yoga Retreats
Information on upcoming Yoga classes
for all ability levels.

180 **Huzur Vadisi, Lycia Region, Turkey**
www.huzurvadisi.com › Courses
Register for courses in a variety of Yoga
styles.

Europa

092–189

092 **Höllbachhof, Bavaria, Germany**
Höllbachhof: www.hoellbachhof.net
› Calendar oder www.jivamuktiyoga.de
› Retreats
Die Yoga Retreats im Höllbachhof werden
häufig vom Jivamukti Yoga Center in
München durchgeführt.

102 **Borgo Iesolana, Tuscany, Italy**
www.yogahikes.com › dates & prices
Über Yogahikes können Sie Yoga- und
Wanderurlaube in Borgo Iesolana buchen.

110 **Il Convento, Tuscany, Italy**
www.il-convento.net › Seminars &
Vacation › Seminar Calendar
Eine Liste aller aktuellen und zukünftigen
Retreats mit Preisen und Kontaktadressen.

122 **In Sabina, Latium, Italy**
www.insabina.com › Retreats
Hier finden Sie Daten und Kontaktinformationen zu allen Yoga Retreats.

132 **Santa Maria del Sole, Puglia, Italy**
www.santamariadelsole.it › Retreats
Eine Liste anstehender Yoga Retreats
(mit Hyperlinks).

142 **Formentera Yoga, Formentera, Spain**
www.formenterayoga.com › Recharge
Retreats › See Schedule
Ein Plan der Yoga Retreats, mit Links für
eine direkte Buchung.

150 **Ibiza Moving Arts, Ibiza, Spain**
www.ibizamovingarts.com › Activities
Buchen Sie einen Wellnesskurs, ein Yoga
Retreat oder eine individuelle Heilsitzung.

160 **Molino del Rey, Andalusia, Spain**
www.molinodelrey.com › Bookings and
Courses
Hier finden Sie Daten, offene Plätze und
Kontaktinformationen für Yoga- und
Wellness-Workshops.

168 **Kretashala, Crete, Greece**
www.kretashala.de › Dates
Ein ausführlicher Zeitplan von Yoga
Retreats mit vielen Angeboten in
deutscher Sprache.

174 **Atami Hotel, near Bodrum, Turkey**
www.atamihotel.com › Activities at Atami
Hotel › Yoga Holidays & Yoga Retreats
Informationen zu anstehenden Yoga
Retreats für alle Erfahrungsstufen.

180 **Huzur Vadisi, Lycia Region, Turkey**
www.huzurvadisi.com › Courses
Melden Sie sich zu Yogakursen der
verschiedensten Stile an.

Europe

092–189

092 **Höllbachhof, Bavaria, Germany**
Höllbachhof: www.hoellbachhof.net
› Calendar or www.jivamuktiyoga.de
› Retreats
Les retraites de yoga du Höllbachhof ont
souvent lieu au centre Jivamukti Yoga à
Munich.

102 **Borgo Iesolana, Tuscany, Italy**
www.yogahikes.com › dates & prices
On peut réserver les retraites de yoga et
les randonnées du Borgo Iesolana par
l'intermédiaire de yogahikes.

110 **Il Convento, Tuscany, Italy**
www.il-convento.net › Seminars &
Vacation › Seminar Calendar
Une liste de toutes les retraites actuelles
et à venir avec leurs prix et les coordon-
nées des personnes à contacter.

122 **In Sabina, Latium, Italy**
www.insabina.com › Retreats
Vous trouverez ici toutes les dates de
retraites et les personnes à contacter.

132 **Santa Maria del Sole, Puglia, Italy**
www.santamariadelsole.it › Retreats
Une liste des prochaines retraites de
yoga accompagnées de liens en hypertexte.

142 **Formentera Yoga, Formentera, Spain**
www.formenterayoga.com › Recharge
Retreats › See Schedule
Le calendrier des prochaines retraites
de yoga avec des liens pour réserver
directement.

150 **Ibiza Moving Arts, Ibiza, Spain**
www.ibizamovingarts.com › Activities
Réservez un cours de bien-être, une
retraite de yoga ou une séance de soins
individuelle.

160 **Molino del Rey, Andalusia, Spain**
www.molinodelrey.com › Bookings and
Courses
Découvrez ici les dates, les disponibilités
et les personnes à contacter pour des
stages de yoga ou de bien-être.

168 **Kretashala, Crete, Greece**
www.kretashala.de › Dates
Un vaste programme de retraites de yoga
avec de nombreux cours en allemand.

174 **Atami Hotel, near Bodrum, Turkey**
www.atamihotel.com › Activities at Atami
Hotel › Yoga Holidays & Yoga Retreats
Des informations sur les prochaines
retraites de yoga pour tous les niveaux.

180 **Huzur Vadisi, Lycia Region, Turkey**
www.huzurvadisi.com › Courses
Inscrivez-vous à des cours de différents
styles yoga.

the relevant hotels, ashrams and centres. Have a look, too, at the webpages of Yoga schools worldwide, which offer retreats through their teachers.

Wie man ein Yoga Retreat bucht:
Hier erfahren Sie, über welche Websites und unter welchen Links Sie am besten die im Buch vorgestellten Orte buchen können. Ansonsten findet man entweder auf den Websites der entsprechenden Hotels, Ashrams und Zentren Termine und Angebote für Yoga Retreats, oder Sie suchen weltweit auf den Seiten der Yogaschulen, die über ihre Lehrer Retreats anbieten.

Comment réserver votre retraite de yoga :
Vous trouverez ici les sites Web et liens vous permettant de réserver de façon idéale les lieux de séjour présentés dans le livre. Sinon, vous pouvez obtenir sur les sites Web des hôtels, âhsrams et centres en question les dates et programmes des retraites de yoga, ou vous consulter dans le monde entier les pages d'accueil des écoles de yoga qui, par l'intermédiaire de leurs professeurs, proposent des retraites.

Central & South America

258–315

Mittel- & Südamerika

258–315

Amérique centrale & du Sud

258–315

© 2009 TASCHEN GmbH
Hohenzollernring 53, D-50672 Köln
www.taschen.com

To stay informed about upcoming TASCHEN titles, please request our
magazine at www.taschen.com/magazine or write to TASCHEN,
Hohenzollernring 53, D-50672 Cologne, Germany; contact@taschen.com;
Fax: +49-221-254919. We will be happy to send you a free copy of our
magazine, which is filled with information about all of our books.

COMPILED, EDITED
AND LAYOUT: Angelika Taschen, Berlin
PROJECT MANAGER: Stephanie Paas, Cologne;
                       Nina Schumacher, Cologne
TEXTS: Kristin Rübesamen, Berlin
FRENCH TRANSLATION: Annick Schmidt, Bergisch Gladbach
ENGLISH TRANSLATION: Robert Taylor, Cologne
DESIGN: Lambert und Lambert, Düsseldorf
LITHOGRAPH MANAGER: Thomas Grell, Cologne
PRINTED IN   Italy
ISBN   978-3-8365-1231-2

The published information, addresses and pictures have been researched with the
utmost care. However, no responsibility or liability can be taken for the correctness
of the details. The information may be out of date due to current changes. In such
cases, please refer to the relevant websites for current prices and details.

Die veröffentlichten Informationen, Adressen und Bilder sind mit größter Sorgfalt
recherchiert. Dennoch kann für die Richtigkeit keine Gewähr oder Haftung übernom-
men werden. Die Informationen können durch aktuelle Entwicklungen überholt sein.
Bitte entnehmen Sie den jeweiligen Websites die derzeitigen Preise und Angaben.

Bien que nous ayons recherché avec soin les informations, les adresses et les photos
de cet ouvrage, nous déclinons toute responsabilité. Il est possible en effet que les
données mises à notre disposition ne soient plus à jour. Veuillez vous reporter aux
différents sites web pour obtenir les prix et les renseignements actuels.

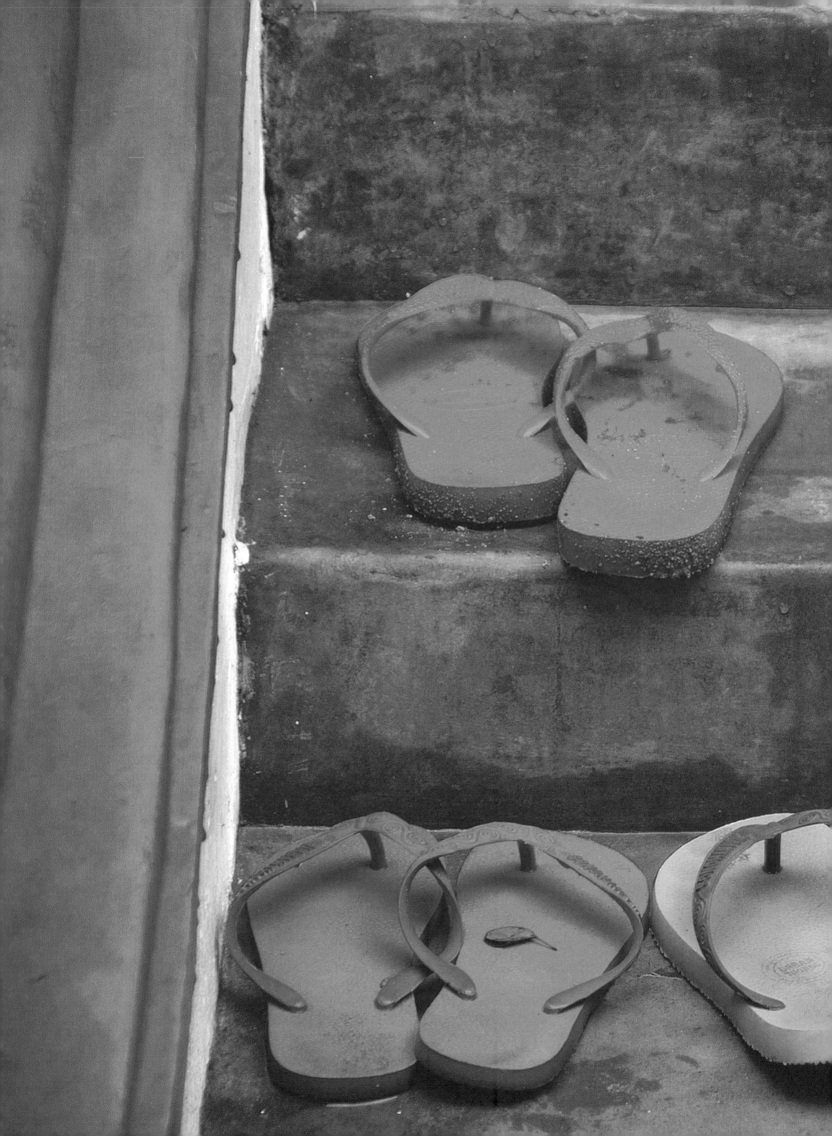